KEEPING THE

ATHLETE HEALTHY

A COMPREHENSIVE GUIDE

By:
Edward H. Nessel, R.Ph, MS, MPH, PharmD

i

Published by Sage Words Publishing www.sagewordspublishing.com

Author: Edward Nessel

Editor: Jake George

ISBN-13: 978-0991501427
ISBN-10: 099150142X

Photo credits:

Cover:
Image credit: http://www.123rf.com/photo_7638349_symbol-of-medicine-abstract-background-3d.html'>maxxyustas / 123RF Stock Photo

Front Cover:
Image credit: http://www.123rf.com/photo_11663980_full-page-of-electrocardiograms-and-heart-disease-illustrations.html'>9and3quarters / 123RF Stock Photo

Chapter 6 Psychology of Aging Charts" Reprinted, with permission, from J.H. Wilmore and D.L. Costill, 1999, *Physiology of sport and exercise,* 2nd ed. (Champaign, IL: Human Kinetics), 547 [or 550 or 552, or 557].

Contents

REVIEWS

"I am a serious and dedicated bicyclist and distance runner who imparts intense training into his daily existence. After reading KEEPING THE ATHLETE HEALTHY, I found its information concise, easy to access, accurate and very helpful, especially for the serious athlete looking for more of a 360 view of how the body responds to vigorous exercise. The author's insights on nutrition and supplements were quite comprehensive and most helpful for me since he appears to be very firmly grounded in this area and is strongly committed to proven therapy and data.

Coach Nessel has put together a treasure trove of real science and practical advice for those wanting to increase their engaging in vigorous exercise to elevate their athletic condition in several sports. His extensive academic knowledge as a pharmacist, biochemist, and physiologist together with his several decades as a coach/trainer imparts wisdom in a balanced fashion. Whether you are looking to improve your race time, keep fit as you get older or just understand your body in a more complete way, this book has something for you. I was also impressed by his breadth of knowledge in both conventional science and in Natural vitamin and mineral supplementation."

J. Todd Wahrenberger MD MPH
Medical Director, Pittsburgh Mercy Family Health Center
Pittsburgh Mercy Health System
249 S. 9th St.

Keeping The Athlete Healthy is an encyclopedic work encompassing the author's expertise in both the medical and the physical. It is written in readable terms, containing everything you'd want to know or didn't know you needed to know about your life as a serious dedicated athlete or, as pertains to most of us, adding sports and vigorous activity as a balance to life. The author has "chops" as a championship coach, swimmer and researcher with the reader benefiting from all three.

Paul J. Kiell, M.D. Psychiatrist, marathon runner and swimmer and erstwhile editor of the *American Medical Athletic Association Journal*

Finally! A go-to manual for athletes of any age, ability level, injured or whole, written in a way I can only describe as incredibly "approachable", yet well documented and authoritative.

As an author with a longstanding reputation for guiding elite swimmers to the Olympic dream, Coach Nessel certainly understands how to shape the powerhouse athlete, but in this publication, his sensitivity to those of us struggling with declining athletic abilities as we advance in age, has renewed my determination to maximize my health. Sensible supplemented eating strategies, pain and injury prevention and treatment, training to build strength and endurance, and emotional considerations in goal setting, has never been easier to understand and to implement, sans hiring your own Olympic trainer!

Thank you Coach for finding just the right words to convince that 10% of my body (brain), to take control of the other 90% (body), while good, better, and best health is still within reach!

Cynthia E. Tilson, RN, BSN, CRNA

Keeping the Athlete Healthy brings to both the novice and seasoned competitor a step by step guide to preparation, training, and maintenance of the athlete. Coach Nessel's unique combination of scientific training in pharmacology, physiology, and biochemistry coupled with his vast experience in preparing world class athletes for competition has resulted in a book that is both comprehensive in scope and yet focused on the real world issues of training. The book guides the reader through a systems biology approach to the complex stress of exercise, the resulting adaptation, and the prevention of injury. This systems based approach integrates sound scientific principles with clear recommendations based upon Coach Nessel's experience as a teacher and coach. As with his previous excellent books, Keeping the Athlete Healthy is concise, well organized, well written, and grounded in an evidence based approach to exercise.

Pope L. Moseley MD MS FACSM FACP FCCP
Distinguished Professor
Regents' Professor
University of New Mexico

"I experienced the amazing range of Coach Nessel's scientific training methods first hand when I asked him to prepare me for the 1500 meter (metric mile) open water swimming leg of the 2013 Pittsburgh Triathlon. I applied his suggested unique swimming stroke techniques, modified weight room routines, diet and supplement knowledge and training physiology over a period of just eight weeks to transform my natural power sprinting abilities into producing a successful distance swim. The Coach knows what it takes to train smart, allowing for increased performance yet preventing illness and injury. I know this comprehensive book will be referred to often to help keep me on the road to future successful training experiences as I age."

Brenda K. Freeman, MD, Consulting Psychiatrist and Medical Director of Alcohol, Tobacco, and Other Drug Services, Pittsburgh Mercy Health System

Hang on to your swim cap, grab your note pad and a cup of Coach N's "Florida cocktail", and dive in for an enlightening read! "Keeping The Athlete Healthy" is a comprehensive and evidence-based discussion of all things athletic, yet much is applicable to everyday life. Though focused on the aging athlete, there is plenty of science to apply to improving the performance of younger athletes. Coach N (Ed), with four decades of coaching swimmers of all ability levels as well as a successful masters swimmer himself, skillfully blends that experience with hard science. His additional background as a pharmacist, biochemist, and physiologist enables him to expertly present and interpret the sea of life and performance enhancement information available in a practical and useable plan. This is a truly amazing and comprehensive manual, to be referred to often as one travels through life – athlete or not. You will want to have your own copy, as I promise you that the pages will be well-worn.

Rosanna Sikora, MD

ACKNOWLEDGEMENTS

This book was a long time coming. As a scientist who always dabbled in sports, I have come to look at the human machine differently than most. My focus has been, and will always be, on the body's ability to adapt. Life is structured such that we must always adapt or fail. Very few of us have gotten through life without a back story where we demonstrate the ability to rise above and solve problems as they develop. Keeping the eyes on the prize has always been innate with me but, like most, I have had positive (and sometimes negative) influences from which to draw.

It is almost a cliché to say that no athlete has ever made it to the rarified elite level alone. Youngsters wanting a piece of the "cake" in their favorite sports must have others who care and nurture their wants and needs. It is the human condition, and thank God for it. I have had many people cross my path through my almost 70 years of existence. I have learned strong lessons from those with a positive attitude and also from those subsisting at the dregs of despair and negativity.

My father often shared his views of life coming to America as a 10-year-old immigrant from the Polish/German boarder in 1920. He was proud of his staunch ability to rise above and make his way in his new homeland. His constant effort was to make his last name one that his whole family could be proud. He never let me forget that. He also imparted probably the best advice I could have ever received growing up and trying to make my own way in this world: "Always do your best... you never know who is watching."

My mother, also a 1920 childhood immigrant but from Lithuania, was quick to assimilate her surroundings and developed a keen sense of the successful in the human condition. She tried her best to make her little Eddie's journey through the impressionable growing years one of worth and consequence. I will always remember her decision as to how to help me swim fast on my first team. "Eat something that swims fast so it will help you do the same." The logic might appear somewhat comical, but with her practical approach to life, it rang true. Having a tuna fish sandwich before swim meets became almost a ritual in the Nessel household.

My parents both wanted to know, why? What was the cause, what would be the effect? How one thing might work better than another. Take note from the good and the bad... all to create a perfect nurturing for the biological scientist I would eventually become. This book is a tribute to their ideals and the inspiration and memories they left behind

INTRODUCTION

A sick or injured athlete is good to no one. The better and, or more dedicated the athlete, the more they become like race horses... You would have to shoot them rather than keep them penned up to heal. I have had to deal with all sorts of human maladies over my 48+ years of coaching and competing and have learned with my "coach's eye" and medical and physiological backgrounds to spot things that offer up bad intentions towards the human condition.

Almost all visits to the doctor's office, physical therapist or the hospital-ER are usually after the fact. It does not take much in-depth analysis to realize the amount of down time and a great physical and emotional distress that can be saved if certain prudent tenets of public health are followed. Much of it is logical but not widely realized. The same goes for many sound physiological principles if they are understood and implemented, and, certainly appreciating the constant respect the physically-active body demands. Of course, accidents and illness can just happen... they come free with breathing and inhabiting the earth, but much can be anticipated, avoided, and somewhat parried to at least lessen the "hit."

KEEPING THE ATHLETE HEALTHY has been formatted to present an easily-understood compilation of what I know and have experienced over the years. Issues that should be considered first concern the ability of the athlete's body to handle dedicated vigorous training and what he or she should expect physically and emotionally as training progresses. The chapters are presented that each can stand alone as council. The second section of the book is dedicated to presenting public health tenets as they relate to sports and the proper care and nurturing of the body. Section three is focused on the thought that it is much wiser to prevent illness and injury if possible than to endure all the problems and time away from the sport while recovering and rehabbing. But, unfortunately, if the athlete does sustain trauma or illness, how best to lessen the result and maybe avoid a second encounter. Several conditions of the body are explained to ensure the best outcome of any potential negative situation no matter what, no matter who. Finally, the last section is dedicated to the 10 percent of the body (the brain) that controls the other 90 percent.

What we believe is what we perceive. No truer words have ever been written than "an ounce of prevention is worth a pound of cure." Everyone involved in athletics; physical education or therapy should have this book available for ready reference.

SECTION I:

PREPARING FOR VIGOROUS EXERCISE... KNOW THYSELF!

It all starts with making sure your desire for physicality matches your innate and developing physiology.

Here, I discuss the need for noting family history, the necessity of knowing what medical conditions might exist and how they manifest, if at all, with vigorous training and competitions. We also need to know appropriate limits which should act as guidelines for a healthy indulgence in sports and intense training. Various ages of participants wishing to push through a challenging physicality will be covered with attendant caveats.

As an overview, topics to be discussed briefly will include blood pressure, anemia (and the opposite... excessive concentrations of red blood cells), asthma, diabetes, heart conditions both congenital (*inborn*) and acquired, the same for errors of metabolism, and various forms of arthritis. Specific subsequent chapters will handle several of these medical conditions in greater detail where necessary as they relate to, and interact with, pushing through the comfort zone.

I take great pains to reduce the important complicated medical and physiological precepts to easily-understood concepts for the non-medical but highly interested reader. Everything is written in understandable English and with an emphasis on keeping the athlete, coach, and, or parent connected with the content. This book is intended to be an easy-to-use guide for reference that can be utilized over and over with each chapter presented as a separate and standalone source of quickly ascertained answers and explanations.

CHAPTER 1

THE PHYSIOLOGY OF BEING IN SHAPE… ADAPTATION AT ITS BEST

Every person who engages in prolonged vigorous movement realizes that with continuous training something happens over time that allows the body to withstand increasingly-demanding physical challenges. What would have sunk your ship in stormy seas just a few weeks ago now presents with calmer water towards your destination. This destination is what every serious athlete and dedicated exercise participant should be striving for throughout their training experience: to be in the kind of shape that allows for a positive ADAPTIVE TRANSFORMATION to occur that matches the physical potential Nature has granted each of us, and then a little more. Climbing the formidable mountain of *being in shape* should be the goal of everyone wanting to be labeled an athlete.

Getting in "shape" is neither easy to attain nor to explain. As you know, the human body is a wondrous machine with many complicated systems able to produce great quantities of energy both quickly and over extended periods of time. This permits the body to adapt to whatever is physically challenging it, and enlarge its capacity to handle increasingly more vigorous exercise. Unlike an automobile engine which has the exact parts needed to produce a certain amount of predicted energy and power, the human body's components can be made to produce more by having them induced more through use of specific physiologic protocols over time. In every instance of adapting to exercise, three main elements, the holy grails of athletic training as I see it, are brought into the picture and must be addressed to a greater or lesser extent depending upon the venue and sport. These elements are *endurance*, *strength*, and *power*. Following the correct pathway to physiologic conditioning is like a professional concert or jazz musician mastering the three main woodwind instruments in proper order: clarinet, saxophone, and flute. The athlete should build endurance, and then go for increased strength and finally, work to capture power.

ENDURANCE

Endurance is where it all starts if the coach/trainer and athlete CORRECTLY approach getting in shape. It takes the greatest amount of time and the most effort to develop all the physiological changes the body needs to build endurance. It is not a simple goal; it is an ongoing process. When speaking of endurance, we must include both the muscular and cardio-respiratory systems. In dealing with muscular tissue, endurance becomes specific to individual muscle groups. When dealing with cardio-respiratory endurance, we speak more of the body as a whole and its ability to sustain extended vigorous physical exercise. This becomes the most important aspect of physical fitness. If physical condition is suspect and fatigue sets in too quickly, muscular strength diminishes as does neuromuscular coordination, concentration, and alertness. To prevent this and to correctly train the athlete, we need to increase the mechanisms required to harvest and utilize energy supplies for prolonged bouts of movement and to concomitantly increase the distribution of nutrients and oxygen throughout the body to sustain total body involvement.

Although fast-twitch muscle fibers are usually larger in size than slow-twitch; slow-twitch fibers can become up to 22% larger than fast-twitch fibers with effective endurance training. What this causes, however, is increased development of endurance fibers at the expense of pure power. Even the subtype of **Fast-Twitch Fibers (Fiia)**, which has more oxidative capacity than the absolute **All-Out Fast Twitch Fibers (Fiib)**, develop more with endurance training. Consequently, the athlete ends up sacrificing all-out power and corresponding speed for enhanced endurance.

Specificity of training will enhance one ability at the cost of another. A sprinter who trains primarily for endurance will cause some fast twitch fibers to switch over to fire more slowly; this will lessen power and all-out speed, but will add THE ABILITY TO PERFORM LONGER. Along with the change in fiber type, a second adaptation occurs with an increase of more than 15% in the number of capillaries innervating muscle fibers which allow for greater exchange of **O**xygen (O2) and **C**arbon **D**ioxide (CO2), heat, wastes, and nutrients between the blood and active muscle tissue. This is an important adaptation; the muscles are then able to contract more efficiently over an extended period of time which delays fatigue.

A third muscular adaptation to endurance training is the increased formation of THE IRON-CONTAINING PROTEIN, *myoglobin*. With appropriate aerobic training, muscle *myoglobin* can be increased in *situ* by up to 80%, allowing for a much better oxygen supply.

The fourth adaptation to aerobic training is an increased number of muscle mitochondria, allowing for increased energy production throughout the working muscles. Again, specificity of training — only those muscles being trained regularly will produce more mitochondria. This is the goal of much of our training: <u>work the main muscle groups needed to power the athlete through the event's requirements,</u> but don't ignore the ancillary groups that can be used to support the whole body through various movements. **Total body development is key to superior athletic performance.**

It takes vigorous exercise to better induce mitochondria to enlarge, multiply, and perform efficiently. But it is important to remember that as the production of mitochondria progresses to where they split and double in amount, those doing the splitting temporarily lose their ability to provide energy. During this time, the athlete may feel sluggish and fatigue more easily. This is only a temporary condition until all the new mitochondria are back on line to contribute to the aggregate energy supply.

The fifth adaptation to occur in aerobically-trained muscle is the enhanced ability to utilize **F**ree **F**atty **A**cids (FFAs) for energy, sparing more of the carbohydrate stores until later in the event or training session for fueling speed.

The cardio-respiratory system's response to endurance-type training is even more encompassing as the major systems adapt to deliver oxygen and energy in greater supply per unit time. The heart's left ventricle chamber gets larger, and the wall thickens to increase the stroke volume, thus the "athletic heart." And, of course, the heart rate decreases during rest and in sub-maximal activity because of the heart's increased efficiency. Several studies have shown that an average of one beat/minute per week is dropped as cardiac condition improves. After six months or more of training, some RESPONSIVE athletes can drop their resting heart rates by 20 to 30 beats per minute or more.

The conditioned athlete also benefits from increased VO2Max (A measure of VO2=Maximum Oxygen Consumption); however, in fully-matured athletes, the highest attainable VO2Max is reached within 8 to 18 months. This indicates that athletes have genetic limits to maximal oxygen consumption.

The respiratory system can be enhanced to a greater percentage increase than cardiovascular function. Though respiration at rest or with easy movement does not increase in functionality from aerobic training, the tidal volume rises consistently at maximum aerobic effort as does the respiratory rate. This is due to increased usage of respiratory tissue, its flexibility in function, increased activity of the intercostal muscles, and increased vascularity for enhanced O2 and CO2 respiration.

A benign side effect of endurance and dedicated training is the observance of what is called *sports anemia*. Upon looking at the athlete's blood test for *hemoglobin* (an important protein carried in the blood that the body produces to transport oxygen where demanded for intense movement) we see the concentration of which becomes diluted giving a false reading of being anemic. What has happened through adaption to continuous intense physical training is the blood volume has increased, which is a good thing. The body does this to create a more extensive amount of circulating fluid that flows more easily to bathe the muscles and carry its nutrients more profusely throughout the body.

But there have been several athletes over the years who were subject to sophisticated manipulative physiology who went the opposite way and intentionally enhanced their blood picture. This is called "blood doping." Feeling they were not truly cheating by doing this since no drugs were consumed, many athletes, mostly seen in the highly competitive European bicycle racing circuit, were in the midst of growing scandals many of which ended in the tragic deaths of experienced cyclists for well-known sponsors. They infused their own increased production of **R**ed **B**lood Cells (RBC) from their intense training to increase hemoglobin concentrations to carry more oxygen. But what they had produced was a too thick and concentrated blood volume which hindered the circulation in many cases and even caused fatalities with clots forming when the blood was forced to circulate rapidly in the midst of intense activity.

STRENGTH

The athlete may ask the trainer or coach, "Why do I need more strength? Why should I devote time and effort to weight training when my focus is endurance?" Of course the answer to that athlete would be, "because a stronger athlete can perform the same tasks with less effort and this translates into less fatigue over time." And as you know, the athlete must also work on areas that are intimately involved with muscle. Connective tissue must be made to adapt to handling increasing resistance from resistance training; tendons must be forced to adapt to handle stronger and thicker muscle fibers that result from this training. Within the first 10 weeks of strength training, the nervous system also adapts by producing more motor-neuronal units.

POWER

Powerful athletes can move through their sport or ACTIVITY-SPECIFIC requirements with speed and grace, and training for power should be as sport specific as possible.

Moving heavy resistance is not enough. Moving heavy resistance quickly but under control is what develops power (with sufficient rest and recovery between power-training bouts, of course).

When pushing the body through bouts of power-generating activity, past the "comfort zone," the athlete is also intentionally creating chemical buffers at the cellular level; ONE OF WHICH, bicarbonate, forms to absorb lactic acid and delay paralyzing acidosis.

Some athletes are just genetically gifted, having a greater percentage of fast-twitch muscle fibers to produce more power. Being the largest fibers in muscle, fast-twitch react the quickest when voluntarily ASKED to contract; however, without a blood supply, the ability to produce energy and remove waste is hindered, AND THUS LIMITED. The slower fast twitch fiber can be INDUCED to HAVE increased blood innervation which allows two things to occur. (1) An increase in the power ability of the athlete ABLE to BE HELD for a longer time. (2) The absolute amount of potential power able to be generated is somewhat diminished. The positive aspect of this is that the increased power produced though not at the absolute maximum, can be held over a GREATER period of time. The athlete then has the ability to pursue the power event LONGER stronger to the finish. Fast twitch fibers also retain their ability to produce power much longer, up to six months, during de-training than slow-twitch fibers which lose their functional aerobic endurance CAPACITY within approximately two weeks of inactivity.

Getting in good condition is a relative thing. Almost everyone has an innate ability to rise to their optimum level, but most who commit to enhancing their physiologic condition will stop short of this. They may fail to see the importance of capturing the elements of endurance, strength, and power. As a result, they will miss the opportunity to achieve an optimally conditioned state.

CHAPTER 2

TO SUFFER PAIN; KNOWING THE DIFFERENCE BETWEEN THIS AND DISCOMFORT

OVERVIEW:

There are several types of pain, all of which can bring the sufferer/endurer to a state of great unease. Pain is one of the most common reasons that patients (athletes, here) seek medical attention or at least guidance from the coaching and therapy staffs with damage to the knee being the largest reason for medical visits. Just being alive qualifies most of us to have had experience with pain in one form, or another and to varying degrees... maybe to help us reach a higher level of existence and grow from it, or to unfortunately "suffer the slings and arrows" about which Shakespeare wrote. The acute and, or chronic physical pain of injury, illness, and constant intense, vigorous training along with the "combat" of competition, and the emotional, deep-stabbing psychological trauma that being alive can eventually bring our way (less if we are lucky, more if we are not) provide the proving ground to build our character and resilience. It has been said that adversity builds character. I believe it only brings out what innate character we have. Pain perception, medically speaking, is a very complex process in which multiple activation pathways are mediated by numerous chemical transmitters in both the periphery (at the sight of injury away from the spinal column and brain) and in the **C**entral **N**ervous **S**ystem (CNS), which comprises the spinal cord and brain.

As to the physical kind of pain which is the main thrust of this chapter, I have often told my athletes, "if you have pain, it means you are still alive so be glad for the feeling." This works most of the time, but not always... especially as it relentlessly mounts through a workout, or a season, or a lifetime. Since I, in my mid-sixties, indulge in the same "tortures" I dish out, dealing with discomfort progressing into pain is almost a daily occurrence when I train. To train sufficiently to induce pain presents a two-edged sword. The body's all-important enzymes and neural and muscle tissues hopefully will adapt the way we want when appropriately stressed out of the comfort zone, but there is the always-present caution that excessive vigorous activity can deplete energy reserves and cause the athlete to suffer excesses where over-reaching progresses into over-training and then into frank athletic fatigue. This is a sure way of putting the athlete in physical harm's way to sustain injury and, or illness which could ruin a serious training schedule. Bad things can happen to an athlete here where the appropriate balance of hard work and the most important part of training, rest and recuperation, are lost during the workout regimen. Sometimes, physically, less is more... and better.

The perception and handling of pain should be led by the individual's motivation and focus at the moment. His present-state physical makeup, his past experience dealing with the actions leading up to pain production during training and competition, and his all-around emotional resilience should all blend like a healthful "cocktail" to produce the desired results. The various causes of pain, their effects on the body and the psyche, and their treatment will be the main topics and take-home points discussed in this chapter.

THE PHYSIOLOGIC MECHANISMS AND DEFINITION OF PAIN

The process of pain transmission from an affected site to its perception in the brain, as mentioned above, involves many neural pathways and neurotransmitters within the central and peripheral nervous systems, either over thin myelinated (protective coating of a fatty-like substance) **A-delta** or non-myelinated **C fibers**. An external stimulus causing the pain activates pain receptors (called *nociceptors),* which then produce an electrical action potential (impulse) that is transmitted along *afferent* (going towards the spinal cord) nerve fibers. These fibers are differentiated by the type of pain they transmit, whether they carry signals *quickly* that delineate well-defined sharp, localized pain (A-delta), or *slower* dull, aching, poorly-defined diffuse pain (C-fibers), and the transmitters included several inflammatory mediators including *prostaglandins, bradykinin, serotonin,* and *histamine.* There are also several peptides such as **Substance-P** that reside within the primary pain fibers signaling the damage to a specific area. The electrical impulse carrying the pain signal then travels to a section (*dorsal horn*) of the cord where pain neurotransmitters such as *glutamate* and *substance P* are released. The transmission then continues up the spine via ascending pathways to higher areas of the brain where it is consciously experienced and deciphered. Once the brain takes hold of these signals it tries to lessen the pain by causing the release of inhibitory stimuli (*endorphins*) through descending pathways down the spinal cord. This mollifying of pain is accomplished through a variety of neurotransmitters including endogenous opioids, *serotonin* (5-*hydroxytryptophan*, 5-HT), *NorepinEphrine* (NE), and *Gamma-Amino-Butyric Acid* (GABA). Researching these chemicals has led to the use of other classes of medications including anti-depressants and anticonvulsants for chronic pain.

The actual substance of pain can be divided into two categories: a. *nociceptive* and b. *neuropathic.* The former is more commonly known as *acute pain.* And it is further categorized as *somatic* and *visceral pain. Somatic* pain usually arises from muscle (spasms, tears, swelling) or other tissue injury... the bane of athletes. It is well localized and is often described as aching, throbbing, or shooting sensations. While visceral pain is often referred from an internal organ, This type of pain (somatic & visceral) is the more common associated with vigorous training and competition and is treated with the usual suspects such as narcotics, **N**on-Steroidal **A**nti-**I**nflammatory **D**rugs (NSAIDS), physical measures and even anti-inflammatory steroids.

Neuropathic pain is physiologically different from *nociceptive* pain, warranting a different approach with different pharmacologic agents for treatment. The mechanism of *neuropathic* pain is more complex and not as well understood as that of *nociceptive* pain. The predominant theory today is that *neuropathic* pain occurs as a result of dysfunction of, or damage to, both the central (brain and spinal cord) and peripheral (rest of the body) nervous systems. There can be a malfunction in the CNS which can lead to several different processes (increased cell firing, decreased inhibition of neuronal activity, and increased generalized sensitization) that are responsible for chronic pain. *Neuropathic* pain is often described as burning, shooting, tingling, and possibly accompanied by numbness. *Hyperalgesia* (the exaggerated response to normally noxious stimuli) and *allodynia* (a painful response to a normally non-painful stimulus) often occur in *neuropathic* pain syndromes. Chronic pain can present as a manifestation of both *nociceptive* and *neuropathic* pain, suggesting the need for a combined pharmacologic approach for optimal treatment.

CHRONIC PAIN AND TREATMENT

This type of pain can become a "resident partner" to a long-standing training regimen, or it can be the remnant of a serious traumatic episode from years previous. And it may also be the most difficult to treat and eliminate. When the pain of an injury lingers past the expected healing time and for longer than three months, it is classified as chronic. And when the psychological component of having to carry the expected daily burden of pain, in varying degrees, follows you everywhere, it can many times become more debilitating than the actual physical component. The Nike Company has utilized a very simple motto, and I believe it has merit: "just do it!" With the appropriate medical and physical therapy having been applied, often, simply moving over an increasing period of time and with increasing effort can lessen the immediate effects of pain. If you choose to do nothing, you will surely be able to do nothing. Usually, chronic pain swells and ebbs like waves out at sea. With the distraction of physical movement and the goings-on of your immediate surroundings and the mental focus needed to keep progressing in a training program, chronic pain can temporarily lessen in overall intensity and duration; it can then rise again either during exercise or immediately after or even be delayed several hours. The threshold of neurological stimulation from the injured site through the central nervous system that actually signals the presence of pain can be temporarily elevated by endogenous (from within) chemicals (*endorphins*) and partially or totally blocked by pharmaceuticals (NSAIDS, *acetaminophen*, true natural and synthetic opioid narcotics). There are also classes of drugs that act outside of their intended use to modify in a positive way the brain's ability to perceive pain. Though these medications might present with side effects that could possibly hinder an athlete to varying degrees and dull the senses, the overall consensus is that if the reduction in constant pain is perceptible and worthwhile, some untoward effects are an acceptable price to pay.

THE USE OF ANTIDEPRESSANTS

This class of drugs has been used for many years to treat pain. The structure of the working chemical molecule in this particular type of medication is called A TricyClic Antidepressant (TCA). Generic names include *amitriptyline, nortriptyline, desipramine*, and *imipramine*. Their role in pain modulation correlates with their ability to increase the amount of circulating inhibitory pain neurotransmitters (*norepinephrine*, NE and *5-hydroxy-tryptophan*, 5-HT) through re-uptake inhibition. The analgesic effect occurs independently of their antidepressant activity since it has been shown that smaller doses work quicker (days vs. weeks) to reduce pain than what is required to act as actual antidepressants. Positive effects for treating *neuropathic* pain have been seen in many studies and are limited by how well the patient can tolerate *anti-cholinergic* side effects (sedation, dry mouth, blurred vision, urinary retention). With this in mind researchers have developed newer antidepressants that have less untoward effects. *Venlafaxine* (*Effexor*) became one of the following generation of antidepressants and released neurotransmitters in varying amounts depending on its concentration in the blood. A popular newer choice, developed in 2004 called *duloxetine* (*Cymbalta*), has showed a good profile for increasing a balanced release of antidepressant and analgesic neurotransmitters and has shown good effects against depression, the *neuropathic* pain of diabetes, and the pain of fibromyalgia. The other *serotonin* uptake inhibitors like *Prozac* and *Zoloft* are good only for depression since they do not release norepinephrine in large enough amounts which are needed for the pain-killing effect.

THE USE OF ANTICONVULSANTS

A few examples of anti-seizure medication (*carbamazepine gabapentin*, and *pregabalin*) have been found useful to treat *neuropathic* and other types of chronic pain. They have several mechanisms of activity which include inhibition of electrolytes sodium and calcium, allowing increases in GABA and inhibition of certain pain receptors (*glutamate*) and work at various sites to block pain transmission to the brain. *Gabapentin* (*Neurontin*) and *pregabalin* (*Lyrica*) are classified as second-generation anticonvulsants and are typically better tolerated with fewer drug interactions than first-generation anticonvulsants (e.g. *carbamazepine*).

TOPICAL THERAPY

With patients suffering a more localized chronic pain syndrome the application of certain medications right to the skin over the troubling area, has proven a workable alternative. If we can derive benefit yet lessen side-effects with local topical pain-killing medication, the efficacious-to-danger ratio becomes quite favorable. The administering of topical NSAIDS has shown much less adverse reactions and has spared the kidneys, stomach, and heart from enduring and suffering potentially serious consequences of usage. Also, the application of *methylsalicylate* or *capsaicin* (a derivative of red chili peppers which blocks the release of the pain transmitter Substance P) in cream form and the localized topical application of a potent anesthetic such as *lidocaine* have proven quite effective with repetitive use.

PAIN FROM ATHLETIC TRAUMA AND SEQUALAE OVER THE YEARS

Ask any athlete, and you will find the medical dictum: "the body never forgets" rings true many more times than not. The higher the level of competition and attendant training, the surer the case for injury development and then the necessary rehabilitation. As an example, there is almost a 100% injury rate in the NFL. This, of course, means that eventually, almost every single player at the highest level in the sport will have suffered a major injury (or series of injuries) that will have a residual effect. Some of my heroes of the gridiron of time past cannot even walk or standalone without support. I am sure that some days even their eyebrows hurt.

IMMEDIATE PHYSICAL TREATMENT OF INJURY

If, say, the knee was to get damaged, the cartilage makes up a good portion of the space of the joint, has good blood supply but no nerve innervation. Therefore, any pain that would result is from collateral damage to tissue surrounding the knee or entering the joint proper. This holds true for any joint having to handle the weight of the body or withstand intense movements. Running and jumping places up to 8 to 10 times body weight on a supporting joint with each "hit" on a hard surface.

There has been a standard protocol for several years that has proved effective for *immediate* treatment of a skeletal-muscular injury. It is called **RICE... R**est, **I**ce, **C**ompression, **E**levation. This is a first-line method of athletic-injury treatment. The closer in time to the injury, the better; certainly within 24 hours of the incident. Heat also has benefit but should be utilized differently. The following chart outlines the recommended treatment with both temperature variants:

Elements of Procedure	Cold/Ice Pack Therapy	Heat/Heat Pack Therapy
TIMING	use immediately and up to 72 hrs. after injury, even after swelling ends	can use as soon as 24 hrs. or after 72 hrs. after swelling
REGIMEN	ice the affected area for 15-20 minutes up to 3-5 times daily, protect skin from freeze burn	apply direct heat up to 3-5 daily; protect skin from heat burn

Elements of Procedure	Cold/Ice Pack Therapy	Heat/Heat Pack Therapy
EFFECTS	decreases blood flow to injury site which decreases inflammatory cells from acting and lessens swelling & pain	increases blood flow to injury and allows for debriding cells to reduce inflammatory site
EQUIPMENT	ice bag, ice cup, frozen gel pack or cool whirlpool bath	dry or moist (best) heating pad hydrocollator pack, heated gel pack, warm to medium-hot bath
PRECAUTIONS	ice packs can be extremely cold and should only be applied over clothing, washcloth or towel, not directly to skin; caution with poor circulation, diabetes, nerve damage or paralysis that allows for skin insensitivity	if hot enough, 1st, 2nd, or even 3rd degree burns can arise; use caution as with cold packs and never while patient sleeps

PHARMACOLOGICAL TREATMENT OF PAIN

The medication treatment indicated for athletic injuries include various choices. Probably the most reached-for and readily-available are the group of NSAIDS... non-steroidal-anti-inflammatory drugs. This class started way back with the discovery by Frederick Bayer in 1899 of the chemical **A**cetyl-**S**alicylic-**A**cid (ASA). Better known as aspirin, science knew that it worked for pain and fever but not how it worked at the cellular level. It took many decades to finally find its mechanism of action, and once this was elucidated, various pharmaceutical houses developed various alterations in the basic active molecule. NSAIDS' main action is to prevent the formation of *prostaglandins,* particularly *prostaglandin* E-2. Local injury or inflammation increases the formation (and its activity) of the enzyme ***CycloOXygenase-2*** (COX-2). This, in turn, leads directly to *prostaglandin* E-2 synthesis with its attendant feeling of increasing pain. *Prostaglandins* can facilitate the transmission of pain signals from the sight of the damage and into and up the spinal cord to the brain due to increasing amounts of COX-2 formation from pain stimuli. So, if we connect the dots, stopping the mediators of pain with readily-available medication, then

16

dealing with pain and injury are easily handled. But, as with most things in life, this sword has two very sharp edges.

Prostaglandins are also needed by the body for protection in several areas. They are needed to ensure the constant formation of protective cells in the stomach to obviate the possibility of bleeding ulcers. They are also needed to ensure adequate blood supply to the internal organs especially the kidneys. When excessive use of NSAIDS is consumed for extended periods, bleeding ulcers and organ failure are very real possibilities. In fact, this class of drugs is the single greatest cause of kidney failure in the United States. And an infamous member of this group, Toradol, has become the bane of the National Football League. Way too many players are on it several times per week throughout their playing careers, especially on game day, where untoward side-effects are now becoming prevalent. The potential for excessive bleeding can also result from this class of drugs as the platelets are bound and made functionless while the drug circulates. When it leaves the body, the platelets are again rendered functional. But this is not as dangerous as aspirin which binds with platelets for their lifespan of about seven to 10 days. Imagine the grave possibility if a player sustains a severe head injury with Toradol circulating through his system... bleeding into the brain.

Interestingly, acute pain usually decreases and even ceases before the body has completely healed because it is so dependent on these inflammatory sensitizers to give out signals of injury. Mother Nature could be making a physiologic mistake here by giving a premature false sense of recuperation and repair to the athlete and coaching staff.

Based on cost, safety, and efficacy, *acetaminophen* (*Tylenol* and others) should be the first choice to treat mild to moderate pain. Adverse effects are minimal if dosages are kept appropriate and **no alcohol is consumed while taking this drug.** This combination has proved deleterious to the liver as have excessively large doses of the drug.

When pain is excessive as with proximity to an injury or when there is an acute exacerbation of pain, the *opioid analgesics* provide the best relief. Most are aware of the sequelae of effects and should be aware of the dangers for excessive and prolonged prescribing. The attendant sedative effect while taking opioids and handling dangerous machinery and driving are a prescription for disaster. The physical and psychological potential for dependency is ever-present and is strongly influenced by dosage, length of time of administration, and the emotional makeup of the patient. Having a single prescriber and pharmacy dispenser can help ensure an appropriate regulatory mechanism to prevent abuse. Though *propoxyphene* (*Darvon, Darvocet*, etc.) and *codeine* have been thought of as not having much potential for abuse, over time and with varying situations, they can, indeed, lead the patient to strongly desire their consumption.

Glucocorticoids present as the most powerful *in situ* (at the site of injury) administration of medication. These anti-inflammatory steroids act to numb the affected area, reduce inflammation and remove it from the injured site, and provide for a sense of well-being even as the injury remains fresh. This can become the "ideal" preparation to get an injured athlete ready for immediate play for an important competition. But not ideal enough to help the athlete heal appropriately over time and with rehab if needed. This class of medication does have a place of purpose if a chronic inflammatory condition flares or lingers beyond sufficient healing time as long as other factors are taken into consideration to allow proper healing over time.

Supplementation with **natural physiologic substances** may help the body withstand debility and pain and help in the total healing process as well, but all studies have not proven conclusively their absolute efficacy. *Hyaluronic Acid* (HA) is a substance in joint fluid that gives it viscosity to act as a lubricant for joint mobility and function. With a chronic inflammatory or osteoarthritic condition of the joint along with the aging process, the molecular weight and concentration of HA is diminished. This allows for bone and cartilage to rub and grind and suffer reduced capacity for appropriate movement. Pain will arise with inflammatory presence. Having HA injected directly into the damaged joint will provide almost immediate effect. Two products, *Hyalgan* and *Synvisc*, are viscous fluids that are administered in a series of injections. The injectable is cleared by the body after only a few days, but pain relief lasts for up to six months. Oral supplementation with HA has shown modest positive effects but only after several weeks of use.

Glucosamine and *Chondroitin* have received much public attention and are being sold almost everywhere there are shelves for such products. Glucosamine is a precursor to *glycosaminoglycans,* an important substance making up cartilage, and chondroitin is a component of the same substance. They have proven efficacy over time, and the pain relief they provide is almost as strong as many of the NSAIDS. In living tissue, these substances can stimulate certain cells to help synthesize *proteoglycans* that make up cartilage and even inhibit an enzyme that can break it down. Whether any of these oral supplements work their claimed miracles in joint tissue is more testimonial than physiological.

Pain comes free with breathing. Most times it is an immediate signal that a definite problem exists right here and now. There are several types of pain that absolutely must not be ignored, and appropriate medical advice should be sought quickly or dire consequences can ensue. Athletic injuries that produce debilitating pain need to be diagnosed and treated with the respect they have garnered over the years. Medications that relieve pain are like blessings from the Gods. They make, at least temporarily, everything all right. What to do with them and how and when to administer them are what good medical care and athletic training are about.

CHAPTER 3

A WEIGHTLIFTING PROTOCOL FOR AQUATIC ATHLETES

OVERVIEW

My overall view for the complete training of competitive swimmers is, in relative importance, to teach them: (1) Proper technique for racing. (2) Inform them of the necessity to develop strength, endurance and power of the muscles, and (3) Expose them to the proper in-pool training to develop total conditioning to meet the demands of the various competitive events. Strength and power have moved up to 2nd place because of the physicality of moving through water: water is 1000 times denser than air and actually increases resistance as one tries to move through it faster. Movement through water requires at least four times the energy as movement on land; in some cases even eight times the energy. Preparing the musculature for this intense demand is something that should not be taken lightly.

The two main types of muscle fibers are: (1) The larger (bulkier) **F**ast **T**witch (FT) fibers which are programmed for powerful movements over a short period of time, and (2) The smaller (thinner) **S**low **T**witch (ST) fibers that have an innate ability to last longer but with less force. Though one is born with a preponderance of one or the other, which usually dictates their talents in athletics, some fibers can be trained to overlap their potential and extend somewhat into the range of the other… fast twitch (FT) fibers can be trained to have more endurance and endurance (ST) fibers can be somewhat trained to have more power.

In addition, proper stretching every day is a must to ensure an adequate **R**ange **O**f **M**otion (ROM), to help heal the muscles from previous training bouts and to prevent injury. It should be standard protocol to stretch before a training session, and a good idea to stretch afterward to help in the recovery of the muscles. In fact, stretching several times a day would not be too much as long as proper form and technique are followed. The most important of which is to allow at least 30 seconds for each stretch. Never let anyone put their hands on you in a stretch; you must do all the movements yourself to prevent possible over stretching and injury.

The use of latex tubing is extremely important. This near perfect piece of equipment can be regulated according to how you feel each day. It allows movements that can pretty much simulate many of the swimming movements. It is easy to pack for travel and rarely presents the possibility of bodily injury.

All movements with weights and latex tubing come under the classification of resistance training. We even use latex tubing in the water to produce both resistive and assistive movements.

WHAT TO DO WITH RESISTANCE TRAINING

- Weightlifting proper should be performed three times weekly; dry land exercises (body-weight movements like crunches, leg lifts, pushups, etc. and latex tubing) should be done 5 days per week.
- The dry land exercises should be done either on the clock (e.g. 30 seconds, 60 seconds, 90 second bouts) or with many (at least 30) repetitions to enhance the endurance factor of the muscles. Early on in the season (the first month), weightlifting should also be done with the consideration of lighter weights and many reps rather than heavier weights with fewer reps… Again to enhance the endurance factor of the muscles.
- As the season progresses into the 2nd month, one of the three weekly weightlifting bouts should consist of using heavier weights and using the "military protocol." This entails doing 12 reps with a moderate weight, then 9 reps with 5 to10 lbs. more, then 6 reps with another 5 to10 lbs., then 3 reps with the same incremental increase, and finally one max rep with 20 to 40 lbs. more than the first set. From 30 to 60 seconds should be allowed for recovery after each set. It is important to try and move the weight with strong bursts of energy, preferably one rep per second to enhance power, not just strength, since power is strength over time, and power is what moves water quickly. If given the choice, I prefer to lift a few hours after practice. I find that a heavy weight training session distorts the feel for the water and does not allow the body to experience a sense of power in the water that we are trying to seek. Many programs have their swimmers do resistive training before swim practice, and this seems to work, but, again, I feel it produces a distortion in the feel of the water. The muscles simply cannot respond to the demands of high-quality swimming the way I would like. If forced to choose, I would forgo the weights for the high-quality swimming as the big meet approaches.
- Once into the 3rd month of training, the emphasis is placed more on power rather than on endurance, though endurance training must not be abandoned. Two out of the three weight lifting bouts are now centered around power lifting. Again, power lifting must entail the individual movements in a one-per-second cadence; taking too long to move a weight will interfere with the neuromuscular adaptation for moving through water in a rapid manner.
- As the big meet approaches, heavy weight-lifting needs to be lessened to allow the musculature time to repair and adjust to "power swimming." The type of day-to-day training in the pool should be altered to enhance the fast twitch muscle fibers and allow for more intense efforts. Faster swimming requires continuous muscular effort of a higher level. There is a need for time to allow the muscles to adapt to the rigor

of high-quality swimming, so resistance training needs to be eliminated. This is especially pertinent as the taper is approached. All weight and resistance training is stopped 10 days out from the big meet. This is sufficient time to allow all physiologic systems to adapt and recover so the best effort in the pool can be put forth.

CHAPTER 4

FROM ENDURANCE, TO STRENGTH, TO POWER IN THE WATER

There has never been an athlete (male or female) I've known, coached, or competed against that did not want to become as strong as possible. The serious competitors all wanted to have the hallmark defined muscle "cuts" of a solid athletic build. My venue, starting in the late 1950's, was the pool where "doing weights" was considered a mistake. It was thought that more developed muscle would inhibit flexibility and get in the way of fast swims; the road to aquatic athletic success, as we were constantly reminded by our coaches, was intensely moving our skinny bodies back and forth doing various swim and kick sets. Then in the early '60's strength training was seen by some visionaries more as an aid than an enemy. A few rising stars began to move free weight and pull on resistance cables to increase their strength and add some muscle endurance so they could move more water longer. This was a simple and logical advancement in swim training. This information soon spread to other sports that traditionally didn't incorporate resistance with their sport-specific training.

Though most aquatic athletes and their coaches didn't realize the absolute differences between endurance, strength, and power and the importance of correct physical preparation and progression to obtain these, they were content to simply add either a few bouts of resistance exercise a week to their in-pool training or an abbreviated session of "dry-land" work on deck each time just before entering the water thinking they were getting one-up on their competition that stayed only in the pool. They were right.

The three elements in this chapter's title succinctly outline the appropriate progression we want the athlete to take. First be able to forcefully move a constant resistance again and again over an extended period of time without getting injured (endurance), then be able to safely move an increased amount of resistance (strength), and finally to be able to move that increased resistance quickly; power equals strength over time. P = Strength time.

Emphasis is placed on leg work since most swim training sessions only afford a minor portion to this. There are advantages to water-stressing the legs that will prove invaluable in close swim races, for the biking and running segments in a triathlon, and as productive cross-training for any athletic adventure that requires leg movement. The importance is that I recommend cutting swim yardage or other training elements, needed, to allocate precious time of a tight schedule to perform these leg-specific water based exercises.

There is also a physiological phenomenon of aquatic training that must be mentioned: sort of a one-way street to increased condition. Training seriously in the water usually produces tremendous benefits for those performing exercises and sports anywhere. Land-

Based exercises only help to a minor degree in water since they cannot nearly measure up to in-pool resistance training for those needing increased endurance, strength, and power in aquatic sports. **The message is clear here**: if you want to max out your physical potential ANYWHERE, you should work the water.

USING THE WATER TO FIRST BUILD ENDURANCE

The normal physiology of muscle activity (as designed by Mother Nature millions of years ago) allows for some muscle fibers to contract while others relax. We also have been endowed with fast-twitch and slow-twitch muscle fibers in varying percentages. The latter produce less force than the former but have more natural endurance since they have a strong blood supply carrying nutrients and oxygen. The fast-twitch fibers contract more forcefully than the slow-twitch, for the most part, but have no blood supply and can only fire for a relatively short period of time before fatiguing from physiologic acidic build-up and *Adenosine TriphosPhate* (ATP) depletion. This evolutionary fact crudely made use of natural basic endurance by giving our ancestors somewhat of a chance to survive an extended dash to the protective trees in nearby forests to escape being food for larger occupiers of the planet with bad intentions toward us. Unfortunately, this UNTRAINED natural endurance is not enough to carry us through today's sport-specific requirements for an extended period of time. And it is an **established** physiologic fact that increasing endurance helps to protect against overuse injury by adapting the connective tissue around the joints and muscles to handle the increased loads of physical exercise we plan to endure. **The wise thing to do first**... Adapt the body by increasing endurance.

*If we bring in aquatic exercise or sports, anything that happens in water requires more than FOUR TIMES THE EFFORT than it does to move on land, yet it spares serious wear-and-tear on the body because of the gravity-free environment water provides. Example: at the world record level it takes longer to sprint-swim 50 meters freestyle (21.64) than it does to sprint-run a 200 meter dash (19.72). For those needing their legs or to increase their general aerobic and anaerobic condition to tackle land-based exercise or sports, **working the legs and various other muscle groups in water is the absolute smart thing to do.**

To begin with, the gravitational pounding against an unforgiving medium (roadbed, ground, dirt, etc.) for hours (and miles) on end will take its toll eventually on almost everyone by breaking down the support structures with acute and, or chronic inflammation especially at the articular (joint) areas. This is not a matter of "if", but of "when." The athlete, of course, must put time on the ground or on the bike if he participates in running and biking; the body still has to be trained to withstand what we expect to put it through. But a wise use of cross-training will spare body parts and enable the athlete to participate that much stronger longer. But I do not recommend running for my swimmers for just such reason as to prevent needless wear-and-tear on body parts more used to a gravity-free environment. I suggest using the mechanical advantage of the bike, in-doors or out, where the negative stresses are shifted away from joint-pounding.

Most training in the pool to build total body endurance requires swimming laps, no getting around that. It is the perfect activity to increase total body condition and to build on the components of becoming powerful. The benefits of the water have even been incorporated into several professional boxers' routines. And swimming with the correct style of fins allows for these benefits to happen even more quickly and to a higher degree for two reasons. (1) **Since the muscle groups of the legs are the single largest to be utilized at any given moment,** putting them through various modes of resistive movement in the water forces the cardiovascular and respiratory systems to reach higher levels of capacity to meet metabolic demand… The heart and lungs do not know you have fins on, only how hard, and fast you are moving through water, (2) unlike air that doesn't change, moving through water releases the phenomenon that **as you travel faster through it, water's resistance increases,** holding you back more. Due mainly to the physical property of water being 1000 times denser than air, doubling your speed through the former causes it to resist your mobility by SQUARED (2 x 2 = 4) the effort, and this occurs only if you streamline and move through it correctly. Fight the water to any degree or add more intentional resistance, and it holds you back CUBED of the effort (2 x 2 x 2 = 8) that means doubling the effort brings on EIGHT TIMES THE RESISTANCE! Anyone not comfortable and experienced in the water can attest to the fact that flailing through it for more than 10 seconds can bring on a great degree of discomfort both respiratory and muscular, usually in that order.

Since forcing the body's conditioning enzymes to produce more *mitochondria* (energy cells) in the vital tissues associated with vigorous exercise is the key to building any increase in the training effect, extending repeated efforts over distances to 300 yards or meters or holding the efforts for four to five minutes elicits the desired adaptive response. This may prove quite daunting to the uninitiated and would drive away most attempting such training. The perceived feeling of being completely out of air in water can humble even the most determined. What works initially is to break the distance or time interval down into segments that allow short recovery periods. During this brief inserted rest, it is more the need to blow off (exhale forcefully) accumulated CO_2 rather than the perceived need to inhale more air that allows for a greater recovery. The effort becomes challenging but doable and can be expanded and made more challenging as condition increases.

Below is a listing of ways to increase resistance in the water to help build cardio-vascular, respiratory, and leg endurance and then to maintain it throughout the training season.

- Using fins and alternating freestyle and butterfly kicks with a kick board in a straight forward (neutral) position for 100 yards/meters; rest 10 seconds, a 2nd 100 with another 10 seconds rest; finally the 3rd 100; no matter how the legs burn each 100 must be traversed uninterrupted and with the same steady cadence held from the beginning. Eventually, the goal is to kick 300 yards/meters straight holding the pace. As condition improves, speed is increased throughout the distance, and two more repeats are added after 30 seconds recovery.

- In deep water, holding the hands continuously above the water line, kicking both freestyle and butterfly at first with NO fins; kicking bout is held for 15- second intervals at first, resting 15 seconds after each, progressing to three by 30 seconds, then 45, then 60; once at this level, USING FINS should bring the athlete to two minutes of straight kicking with several repeats after 30-second recoveries.
- "Water-walking:" performed both with fins and without; this is not typical kicking as would be practiced with swim strokes; this entails quick, smooth alternating repetitive movements of the legs raising the knees up as high as possible toward the chest and then kicking back away from the body with the bottom of the feet pressing against the water; performed on the stomach and on the back with hands folded in a praying position; this works not only all the muscles of the legs but also serves to stretch and develop the hip-flexors. It is the most inefficient way to move through water, but the one that brings out the training effect of leg endurance the most. One length of "water-walking" is equivalent in metabolic demand to three to four lengths of traditional swimming or kicking. One-length repeats of 25 yards or meters are worked with 15-30 seconds rest per length; the use of fins requires doubling the distance.
- Lastly, the athletes are tied to fastened sturdy latex tubing and are asked to kick with fins against its force starting for 15 seconds. The goal is to continue the kick and hold a set distance from the starting wall while stringing the 15-second segments together to continuously move against the pull-back of the tubing for up to two minutes. A further benefit is derived here: preventing the "cocoon effect."

Normally when the brain perceives movement it expects movement, either forward, backward, or side-to-side; but when the tubing is fully extended there is no longer forward movement, so the brain starts to "short-circuit," and the athlete may panic and feel that he is being swallowed or smothered by the water. If handled properly, this builds mental toughness and the aerobic condition to withstand this most demanding of stresses.

PROGRESSING FROM ENDURANCE TO STRENGTH

To train for increasing strength, every workout procedure listed above needs to be handled in demanding fashion. We are less concerned with how long we can hold an exercise than how much resistance we can overcome during a designated length of time.

- To further increase resistance; the board is placed in front of the swimmer half submerged with the rounded end up resembling a "tombstone." This DOUBLES frontal resistance. Then we increase resistance by FOUR TIMES the original by placing the kickboard half submerged sideways, so it resembles a "snowplow." A typical exercise bout calls for using one type of kick, alternating the kickboard positions, one length of each: neutral, "tombstone," and "snowplow." The speed of the kick is held constant while the resistance is increased. This is repeated four times with a 30-second rest in between bouts. Another exercise demands that all three lengths of the pool are traversed using the "tombstone" configuration, 30-second rest, then three lengths using "snowplow;" three lengths holding the board in neutral position, finally one length each way with the board. Constant speed is something that must be maintained or attempted.

- Deep-water kicking is now performed holding a medicine ball with both hands out of the water; recommended starting weight is six pounds for a duration of 20 seconds; this is attempted four times with a 20-second rest in between. As strength increases and condition rises, slightly heavier medicine balls are used topping off at 10 pounds while holding the kicking bout for up to 60 seconds. Fins are to be used for free and fly kick but those wanting to train breaststroke kick must do it sans fins. Upper body strengthening is a welcomed "side-effect" of supporting the ball above the water line.
- "Water-walking" with a medicine ball overhead should be done with fins except those wanting to work the breaststroke kick; the already taxing demands of this exercise are magnified by four holding the ball above water. Water-walking forwards on the belly holding the ball up is called "presentation" and is the absolute hardest exercise to do; more than twice the difficulty of "walking" on the back. Stress is placed on the arms, shoulders, trunk and legs and is magnified as the athlete moves down the lane.
- Kicking against the pull of latex tubing with an increasing intensity up to a predetermined point in the pool over a designated length of time, then stopping and allowing the tubing to pull back the swimmer to the starting point; repeating this bout after 30 seconds rest for a total of five.

GOING FROM STRENGTH TO POWER

Now we are least concerned about holding an exercise for time; rather, we want to move whatever resistance is in our way as quickly and POWERFULLY as possible. Short bursts of intense energy are required, and the fast-twitch muscle fibers are tapped in repeated bouts, each after adequate recovery. Per unit time, this type of training is the most demanding and is correctly reserved for the last position in the progression. * You cannot be powerful unless you have endurance and strength in place. Go for power too soon in the training scheme, and injury is more than likely to occur. **THERE IS NO SHORT-CUT TO POWER**

Our goal is power. It is a prolonged and challenging process to attain it. If things go well, the athlete will perform up to his potential. But we know how hard he has worked to make it all look so easy.

CHAPTER 5

THE CARE AND NURTURING OF THE BREATHING PROCESS

There are several things in life we simply take for granted; you do not need intense mental effort nor demand of dedicated focus to figure them out. One of these things is the main topic of the presentation. We as a species have acclimated appropriately to our environment and even more closely to our immediate ambiance. This is the way the human element has always functioned, and it is mostly directed by the way we live our lives. The human body is the most miraculous machine ever, and after so much effort to study its functions, we still don't know very much. Biological scientists are continuously engrossed to peel back and expose the hidden reasons for how and why the body acts, reacts, and adapts to its surroundings and changes in immediate conditions. If we stay in our comfort zones, for example, we expect very little challenge to be created in the body's functioning. But if we push ourselves into areas of serious physical challenge, we then see much of our efforts to endure this challenge consume much of our deep energy reserves and mental toughness. Things occur to either allow adaptation or failure. And the single most important adaptation we can work to achieve, in my opinion, is the reliance on our ability to exchange air adequately as our ever-increasing need for oxygen drives all metabolic processes and takes over our very existence in sport and exercise.

We have come to consider this a natural right of our very being. Compromise our breathing ability, even a little, and the body will respond dramatically in kind. Nature has provided for us to adapt, even thrive on what the earth offers up: only 21% pure oxygen at sea level. Most of the rest of our ambient air mixture has non-physiologic nitrogen (78%) with minute' amounts of trace gases. But our physiology can only work with oxygen. Our biochemical reactions are geared to how much $O2$ can we inhale, absorb and chemically-turn into bio-friendly compounds to enable quality muscular activity. This is such an important process that the main computer of our body, the brain, is brought in almost immediately to control our perception of where we are moment by moment with regard to how much oxygen is available and our ability to utilize it.

THE BRAIN'S INVOLVEMENT IN THE BREATHING PROCESS

With any serious attempt at athletics or intense physical exercise, it is the brain that takes control of our bodies. Nature gave it the software to quickly perceive our ambient oxygen supply ranging from everything is all right to there is absolutely not enough to go on. (This is an important concept which will be discussed below: "what we perceive is what we believe.") The brain's respiratory center is given such importance that it continues to function allowing us to exchange air even when other controlling centers begin to shut down under the increasing influence of alcohol and, or drugs. But it is not infallible. With sufficient damaging dosages of central nervous system depressants, the ability to breathe becomes labored and eventually can be inhibited enough to bring about suffocation.

This 10% of our body mass (the brain) absolutely influences the other 90%. And the controlling segment of the brain that is the center of all this activity is next to the respiratory center and is called the *amygdala*. It is strongly stimulated by the presence of (CO2). The more this compound builds up in the body, the stronger the *amygdala* " screams" stop. The participant's perception proceeds quickly from "I feel okay," to "I don't feel okay," to "I think I am going to die." Often-times panic ensues with enough *amygdalal* stimulation. And this is manifest to a greater degree in the water than on land since humans are all born land-based beings, the water presenting as a foreign and ever-threatening medium through which swimmers choose to move. With very few exceptions (example: the appendix) Nature does not waste much time and energy providing body parts or biochemical reactions that do not have protective or activating functions. The *amygdala's* main activity is to sense threatening or exceptional conditions that are perceived to be interfering with the body's ability to easily move, and this perception is centered around the need to obtain as much oxygen as quickly as possible.

Since it is intuitive that our perceptions command our beliefs, to feel we are out of air causes us to work the inhale more than the exhale. With intense exercise or movement, this perception can become all-controlling; to the point that it absolutely influences what we do and how long we do it. The uninitiated or untrained athlete would show great distress with a marked grimace and veins popping from the neck desperately trying to inhale as much air as quickly as possible. This painful distortion of facial features and labored air-exchange produce what is called the **"dragon-breathing syndrome;"** all this because of the intense feeling of being out of air. Since physical law states that two things cannot occupy the same space at the same time, if forcefully exhaling the "stale" air with its carbon dioxide load is the process taught and learned, the ability to inhale adequate "fresh" air becomes easier and more successful since there is now room in the lungs. If the brain can be "schooled" to handle this situation, then the athlete would be able to push past this limitation of perceived air distress. This approach has now even come to rule present-day Navy SEAL training.

THE PHYSICAL ASPECTS OF HARNESSING AMBIENT AIR

There are many influences that come into play when working the breathing processes... what I call sufficient or insufficient "air-exchange." Our health can change quickly when encountering diseases of varying intensity that affect respiration.

While studying pathology in graduate school, my professor once opened a lecture with the question of how many of us smoked cigarettes and how many consumed alcohol on a regular basis. He then offered up a comment that if we knew what was out there waiting to "get" us, we would all hide in a cave, until we found out what was waiting for us in the cave.

Interpretation: there is no safe place to hide so we better act appropriately and work to attain and maintain the best possible quality of health we can. Our health can be greatly influenced by our life styles and ambient surroundings. The intuitive activity of every athlete or participant in vigorous exercise is centered around the most important of life's processes: keeping the air exchange accessible and in good working order no matter what we choose to put our bodies through. The body must always be in a state of adequate hydration for general health; so should the air we breathe.

We move faster; we breathe faster. The more intense the movement, the more intensely the body must satisfy the inevitable increase in demand for oxygen-laden air. When the quality and, or quantity of ambient air changes such that the body must acclimate, there is an immediately added stress to pulmonary functioning. The scandalously poor air quality in China for the 2008 Games placed great stress on many of the Olympians, some of whom were forced to endure breathing difficulties over extended time and great distances. There is almost always an obvious delay in the appropriate response to handling diminished air quality or quantity. When air becomes cold and dry as in winter months at northern latitudes, the quality of the air exchange is diminished due to lack of soothing warm moisture. If the home or place of activity becomes heated and, hence, dried to contain less than 50% humidity the nasal passages and bronchioles begin to dry out; mucous usually thickens, further interfering with an increased need for quality air exchange. The dry cotton-mouth feeling inhaling excessively dry air is just an early warning sign of the need for more moisture. The participant in sport or exercise should always hydrate before, during, and after an intense, concentrated effort. Indoors at a chlorinated pool always demands adequate hydration; same for exercise in the heat or extremely dry conditions. Most don't realize you sweat and lose physiologic moisture even in the water. And this can set up the athlete to become more susceptible to respiratory infections and irritants since the linings of the breathing tubes lose their ability to keep the mucus thin and flowing. Irritation over time leading into inflammation of the breathing process could develop into **Exercised-Induced** *Bronchospasm* (EIB), athletic asthma and diminished air flow when most needed. The best and most immediate form of treatment would be the use of a hot-steam or warm/moist air vaporizer. Many physicians recommend the use of a cool-mist unit, but this is mostly for the reason of preventing the possibility of getting burned from the steam. Bacteria, molds, and viruses can more easily be transmitted and spread all over with cool mist equipment. The hot, soothing moist air from a steam-producer is sterile when it comes out of the unit and provides a better condition all around for the person seeking safe humidified air.

As we age, our lungs lose elasticity and the ability to exchange increasing amounts of inhaled air into our circulatory system. This markedly diminishes that which needs to be carried to where it will do the most good: the vital organs and the skeletal muscles for immediate movement. The total amount of air in the lungs, for the most part, remains the same but during the aging process the amount of oxygen-laden air for physiological use declines. The residual, or "dead air" increases over time and cannot be relied upon to deliver oxygen for our biochemical needs. We normally would have to endure what our lungs can provide with active exchangeable air. Expected decline in an aging healthy person is between eight and ten percent per decade. But this degradation can be cut in half with proper training and appropriate energy-supplementation. Inducing our physiology with the physical aspect of certain training sets to increase a specific group of enzymes involved with upgrading our VO2Max capacity (the facility to extract oxygen from our inhaled air) should be the goal of every quality coach and athlete for maximizing oxygenation of the active body. It is time-consuming and requires the right type of training over many months from someone familiar with inducing this type of pertinent physiology. The end result will hopefully be what every athlete seeks: being able to strongly finish races.

Training at altitude has its positive effect on causing the body to increase its oxygen transport and utilization systems, but this, too, takes dedication over several weeks to months to induce the proper adaptation for increased oxygen-usage. The protein complex in the blood that is mainly involved with this shuttling of oxygen to where it is needed quickly and consistently is *hemoglobin*. We have all heard of those athletes (so inclined as to give up the sportsman's code to win at all costs) who have been seen to instill their own concentrated hemoglobin back into their circulation with intent to maximize oxygen-carrying capacity without having to worry about certain markers (drugs or foreign bodies) showing up that would indicate a cheating protocol on blood tests. But if the hemoglobin is way too concentrated as compared with laboratory guidelines, it would indicate nefarious intentions. Also, as with many things in life, there is a strong potential for abuse and dangerous outcomes. The excess heme can thicken the blood and hinder its movement with the formation of clots. The dangerous sequelae are obvious if this develops. Is winning or improving performance possibly worth this risk... Not on your life!

And, of course, the obvious: inhaled irritants can wreak havoc on the breathing process. United States Swimming has banned smoking near pool decks and in venues. Many colognes and perfumes also have irritating properties, as does traffic exhaust that seems even more disturbing because water has a unique physical property of drawing fumes to it and concentrating these vaporous compounds right where the swimmers need air. And it is not just human athletes that can be affected by poor air quality as mentioned above with the Beijing Games. When brought to race during certain months in the Tri-State Metropolitan area (New York, New Jersey, Connecticut) having the air cool, dry, and laden with particulate matter from pollution, thoroughbred horses were often seen to bleed from their noses after several days of running. The body can often overcome this type of insult if it is infrequent, but not if continuous exposure becomes the norm. There will be a price to pay for having to continuously and forcefully exchange unhealthy air such that our breathing apparatus becomes compromised, and performances will definitely be diminished.

There have been a few physical procedures that have been and are still being utilized to hopefully aid in the breathing and recovery processes. But these simply don't provide for the benefits they were hoped to receive. The breathing in of pure oxygen to help recovery is, for the most part, useless. In the past we have seen professional football players on sidelines, to name one sport, mask-over-face inhaling from oxygen tanks. The body can NOT store oxygen, and it cannot increase its ability to immediately carry oxygen to demanding tissue, even at mild altitude. If the athlete thinks inhaled pure oxygen is his salvation, he is being incorrectly advised; rather, it is his physiologic condition and training that needs to be brought into question. His preparation for intense repeated movement simply has been improper and inadequate.

Also, the use of pinched breathing snorkels while swimming to supposedly increase the resistance to inhalation requiring more power of the breathing apparatus when under physiologic stress has proven to be non-beneficial. This still seems to be a very popular training mode for many programs. But in actuality, it is a waste of time and energy. This apparatus does not increase the strength and endurance of the *intercostal muscles* (between the ribs) to help the athlete inhale more air with each breathing cycle. The breathing muscles are exercise adequately through regular and dedicated training. Rather, the exact opposite is what should be stressed. It is the EXHALE rather than the inhale that aids the process of air-exchange more thoroughly and efficiently as explained previously.

THE PHYSIOLOGICAL AND BIOCHEMICAL ADAPTATIONS TO BETTER UTILIZE AMBIENT AIR

As touched upon above in the physical aspects of breathing, the actual cellular-level biochemistry and physiology that is driven by the quality of the breathing process can and should be stressed such that the body will consistently benefit from enhanced air-exchange to more strongly finish races. As I am fond of saying to my athletes: "It's not how far you swim, nor how fast you swim; rather, it is how far can you swim fast?!" What has been shared so far is how we utilize our ambient air initiated with the natural procedure of inhalation. With the science of physiology and the concomitant biochemical study of the processes within our bodies, sophisticated and daring experiments from the lab to the athletic venue have shown that remarkable adaptations can be developed to enhance how the body can utilize its air supply over time and distance. This now brings in the concept of **enzyme-induction**.

It is the wise coach, biological scientist, and dedicated athlete who combine to form a winning combination in establishing pertinent protocols for enhanced air-utilization. All around exchange of information from experimental results with observant notation can bring about amazing results. But there first must be a desire to understand what goes on inside the body. As such, know that all major biochemical processes are influenced by enzymes and enzyme groups. And there are several that need to be induced to produce a quality athlete.

Enzymes are protein compounds that act as catalysts and drivers of how the body reacts and adapts to various types of physiological stress. The enzyme group that governs **aerobic capacity** or **maximum oxygen consumption** (VO2Max) is an extremely important one. If the body cannot extract sufficient amounts of oxygen for its needs from inhaled air over time and distance, quality movement will be short-lived, and performances less than stellar will be seen in mid-distance and distance events.

VO2Max is influenced by size and mass of the athlete more with land-base and weight-bearing activities (with bigger usually allowing for greater values) than with gravity-free and non-weight bearing activities such as swimming and cycling. In the latter types of exercise, the extracted and consumed amounts of oxygen per unit time are more concerned with the ability to simply extract the needed amounts of oxygen from ambient air than the actual size of the athlete. BUT, we also must not discount the actual physical dimensions of the athlete with regards to actual lung size and subsequent usable oxygen transfer to demanding organs and tissues. Maximum increase in capacity for oxygen extraction and utilization from the ambient air is the goal for building aerobic capacity and is usually optimized by 8 to 12 weeks of appropriate training where distances of repeat 300 yards or meters have been shown to provide adequate physiological adaptation along with relatively short rest intervals at 75%-80% perceived effort. Even lesser distances can be utilized appropriately to enhance this capacity as long as work and rest segments are correctly used in tandem. Keep in mind that even the 100-meter distance for each swimming event, and its equivalent on land in time and energy cost (a 400-meter run) takes enough time and consumes enough energy to require an important percentage of aerobic capacity.

So once the body has been adapted to inhale and absorb increasing amounts of oxygen-laden air, what next in the chain of functions is necessary to allow ever-more intense biochemical activity to proceed smoothly? The body has to have receptors available to grab hold and direct newly-arrived oxygen to where and how it can do the most good... producing prodigious amounts of energy for maintaining speed and power.

The answer is the extremely important production of *mitochondria* throughout the skeletal musculature and vital organs. These organelles (small parts or subdivisions of organ tissue) are the only substances that can produce energy and manufacture the fuel for movement: (ATP). The more of this we have in store and able to quickly make available, the stronger, longer, faster the athlete can move. Again, there are training sets to produce more and more of this vital substance along with newly-discovered energy supplements. The appropriate utilization of both can combine to produce still sought-after optimum results.

CHAPTER 6

THE PHYSIOLOGY OF AGING

OVERVIEW

There are several aspects to physiologic aging that can interact to diminish the body's ability to perform vigorous activity. It is the intention of this writing to delineate those aspects and assess what, if anything, can be done to delay, stop, or even reverse the negative effects of time on the human body.

It seems that today athletes of all ages and abilities are on a quest for optimum performance in their chosen athletic endeavors. More so than ever, age is becoming of secondary importance... Allowing one to compete in the next older bracket, or more remarkably, in open competition as evidenced at the 2000 Olympic Games, but without diminished performance. Opportunities are more available now than ever for older athletes (now called Masters or Senior athletes) to compete in various sports activities ranging from marathon running, to swimming, to cycling, to weight lifting.

However, although these older athletes exhibit strength and endurance capacities far greater than those of untrained people of similar age, even the most highly trained older person experiences a decline in performance after the fourth or fifth decade of life. (1)

In modern societies, the level of voluntary physical activity begins to decline soon after people reach adult maturity. Included in trying to reduce stress as we age is the reduction in muscular effort. Modern technology has afforded us the fact of life that things are now much less physically demanding. Considering the above, one wonders why some older individuals choose to remain physically active when the natural tendency is to become sedentary.

It is common knowledge, at least to those who are generally aware of what it takes to feel physically sound, that repeated vigorous activity is extremely important to maintaining robust health into advanced age. But to distinguish the differences in physiologic parameters due to **chosen** reduced activity (as seen with many as they get older) and advancing age proper, one need only to study Masters competitors, regardless of their chosen sport. It is all too obvious that, as we age, we need more rest between work bouts as compared to younger athletes. Even at a high level of conditioning, the older athlete requires more recovery time to engage in a repeat maximum effort than a younger athlete.

Of course, there is another element that should be addressed regarding one's ability to develop and retain aerobic and anaerobic capacities regardless of age. That element is simple genetics. It has been shown that "picking the right parents" and being the recipient of a great mix of DNA can influence up to 50% of an athlete's ability to perform at a superior level. (2) Those such blessed and devoted to continuous hard work to maximize their athletic potential are the ones we usually see representing the USA at the Olympic Games. How much they retain is in their hands, however, due mainly to how much they choose to exercise vigorously throughout their later years.

Parameters to be discussed and illustrated will include sports performance comparisons by age, respiratory changes with aging, cardiovascular changes with aging, changes in strength with aging, body composition with aging, trainability of the older athlete, and how training can delay the decline in exercise performance.

SPORT PERFORMANCE

Records in running, swimming, cycling and weight lifting suggest that we are in our physical prime during our 20's or early 30's. Although older **runners** have achieved some exceptional records, running performance in general declines with age, and the rate of this decline appears to be independent of distance. **Longitudinal studies** (testing the **same athletes** repeatedly as they age) of elite distance runners indicate that, despite a high level of training, performance in events from the mile to the marathon **declines** at a rate of about **1% per year** from age 27 to 47. (3,4) It is also interesting to note that in a **cross-sectional analysis** (results of **different athletes** representing the various age groups) American records for both the 100-meter and 10-km runs also decrease by about 1% per year from age 25 to 60. **Beyond age 60,** however, the records for men slow by **nearly 2% per year.** Another cross-sectional sprint-running test of 560 **women** between the ages of 30 and 70 revealed a steady **decline** in running velocity of **8.5% per decade (0.85% per year).** The patterns of change are about the same in both sprint and endurance running performances. (see figure A)

A study of past national masters **swimming** championships (1991-1995) shows that, for the 1500-meter freestyle, both men and women **slowed steadily from age 35 to about 70, after which swimming times slowed down at a faster rate.** Additionally, the **rate and magnitude of the declines** in both the 50-meter and 1500-meter freestyles were **greater for females than males** (a possible strength component here). (5) Another analysis shows a comparison of U.S. Masters **swimming** records in the 100-meter freestyle; the times get slower by about **1% per year** for both men and women from age 25 to age 75. But because success in this sport depends on skill as well as on strength and endurance, some U.S. Masters swimmers have achieved their personal best performances at 45 to 50 years of age.

Cycling performances are best seen in the age range of 25 to 35. Male and female cyclists' records (40-km distance) drop at about the same rate with age; an average of 20 seconds (0.6%) per year. The U.S. national cycling records for the 20-km distance show a similar pattern for both sexes. For this distance, speed decreases by about 12 seconds (0.7%) per year from age 20 to nearly age 65. (6)

In general, **maximal muscle strength** is achieved between the ages of **25 and 35.** Beyond that age range, the ability to LIFT WEIGHT declines at a steady rate of about 1.8%

per year. Of course, as with other measurements of human performance, **individual strength varies considerably.** Some individuals, for instance, exhibit greater strength at age 60 than people half their age.

Thus, to summarize the above: (a) records in running, swimming, cycling, and weight lifting indicate that we are in our physical prime during our 20's and early 30's; (b) in all of these sports, performance generally declines with aging beyond our physical prime. However, with swimming, which relies heavily on skill, some older athletes attain their personal best performances in their 40's and 50's; most athletic performances decline steadily during middle and older age, primarily due to decrements in endurance and strength. (7)

Now we will look at the specific parameters which tear at us through the years and act to cause inevitable declines in athletic performance...

CHANGES IN CARDIORESPIRATORY ENDURANCE WITH AGING

To a large extent, changes in endurance performance that **accompany aging** can be attributed to **decrements in both central and peripheral CIRCULATION.** Measurements of cardiac output and limb blood flow are not easily performed, so early studies of the effects of aging on the physiology of endurance exercise examined **maximum oxygen uptake (VO2Max), which correlates well with maximal cardiac output.** (see Table 1) More recently there have been effort's to measure blood flow and oxygen exchange in the leg muscles of exercising older subjects, but these studies are limited in number, so for the most part **the explaining of the decline in endurance performance is limited to changes in maximal oxygen uptake (aerobic capacity).**

STUDIES OF NORMALLY ACTIVE PEOPLE

The first studies of importance and relevance regarding the aging process and physical fitness were done in the late 1930's. (8) What was ascertained from these studies was the fact that **maximal oxygen uptake in normally active men declined steadily from age 25 to age 75 at about an average of 1% per year** (see Table 2), **which is the same rate of decline seen in endurance running, swimming, and cycling performances.** More recently, a review of 11 cross-sectional studies, most involving men under age 70 examined the rate of decline in **VO2Max** with age; these showed a decrease of from 0.8% to 1.1% per year. (9) In the few longitudinal studies performed in this area (10,11,12), a wide range of decline in aerobic capacity was seen, but these variations can be attributed to the subjects' different activity levels and ages at the beginning of the studies. Nevertheless, the rate of decline in **VO2Max** is generally agreed to be approximately 10% per decade or 1% per year **(0.4ml)** per year in relatively sedentary men.

kg min

Some studies have shown that, on average, women demonstrate a lower rate of VO2Max decline with age **(0.2 to 0.5ml)** per year than men. (8) While others show no difference. (13,14)

But there is one variable many women have over men. Due to their less consistent physical activity as they grow into maturity, many women not involved with sports or training start their decline in VO2Max earlier (late teens) than men (mid-20's).

To provide a more accurate comparison of VO2Max values in men and women, simply comparing values with the increased body weight component as one ages is inadequate and will give inappropriately-low values of aerobic capacity. One should use actual readings of **Liters/min of oxygen uptake rather than the relative reading with the increased body weight component** to get a more appropriate comparison of aerobic capacity with aging. Also, comparisons of such aerobic capacity values do not take into consideration the interval's initial **VO2max** values. For example, a decline of *0.5ml/kg per minute* in someone with an initial value of *30ml/kg per minute* would have a greater impact than in someone with a value of *50ml/kg per minute.* It would be better (and more accurate) to compare groups of people in terms of their percentage change in *VO2max,* which can be calculated as follows:

$$\textit{\% Change} = \frac{\textbf{VO2Max-Initial VO2Max}}{\textbf{Initial VO2Max}}$$

Using this formula, it has been shown that both men and women lose about 1% per year in aerobic capacity. This decline is caused primarily by a reduction in maximum heart rate and stroke volume. These reductions decrease cardiac output, which then limits oxygen transport to the muscles.

STUDIES OF OLDER ATHLETES

Scientists at the Harvard Fatigue Laboratory have done some longitudinal studies on former elite runners encompassing about 30 years. What information that came out of the study showed that runners who did not continue to train during middle age showed much larger declines in aerobic capacity (43% decline on average from age 23 to 53) than those who "stayed in shape." (15) **These facts seem to prove that prior training offers little advantage to endurance capacity in later life unless a person continues to engage in some form of vigorous activity.**

Another study observed that over a 10-year period, older track athletes (ages 50 to 82) who continued to train and compete were able to maintain their VO2Max values at a fairly high level, whereas those who reduced their training showed a significant decline in aerobic capacity. (16) The main premise from this study emerged to show that, as one passed middle age, vigorous training was the main component to keeping Father Time (aerobic capacity in this case) relatively in check, or at least in slowing down his agenda for us all. However, other changes were the same for both groups: (a) maximum heart rate decreased by about 5 to 7 beats/min per decade; (b) body weight increased from an average of 154 lbs. to 164 lbs.; body fat increased significantly from about 13% to over 18%.

More recently, longitudinal studies of older runners and rowers have reported a decline in aerobic capacity, cardiovascular function, and changes in muscle fiber composition with aging. (17,18,19,20) These athletes were studied for as long as 28 years during which time some continued to train for competition, and others became quite sedentary. Those athletes who trained hard experienced a 5% to 6% decline in *VO2Max* per decade. Those who stopped training when young experienced nearly a 15% decline in aerobic capacity per decade… The combined effects of reconditioning and aging.

It is now commonly accepted that **reducing the effects of aging (on endurance) depends to a great extent on the individual's training adaptability,** a fact found to be as much dependent upon **genetics as hard work.** It also appears that highly intense training has a slowing effect on the rate of loss in aerobic capacity during the early and middle years of adult life (30 to 50 years of age), but less effect after age 50.

RESPIRATORY CHANGES WITH AGING

In dealing with the lungs and ancillary anatomy (chest wall and respiratory muscles) as one ages, it seems that simple loss of lung tissue elasticity and attendant stiffening of the chest wall are the prime factors in reduced respiratory capacity, demanding more effort and energy to breathe. This occurs almost universally in sedentary people as they age.

What is seen from all this is a reduction in both **Vital Capacity (VC)…** The total volume of air expelled after maximal inhalation and forced expiratory volume in one second (FEV 1)… The greatest volume of air exhaled in one second. These decline linearly with age beginning as early as 20 but usually as one approaches 30. While these decrease, **R**esidual **V**olume (RV)… The amount of air that cannot be exhaled… Increases and the **T**otal **L**ung Capacity (TLC) remains unchanged. As a result, the ratio of the residual volume to the total lung capacity (RV) increases, TLC Meaning that less air can be exchanged. In our early 20's residual volume accounts for 18% to 22% of the total lung capacity, but this increases to 30% or more as we reach age 50. The absolutely damaging habit of smoking accelerates this increase.

These changes are matched by changes in maximal ventilatory capacity during exhaustive exercise. **Maximal Expiratory Ventilation (VE max) increases until physical maturity then declines with age.** VE max values average about 40 L/minute for 4 to 6 year old boys, increases to 110 to 140L/min for fully mature men, then drops to 60 to 80 L/min for 60 to 70 year old men. Females follow the same general pattern, although their absolute values are considerably lower at each age, primarily because of smaller stature.

During middle and older age, endurance training reduces the loss of elasticity in the lungs and chest wall. As a result, endurance-trained older athletes have only slightly decreased pulmonary ventilation capacities. Decreased aerobic capacity among these older athletes cannot be attributed to changes in external respiration. Also, during strenuous exercise, both normally active older people and athletes can reach nearly maximal arterial oxygen saturation (97%). (21) Thus, neither changes in the lungs nor in the blood's oxygen-carrying capacity appear to be responsible for the observed drop in **VO2Max** reported in aging athletes. Rather, the primary limitation is apparently lined with oxygen transport to the muscles. Aging results in a general decrease in maximum heart rate and stroke volume, which lower maximal cardiac output and blood flow to the exercising muscles. In addition, it is generally the case where less oxygen is extracted by our muscles as we age.

CARDIOVASCULAR CHANGES WITH AGING

In general, cardiovascular functions diminish as we age. One of the most notable changes that accompanies aging is a decrease in **M**aximum **H**eart **R**ate (HR max). Whereas children's values frequently exceed 200 beats/min, the average 60-year-old has an HR max of approximately 160 beats/min. **HR max is estimated to decrease slightly less than 1 beat/min per year as we age with the average HR max for any age calculated by the formula: HR max = 200 - age.** However, this equation is, at best, only a good approximation for the AVERAGE population; there can be individual variation with as much as + or - 20 beats/min or more.

The reduction in **HR max** with age appears to be similar in both sedentary and highly trained adults. At age 50, for example, normally active men have the same **HR max** values as former and still-active same-aged distance runners. This reduction in **HR max** might be attributable to morphological and electrophysiological alternations in the cardiac conduction system, specifically in the *Sino-Atrial* **(SA) node** and in the **Bundle of HIS**, which could slow cardiac conduction. (22) Also, the heart becomes less sensitive to the body's chemical stimulation (with catecholamine's, like *adrenaline*).

Another parameter negatively influencing aerobic capacity is the decrease in **S**troke **V**olume (SV max)… the maximum amount of blood pumped out with each heartbeat. This is due primarily to increased total peripheral resistance from reduced pliability ("hardening") in the arteries with aging and to possible reductions in left ventricular (the main chamber of the heart that pumps blood to the body's organs) contractility.

The decrease in *VO2Max* with aging and inactivity then is largely explained by decreases in Cardiac Output (CO = Heat Rate x Stroke Volume), along with the body's lessened ability to extract oxygen from the blood supply.

When compared to sedentary men of the same age, those who were consistently active had higher *VO2Max* values because they had greater stroke volumes and thus also greater maximal cardiac outputs. But as stated above, as an inevitable part of aging, regardless of present condition, an older athlete will have less of all three important cardiac output functions than a younger athlete. Cardio-vascular reconditioning that accompanies reduced activity aside, it is the combination of increased peripheral vascular resistance (inhibiting blood flow to muscles, etc., increased body weight, and age-related negative changes in the respiratory and cardiovascular systems that combine to decrease *VO2Max* in men by about 10% per decade after age 25. But if the body composition and physical activity are kept constant, deterioration due to the aging process in and of itself results in a *VO2Max* decline of only about 5% per decade. (see Table 1)

Some research indicates that older athletes who train with the same intensity and volume as their younger counterparts can have as little as a 1% to 2% decrease in aerobic capacity per decade until age 50. After age 55, reduced cardiovascular capacity will eventually slow down even these remarkable athletes.

CHANGES IN STRENGTH WITH AGING

The level of strength needed to meet the daily demands of living remains unchanged throughout life. However, a person's maximal strength, generally well above the daily demands early in life, decreases steadily with aging, The ability to stand from a sitting position, something we all take for granted, is compromised at age 50, and by the age of 80, becomes impossible for some. (see Figure B, a) Another example of a physical requirement that most take for granted is the opening of a sealed jar. When set at a specific resistance, this task can be accomplished by 92% of men and women in the age range of 40 to 60, but after age 60, the **failure rate** becomes 68% and by the age range of 71 to 80, only 32% can open the jar! (21)

As can be seen from Figure B, b, similar data describe leg strength changes with aging in men. Knee-extension strength in normally active men and women decreases rapidly after age 45 to 50, but strength-training the knee extensor muscles enables older men to perform better at age 60 than most normally active men at half that age.

Age-related losses of muscle strength result primarily from the substantial loss of muscle mass that accompanies aging or decreased physical activity. Sedentary older adults can show both a large loss in muscle mass and an increase in subcutaneous fat.

It has also been found that swimming, generally noted by the average sports enthusiast as exercising most of the muscle groups equally, actually does not. When tested with CT scans, swimmers who did **not** train with weights **nor** did dry-land exercises, had a dominance of triceps (back of the upper arm) muscle development at the expense of the biceps (front of the upper arm). Those who swam **and** trained with weights or did dry-land exercises developed a balance of the opposing muscle groups.

It has been concluded from numerous studies covering a period of over 20 years that the amount or intensity of activity or perhaps both might play an important role in fiber-type distribution with aging. (23, 24) The apparent **increase** in **slow-twitch (ST)** muscle fibers with aging and, or disuse are due to a **decrease** in the number of **fast-twitch (FT)** fibers.

Though the precise cause of this is unclear, it has been suggested that the number of **FT motor neurons decreases during aging,** which eliminates innervations of these muscle fibers. **Fibers that cannot be activated, gradually atrophy and eventually become absorbed by the body.**

An additional factor of aging and muscle fiber function comes into play with the observation that with advancing years, the maximum discharge rate of the motor-neuron unit is distinguishably less than with the young. This causes strength reduction due to an impaired ability to fully drive the surviving motor units. (25) In addition, **with aging, the nervous system's ability to process or detect a stimulus is slowed,** thus delaying a response to the muscles, though people who remain physically active are only slightly slower than younger active individuals.

Documentation from numerous investigations has shown that a **decrease in both number and size of ST and FT muscle fibers occurs with aging.** Research indicates that approximately 10% of the total number of muscle fibers are lost per decade after age 50, which can, in part, explain the muscle atrophy that occurs as we age. (26)

It was thought for some time that **any** type of training would have an effect on preserving the musculature, but **what is now known is that only strength training can preserve, even enhance, the cross-sectional area (increase in thickness) of the trained muscles no matter what the age.** Endurance training had a negligible effect in this area. But endurance training was shown to cause a positive adaptability by maintaining an adequate capillary supply to the muscles and an adequate positive stimulus to the oxidative enzymes there, thus allowing for only a 10% to 15% decline from younger athletes…all of which suggests that **the aging process has little effect on skeletal muscle's adaptability to endurance training.**

BODY COMPOSITION AND AGING

There are three things that mainly affect how much fat our bodies accumulate as we grow and age: (1) how much and what we eat, (2) how much and how intense we exercise, and (3) our individual heredity. Body-fat composition from early age is dictated to a great extent by how many fat cells are present in our constitution and how full of fat they become. If one has a tendency to be overweight and goes on a diet, the fat cells do **not** disappear; they merely shrink in size. The end result is a thinner person with less body fat, but the caveat here is that if caloric intake exceeds expenditure, the fat cells will just fill up again and produce the same overweight condition. Also, many people just reduce calorie intake when they want to lose weight; they do **not** add lean body mass (muscle) with exercise, so we may see a lighter (in weight) person, but not necessarily one who is relatively leaner.

Beyond age 30, the body has a normally-reduced ability to mobilize fat that adds to the propensity of weight gain. This, coupled with the gradual decrease in lean-body mass from lessened physical activity, allows for an increased percentage of total body fat.

As one might anticipate, the body fat content of physically active people is significantly lower than that of age-matched sedentary people. Highly-trained male and female runners at an average age of 45 years, for example, have been reported to average 11% and 18% body fat, respectively… considerably lower than those reported for sedentary people of similar age: 19% in men and 26% in women. Interestingly, older competitive swimmers (average age of 50 for men and 43 for women) have less body fat than age-matched sedentary people, yet these athletes are fatter on average than a group of equally fit distance runners… males having 15% body fat and women 23%. This is due, in part, to the gravity-free environment of the water and to the supine position of the body while swimming... both allowing the body to exercise vigorously but at a lower heart rate and, therefore, with less caloric consumption per unit time.

Though we see that athletes of any age are leaner than their less active counterparts, older ones, for the most part, have substantially more body fat than younger athletes.

TRAINABILITY OF THE OLDER ATHLETE

Despite the decrements associated with aging, older athletes are capable of exceptional performances. Their ability to adapt to endurance and strength training is well documented. Recent studies have shown that improvements in VO2Max with training are similar for younger (ages 21 to 25) and older (ages 60 to 71) men and women. (27, 28) Though the baseline readings for VO2Max were lower for the older athletes, the absolute increases with training were similar.

In other words, the **trainability** of the older athlete was similar to those much younger. This can be explained by the fact that **in older individuals there was greater improvement in the muscles' oxidative enzyme activities, whereas improvement in younger people is largely due to increased maximal cardiac output.** But to put this into perspective: this does **not** mean that endurance training can enable older athletes to achieve the performance standards established by younger athletes.

Loss of strength might be attributed to a combination of aging and reduced physical activity that produces a decline in muscle function. But although it is difficult to compare the adaptations to strength training of younger and older people, aging appears neither to impair the ability to improve muscle strength nor to prevent muscle hypertrophy (large mass).

In essence, then, the scientific literature has shown that, though we cannot halt Father Time and his inexorable march toward our decline with aging, we can fight back to a large extent by taking up the cause of regular endurance training, strength training, and proper and appropriate nutrition (for weight control).

Youth may be wasted on the young, but a wise person of years need not be envious; he can make the best of his existence and enjoy a healthy and vigorous life. (29).

The following four images are Reprinted, with permission, from J.H. Wilmore and D.L. Costill, 1999, *Physiology of sport and exercise,* 2nd ed. (Champaign, IL: Human Kinetics), 547 [or 550 or 552, or 557].

Table 1					
Changes in Aerobic Capacity and Maximal Heart Rates With Aging in a Group of 10 Highly Trained Masters Distance Runners					
			$\dot{V}O_2$max		
	Age (years)	Weight (kg)	(L/min)	(ml · kg^{-1} · min^{-1})	HRmax (beats/min)
	21.3 (±1.6)	63.9 (±2.2)	4.41 (±.09)	69.0 (±1.4)	189 (±6)
	46.3 (±1.3)	66.0 (±0.6)	4.25 (±.05)	64.3 (±0.8)	180 (±6)

Note. Values are ± SE.

Table 2		
Changes in $\dot{V}O_2$max Among Normally Active Men		
Age (years)	$\dot{V}O_2$max (ml · kg^{-1} · min^{-1})	% change from 25 years
25	47.7	—
35	43.1	-9.6
45	39.5	-17.2
52	38.4	-19.5
63	34.5	-27.7
75	25.5	-46.5

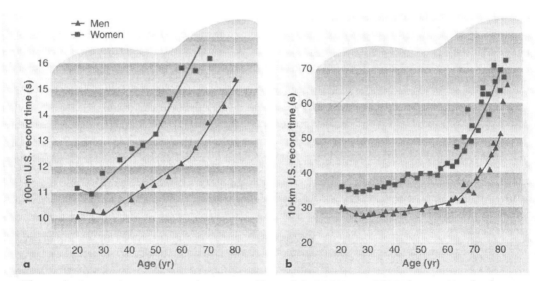

Figure A Change with age in men's and women's world records for (a) 100-m and (b) 10-km runs. Note that these running records slow at a much faster rate after the age of 50 to 60 years.

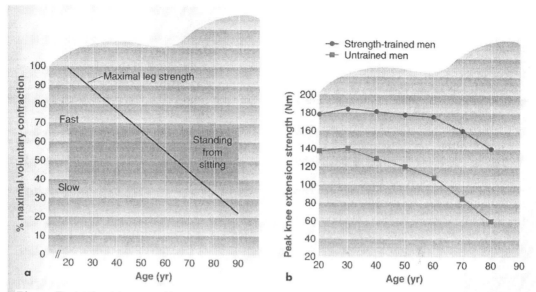

Figure B   (a) The ability to stand from a sitting position is compromised at age 50, and by age 80 this task becomes impossible for some people. (b) Changes in peak knee extension strength in untrained and trained men at various ages. Note that older men (e.g., 60 to 70 years) who strength-train can have knee extension strength equal to or greater than individuals who are only a third their age. MVC = maximal voluntary contraction.

REFERENCES

1. **Physiology of Sport and Exercise, 2nd Ed.,** 1999, Wilmore, Jack H. & Costil, David L; Human Kinetics, p. 546

2. **Exercise and Sport Sciences Reviews, 20,** 1992, Bouchard, C; Genetics of Aerobic and Anaerobic Performances; pp. 27-58.

3. **Scandinavian Journal of Medicine and Science in Sports, 6,** 1996, Trappe, S.W., Costil, David L., Goodpaster, B.H.; Calf Muscle Strength in Former Elite Distance Runners; pp. 205-210.

4. **Journal of Applied Physiology, 80,** 1996, Trappe, S.W., Costil, David L., Aging Among Elite Distance Runners: A 22-Year Longitudinal Study; pp. 285-290.

5. **Journal of Applied Physiology, 82,** 1997, Tanaka, H. & Seakes, D.; Age and Gender Interactions in Physiological Functional Capacity; Insight from Swimming Performances; pp. 846-851.

6. **Physiology of Sport and Exercise, 2nd ed,** 1999; p. 548. **Ibid;** p. 549.

7. **Arbeitsphysiolgie, 10,** 1938, Robinson, S; Experimental Studies of Physical Fitness in Relation to Age; pp. 251-323.

8. **Federation Proceedings, 46,** 1987, Buskirk, E.R. & Hodgson, J.L., Age and Aerobic Power: The Rate of Change in Men and Women; pp.1824-1829.

9. **Journal of Applied Physiology, 35,** 1973, Astrand, I., Reduction in Maximal Oxygen Intake with Age; pp.649-654.
10. **Federation Proceedings, 44,** 1985, Dill, D.B.; Aerobic Capacity of D.B. Hill, 1928-1984; p. 1013.
11. **Journal of Cardiac Rehabilitation, 5,** 1985, McKeen, P.C.; A 13-Year-Follow-Up of a Coronary Heart Disease Risk Factor Screening and Exercise Program for 40 to 59-Year-Old Men; pp. 10-59.
12. **Biology in Sport, 2,** 19856, Cempla, J.; Decrease of Maximum Oxygen Consumption in Men and Women During the Fourth to Sixth Decades of Life, in the Light of Cross-Sectional Studies of Cracow Population; pp. 45-59.
13. **Acta Physiolgica Scandinavica, Suppl, 125,** 1957, von Dobeln, W.; Human Standard and Maximal Metabolic Rate in Relation to Fat-Free Body Mass; pp. 37-79.
14. **Journal of Sports Medicine and Physical Fitness, 7,** 1967, Dill, D.B.; A Longitudinal Study of 16 Champion Runners; pp. 4-27.
15. **Journal of Applied Physiology, 62,** 1987, Pollack M.L.; Effect of Age and Training on Aerobic Capacity and Body Composition; pp. 725-731.
16. **Medicine & Science in Sport & Exercise, 28,** 1996, Hagerman, F.C.; A 20-Year Longitudinal Study of Olympic Oarsman, pp.1150-1156.
17. **Journal of Applied Phys., 82,** 1997, Pollock, M.L.; Twenty-Year Follow-Up of Aerobic Power and Body Composition of Older Track Athletes, pp. 1508-1516.
18. **Journal of Applied Phys., 80,** 1996, Costill, D.L.; Aging Among Elite Distance Runners: A 22-Year Longitudinal Study, pp.285-290.
19. **American Journal of Phys., 271 (40),** 1996, Widrick, JJ; Force-Velocity and Force Power Properties of Single Muscle Fibers from Elite Master Runners and Sedentary Men, C676-C683.
20. **Provost Lecture Series, 1990,** Saltin, B.; Aging, Health, and Exercise Performance, Muncie, IN: Ball State University.
21. **Federation Proceedings, 38,** 1979, Lakatta, E.G.; Alterations in the Cardiovascular System that Occur in Advanced Age, pp. 163-167.
22. **Journal of Applied Phys, 78,** 1996, Costil, D.L.; Skeletal Muscle Characteristics Among Distance runners: A 20-Year Follow-Up Study, pp. 823-829.
23. **Scandinavian Journal of Medicine & Science in Sports, 6,** 1996, Costil, D.L.; Calf Muscle Strength in Former Elite Distance Runners, pp. 205-210.
24. **Journal of Applied Phys.,79,** 1995, Kamen, G.; Motor Unit Discharge Behavior In Older Adults During Maximal-Effort Contractions, pp. 1908-1913.
25. **Journal of Neurological Science, 84,** 1988, Lexell, J.; What is the Cause of the Aging Atrophy? Total Number, size, and Proportion of Diff Fiber Types Studied in Whole Vastus Lateralis Muscle from 15 to 83 Year Old Men, pp.275-294.
26. **Journal of Applied Phys., 71,** 1991, Kohrt, W.M.; Effects of Gender, Age, and Fitness Level on Response of VO2Max to Training in 60-71 Year Olds, pp.2004-2011.

27. **Journal of Applied Phys., 66,** 1989, Meredith, C.N.; Peripheral Effects of Endurance Training in Young and Old Subjects, pp. 2844-2849.
28. **Journal of the American Medical Association, 262,** 1989, Paffenbarger, R.S.; Physical Fitness and All-Cause Mortality: A Prospective Study of Healthy Men and Women, pp. 2395-2401.

All graphs, charts, and tables were taken from Physiology of Sport & Exercise, 2nd edition, 1999, Wilmore & Costill.

CHAPTER 7

WHY IT MAKES PHYSIOLOGIC SENSE TO WARM UP AND COOL DOWN

Unless you are an experienced athlete or someone exposed to same, there is a better than even chance your warm up/cool down ritual might be lacking in content and extent. Logic would dictate that SOMETHING be done to prepare for vigorous exercise. But, what, exactly? And how much? And when? And, of course, why? The WHY is very important, for I have found that teaching and EDUCATING directly correlates with understanding the reasons for it. Once understood, the athlete will most always respect the importance in the training regimen that this protocol renders and institute it as equally important as the training sets themselves.

If you do not partake of these preparatory and recovery activities, you are at greater risk for injury, and you will simply not perform up to your potential. The body must be prepared, conditioned if you will, to summon its energies and mobility for intense physical activity if you want a quality effort, and it is wisest medically to afford the body adequate time and ability to approach recovery even during a training session or between repeated competitive efforts.

Of major consideration is the allowance of the musculature's full range of motion for the different body movements per event. To stretch the muscles when "cold" is to ask for trouble. Muscles have but one action: to contract with force. If they are asked to perform this activity with no opportunity of easy sport-specific preparatory activity and the concomitant increase in blood flow *in situ* (at the site), their range of motion and the force produced will usually be diminished. We want long powerful movements to allow the covering of distance per stroke, step, throw or leap to be as much as our trained bodies can muster. Also, muscle fibers, when properly trained over time to become powerful, usually develop more force than the connective tissue (tendons) to which they are bound. Not allowing them adequate warming and not having them sufficiently elongate to their full range of motion can produce an environment for muscle and tendon tears when immediate demand is sought. But the body actually tries to prevent its muscle fibers from stretching. It develops an inhibitory stretch reflex which tries to keep the fibers of muscle in their steady state of length thinking if the fibers are stretched; imminent damage will ensue. To effectively stretch muscle, one has to hold a static (non-movement) stretch for as long as 30 seconds to break this inhibitory reflex. Best if the muscles have been somewhat pre-warmed with easy movement. After about 20 seconds the athlete can feel the resistance to the stretch ease up, and a comforting sense of elongation and relaxation of the muscle begins. Sometimes, with really tight muscle groups or in a cold environment, multiple 30-second stretching bouts work best to bring about the desired elongation. Of course, there is a two-edged sword in place here: if the muscles are stretched just before use, they can become weakened by as much as 30%. And because of this, many coaches and athletic trainers are now having their athletes forgo stretching altogether as long as the easy and sometimes prolonged movements in a prescribed warm up make the athlete feel ready to compete. It has been demonstrated that if the athlete's muscles are kept warm, a stretch session can have its desired effect for up to two hours. Thus, stretching along with a prescribed warm up about 45 to 60 minutes before vigorous activity should not contribute to weakening the musculature, yet allow for optimum movement.

The second, and medically more important reason to warm up and cool down encompasses the cardiovascular system. The heart and blood vessels must be conditioned appropriately with progressive increases in the demands placed upon them to fulfill the needs of increasing physical activity. Heart rate and blood pressure need to be increased to have the physical being ready to go when the athlete needs to perform. There are no absolute set distances to be covered during a warm up, but physiologic consensus has shown that the older the athlete, the more the need for the warm up and the longer it needs to be. The greater the muscular development, the greater the need for the warm up. The more intense the upcoming athletic effort, the greater the need for a sufficient warm up. The colder the environment, the longer and the more important the progressive warm up needs to be. An injured athlete is good to no one, and sustaining a muscular or tendon tear because of insufficient time and thought to complete an appropriate warm up is an absolutely avoidable circumstance. If approaching intense physical activity or competition in the next 30 to 60 minutes, faster and more intense short-burst efforts are recommended in the prescribed warm up to present a "memory" of speed and power for the neuromusculature. To allow sufficient time for the body to recover from this increased movement, an absolute minimum of 20 minutes must be factored into the protocol. If less time is allotted, the body cannot recover sufficiently to have it pristine and ready to go. We see a buildup of a muscular acidic (lactic) environment and a depletion of *glucose* and ATP which presents as a concomitant diminished immediately-available energy reserve... all athletic hazards.

This building into speed is important for another reason. There is a small, but growing segment of the athletic world, especially swimmers, who would benefit greatly from a certain type of warm-up: the exercise-induced asthmatic who needs to lessen certain irritating chemicals released into the bronchiole tree upon vigorous activity. We see this also in land-based asthmatic athletes exposed to cold air. Balancing short, rapid movements apropos to the specific sport with adequate rest for air-recovery allows for the secreting of these chemicals and their depletion over time. Some chest discomfort and possible coughing are typical signs of the chemicals at work but eventually the symptoms subside. This ritual, though not pleasant, could make a big difference in the ensuing athletic event if it does not negatively affect the emotions of the participant. The experienced and, or well-coached athlete can come to utilize this fleeting feeling of air challenge to his or her advantage knowing that in a few minutes the body's ability to exchange air sufficiently will be up and present. Of course, most who endure "athletic asthma" are or should already be on prescribed inhalation and oral medication. The best pharmacology and physiology dictate that the inhalation medication needs to be administered at least one hour before need. This would most often coincide with the beginning of the warm up protocol. The oral medication is usually prescribed for a single dosage every 24 hours.

Cool downs have their own importance both athletically and physiologically, which often coincide.

They can vary in intensity and duration from absolutely passive, gently active or moderately active. Passive cool downs are least efficient and effective. Just resting will eventually get your air back, but it sometimes takes extended time and won't accelerate muscular and physiologic recovery. The athlete will still be under the PROLONGED influence of the negative effects of vigorous exercise (elevated blood pressure, heart rate, and blood and muscle-fiber lactate with early soreness). Gentle recovering activity provides a bit more response to intense activity but may still not allow appropriate or desired amounts quick enough for repeated efforts. Moderate recovering activity (about 50% to 60% effort) provides the best method for bringing the body "back down to earth." The exact muscular movements must be utilized in this protocol along with other easier movement to extend the cool down procedure enough to be of benefit. Since lactic acid rarely travels more than a few cells away from the ones just used in athletic activity, they need to use the built-up acid as fuel to accelerate recovery. At the moderate percentages listed above, most of the time no more lactate will be produced but the already-in-place acid will be directed to the liver and oxidized to pyruvate for use as new fuel after the recovery. Examples of this type of cool-down recovery would be: for swimmers: a straight 200 swim mixing what was just raced with freestyle. If the freestyle were raced, then only freestyle should be used at moderate pace. Then 4 x 50 yards/meters one length each of the racing stroke and freestyle and finally 8 x 25's alternating free with what was just raced... all done at MODERATE intensity so as not to create more lactate that we are trying to remove quickly. With land-based racing, it is more about time in recovery than distance. A workable time in cool down recovery mode would be between six to eight minutes. If the athlete feels he/she needs more, then, of course, more is taken until a sense of adequate homeostasis is retrieved.

There is also need for short bouts of recovery in between sets or with extended intervals while training. The mechanism of choice here is to bob up and down in the pool at the finish walls. INHALING while getting the HEART ABOVE THE WATER LINE (out of the water) then EXHALING while the HEART IS BELOW THE WATER LINE acts as a "poor man's" CPR... the body responds by lowering its heart rate, respiration, and blood pressure rather quickly affording the athlete a definite sense of quick recovery. Some of my swimmers would not be able to satisfactorily complete certain demanding intervals without this mini-cool down protocol.

Moderately-active recovery is the most complete and allows for the best return to base-line. Allowing an easy few laps after the bobbing-up-and-down ritual affords even more complete recovery for even more demanding upcoming sets. This is emphasized over and over to my athletes to reinforce the importance and the absolute need for a proper cool-down. I also recommend that if the athlete is to include stretching in his training and competing regimens, it produces even more benefit AFTER the exercise bout than before.

Every one of my training sessions concludes with at least a 200 yards/meters cool-down at moderate intensity. As we age, this protocol has another serious physiologic benefit. In swimmers and runners and cyclists, blood tends to pool in the legs that can create a blood volume deficit or slight vacuum through the heart. Cardiac irregularities with *syncope* (fainting) have been seen because of this. Moving muscle for several minutes will push pooled blood from the lower extremities back to the heart to obviate this potential for serious cardiac involvement.

CHAPTER 8.

SUDDEN DEATH IN ATHLETES

SUDDEN, DEATH IN ATHLETES... I cannot think of any grouping of words, large or small, which can bring us more quickly to an awareness of our own mortality. Even the most hearty and successful athletes would be psychologically hard-pressed to ignore these words when encountered.

I have experienced someone's sudden death during, or shortly after, athletic involvement four times in 12 years, the last being a 19-year-old female (on my masters team) who died suddenly just a few hours after practice. She was young, vigorous and seemed in perfect health with no overt physical complaints. She was always able to complete the daily workouts and really seemed to enjoy the time she spent training.

All four (three male and one female), ranging in age from 19 to 63, had one thing in common: they were all well-trained over a period of years and proficient in their chosen sport.

None of what follows is intended to frighten; rather, it is intended to enlighten. Try hard not to become like me, a card-carrying hypochondriac who "suffered" every disease he studied in pathology. It got so bad that my wife would say: "What are we dying from this week, dear?"

If any of the facts or symptoms which follow seem pertinent to your personal situation, it would be wise to consult with your physician. Most of the time the good news heard from the doctor is more than worth the time and expense taken to seek it out, and just in case there is a potential danger, the prevention of tragedy is priceless. And please keep this in mind as we progress into the chapter: though sudden death is both dramatic and traumatic to all who experience it, in the grand scheme of things relating to the general population, it is a very rare occurrence. But if, for several reasons, you are a prime candidate for a massive heart attack ("acute myocardial infarction," as a medical examiner would call it), even if you are very fit and active, you are more likely to trigger that event during vigorous activity.

Sudden death is defined as death which is unexpected, not due to trauma, and occurs within six hours of the onset of symptoms. (This definition excludes heat-related death, although heat stroke can be fatal.) The underlying cause is usually considered to be structural heart disease, although, at autopsy, several patients may be seen with no easily-diagnosable condition. (1)

Cardiovascular disease associated with exercise-related sudden death is best divided, for physiologic reasons and ease of presentation, into two categories based on age, with 30 years old being the demarcation...

SUDDEN DEATH IN ATHLETES 30 YEARS OLD OR YOUNGER

Under age 30, congenital (from birth) abnormalities of the coronary arteries and *Hypertrophic Cardiomyopathy* (HCM) are the two most common causes of sudden death in athletes. (2, 3, 4) With the former condition (7) several different "arrangements" of the coronary arteries have been observed, most often with the left main coronary artery... which feeds the major portion of the left ventricle (pumping chamber of the heart)... arising from the right side, giving it a twisted and tortuous path to its ultimate destination. This condition is very rare, but the fact that such abnormalities are the second leading cause of unexpected cardiac death in young athletes reflects the difficulty in their detection. Indeed, the first sign of a congenital coronary artery anomaly is usually sudden collapse and death on the playing field. (5)

In *Hypertrophic Cardiomyopathy* (HCIVI), we see the most common cause of sudden death in young athletes as an unexplained thickening of the heart affecting principally the left ventricle (pumping chamber of the heart); the degree of enlargement and thickening, which is often familial, can go to the extreme, thereby preventing the heart from filling with enough blood to deliver it where and when needed upon increased demand from vigorous activity. Because of this impaired delivery of blood and oxygen (especially to the heart itself), cardiac arrest occurs due to the development of incorrect electrical rhythmicity... the heart simply cannot beat in proper sequence and "short-circuits" itself. Obviously, since involvement in athletics can be quite demanding physically, the risk of sudden death in individuals with this condition needs to be addressed by correctly diagnosing them and then having them excluded from participation in competitive sports. Unfortunately, diagnosis of this malady during routine pre-participation evaluations can be difficult.

With proper questioning, approximately 60 percent of positive cases will provide a history of chest pain, dizziness, fainting, or fatigue, particularly upon physical exertion. And one in five will have a family member with this disease. (6,7) The medical history, with attention to these details, is therefore *mucho importante`*.

Also, the actual physical examination with this condition can, at times, be deceptively benign. But an experienced sports-medicine internist or cardiologist would know the procedures to differentiate a harmless murmur (extra cardiac sound) from a dangerous one, and be able to distinguish dangerous cardiac enlargement and thickening (by use of an **Electro-c**ardiogram (EKG) or sound -(echo)- cardiogram) from the so-called "athlete's heart."

Myocarditis, or inflammation of the heart muscle itself, can also cause *sudden* death, especially when combined with vigorous exertional effort. Without symptoms or signs suggestive of myocardial (heart) involvement, the diagnosis of this condition is exceedingly difficult, if not impossible, to make. Of the identifiable causes, viruses such as Coxsackie B and echovirus are the most common microorganisms found on site. (8) To restrict participation on the basis of a low-grade fever, or to recommend evaluation of such non-cardiac symptoms by a cardiologist is both impractical and unrealistic. Many athletes "play through" a cold or mild fever, especially if they are highly competitive. But for the athlete who presents with more serious symptoms of possible cardiac compromise such as difficult breathing, fatigue, palpitations, chest pain, dizziness, fainting, cough, neck vein distension and fever, participation should be restricted.

Reggie Lewis, 27, of the Boston Celtics and NCAA All-America Hank Gathers, 23, are two examples of great athletes finally succumbing to chronic *myocarditis*, among other cardiac ailments. Playing with this condition for some time but ignoring the associated cardiac warning signs, they were tragedies just waiting to happen.

Another condition that can negatively affect the functioning of the heart early on is Marfan's Syndrome, It is not as common as those described above, but is seen enough in the population to warrant consideration as a potential killer of athletes. Individuals with this disease are at risk for sudden death due to the rupture of the main artery (the aorta) which leaves the heart. The syndrome has many facets and signs and should be considered if the athlete presents, during a pre-sports physical, with abnormal sounds in the cardiac rhythm due to valvular damage, extra-long fingers, shallow, inwardly curved chest, scoliosis (improper curvature of the spinal column), hyper extensible joints, (7) above average height, eye involvement with lens dislocation and near-sightedness, Since the disease is progressive, an early sufferer may be able to partake in a certain sport depending upon cardiac evaluation, but intense monitoring is a must to prevent tragedy.

There is one more defect that at one time contributed to sudden death in athletes. Congenital aortic stenosis (narrowing of the valve leading from the left ventricle to the aorta) was often mentioned in the older literature on this topic. However, these individuals are now screened out of intense competition by the loud murmur which is heard, ease of diagnosis by echocardiography, and subsequent prohibition from competitive athletics.

To sum up for the younger athlete and to put things into perspective: the National Institutes of Health estimate that 200,000 competitive athletes under the age of 30 would have to be screened in order to find ten with congenital heart disease capable of causing sudden death, of whom only one would die. (6) Hence, *a careful family and personal history followed, if necessary, by a thorough physical examination* remain the most effective and appropriate means of screening young athletes for risk of unexpected cardiac death, especially with the fact that there are about 4 million competitive high school-age athletes (grades 9 thru 12), 500,000 collegiate competitors, and over 5000 who earn their living in professional sports.

It is incumbent upon the athlete to be aware of and report any repeated ill feelings while engaged in vigorous exercise. A famous runner and author, Jim Fixx, some years back, had such repeated ill feelings (chest tightness and pain) but foolishly chose to "run through" them. At the height of his popularity, he succumbed to a massive coronary while running; in his early 40's and with an athletic build, the cause at autopsy proved to be occluded coronary arteries... the result of a familial propensity toward extremely high blood fats (*triglycerides*).

It must be recognized, however, that certain anomalies that pose such risk are difficult or even impossible to detect in the casual pre-participation assessment. Still, awareness of abnormal findings on history and, or examination that indicate risk for sports play is important in minimizing the incidence of sudden death.

SUDDEN DEATH IN ATHLETES OVER 30 YEARS OLD

By far the most common cause of sudden heart death over age 30 is *coronary atherosclerosis* (narrowing of the artery due to deposition of blood fats and calcium) (9, see fig 3), and the artery usually involved is the left anterior descending coronary artery, otherwise known as the "artery of sudden death." Because most deaths occur after the age of 30, this is the most common overall cause. But even here, the majority of sudden cardiac deaths occur during daily activities and not with exercise. (10) One of the world's leading authorities on the topic, the late Ernst Jokl, MD, stated that death during exercise is usually not due to exercise per say. (12) This bodes well for exercise in general, and it has been proven not to be the dangerous activity many would have us believe.

But not so fast. If we are playing with statistics, we need to include and analyze The National Institutes of Health estimate that, for men OVER age 30, it would take a group of 10,000 asymptomatic athletes to screen out a subgroup of 100 with risk factors of dying 18 times that of the rest of the population. (11) Suddenly the numbers become a bit more emphatic. The combination of stress, genetics, poor dieting, drug or alcohol abuse, no exercise, intermittent exercise, or excessive exercise all OVER TIME can play havoc on the "innerds of the body, especially the coronary arteries." (13)

Though statistics has shown that it would take hundreds of thousands of hours of vigorous exercise to produce one cardiac death in the general population, there are many who suffer overt cardiac illness, but are snatched from the clutches of death with modern heroic medical procedures. (14) They may get the scare of their lives, and they may be left with varying degrees of cardiac debility, but many get a second chance at staying alive.

- Dr. Philip Ades, Director of Cardiac Rehabilitation at the University of Vermont, has developed the questionnaire below for competitive athletes:
- Has it been more than two years since you had a physical examination that included a blood pressure reading and listening to the heart?
- Have your parents or has a physician ever told you that you have a heart murmur?
- Have you experienced chest pain or fainting within the past two years?
- Has anyone in your family died suddenly at a young age (under 35)?
- Has a physician diagnosed anyone in your family with an abnormally-thickened heart or Marfan's Syndrome?
- Do you use or have you ever used cocaine or *anabolic* steroids?
- Has a physician every disqualified you from athletic competition? Especially important for older athletes:

- Does your family (parents, grandparents, brothers, sisters) have a history of coronary artery disease, including heart attack, bypass surgery, or angina before age 65?
- Do you smoke, have high blood pressure, high cholesterol, or diabetes? (15)

As you can see from the above questions, genetics, life style (present and in the past), and medical history all play a role in forming one's present state of health.

Kenneth Cooper, MD (the Father of aerobics) advises maximal exercise stress testing for anyone over 40 who wants to exercise vigorously. At his Aerobics Institute in Dallas, careful attention to testing technique has lessened the false positive rate. Most cardiologists agree that exercise stress testing should be done on anyone over 40 who wants to exercise vigorously who has two or three of the following cardiac risk factors: elevated blood fats, diabetes, high blood pressure, cigarette smoking, excess alcohol intake, physical inactivity, and positive family history.

In addition to the standard EKG, the stress testing can monitor for heart rate, blood pressure, and abnormal rhythms that may not show otherwise. Non-invasive techniques, such as thallium scanning or echocardiography (ultrasound), can be added to improve accuracy and to diagnose valve and heart muscle problems.

In an interview taken from the American Medical Athletic Association Quarterly, John Cantwell, MD, cardiologist and Program Director, Georgia Baptist Medical Center, Atlanta, states:

- Even highly fit people can have coronary disease, which may be asymptomatic.
- Screening treadmill tests at periodic intervals are worthwhile, especially in those over age 40 who compete.
- A low HDL (high density lipoprotein... the "good kind of fat") may be an important coronary risk factor, even when the total cholesterol is under 200mg/dl.
- Based on our experience in cardiac rehabilitation, sudden collapse while active is usually an electrical event (ventricular tachycardia leading to fibrillation) in the setting of underlying coronary disease, rather than an acute myocardial infarction (tissue destruction).(1 6)

The following is a brief list of warning symptoms (that can vary from patient to patient) of possible coronary involvement or stroke. Many times they turn out to be benign, but the patient should not make that decision. If the distress seems to build or does not dissipate in a reasonable period of time, getting to a medical facility ASAP could prove life-saving.

- Pain becomes severe in the exact center of the chest (as if an elephant were sitting on you).
- Pain radiating usually down the LEFT arm, sometimes all the way to the fingers. (called "referred pain")
- Pain occurring in the LEFT side of the jaw. (also called "referred pain")
- A severe case of what fools like indigestion leading into nausea.

- Sweating, yet clammy cold skin (may be aggravated by panic of what may be happening).
- Difficulty in breathing or catching one's breath or the ability to talk.
- Sudden severe pain in the head with tingling or paralysis on one side of the body.
- Blurred vision or what appears to be half vision as if your eyelids were closing.
- Difficulty in speaking or forming words.

SUDDEN DEATH IN ATHLETES: REGARDLESS OF AGE

All of what I've written above has either been the result of unfortunate congenital or genetic developments (certainly beyond the control of the victim) or the result of an ignorant (to proper heart-health) or foolish lifestyle. But there is one area that is the most frustrating of all: that of dangerous drug abuse, especially in athletes... people who should know better, but are seduced for whatever reason by the prospect of taking something simple to produce (in their minds) extraordinary performances. Many athletes from good high school quality to proven professionals have tried to get an edge on their opponents and their sport by repeatedly taking dangerous stimulants and steroids.

Is it fear or self-doubt that steers these highly-driven people to try almost anything to get to that higher level of performance? Is it a falsely-perceived necessity to "level the field" in a win-at-all-costs, drug-contaminated sport? Is the pressure so great in some areas and for some people that they succumb to any and all temptations to get one-up on the competition? Loaded questions? Yes, and, unfortunately, true.

It has been a few years now since the following tragedies occurred, but three sports come to mind regarding drug abuse and the untimely deaths of famous athletes. Two famous football stars succumbed to the effects of steroid abuse: Lyle Alzado with an inoperable brain tumor, trying to make a comeback at age 42 with the Denver Broncos, and John Matuszak (recently retired from the Oakland Raiders) with a cerebral hemorrhage. In competitive cycling, a few Europeans died of strokes and heart attacks (while racing) from stimulant and steroid ingestion. And probably the saddest and most infamous of all, Len Bias, 21, the quintessential collegiate basketball player of his time... already signed to the Boston Celtics.. .suffering a fatal coronary from long-time use of cocaine while on the court. Autopsy of Bias showed he had several small heart attacks (*myocardial infarcts*) over a period of time. Self-inflicted, self-destructive, unnatural behavior producing sudden untimely deaths in supposedly superb physical specimens... It just doesn't make sense!

EMERGENCY TREATMENT OF CARDIAC ARREST

As can be seen from the text above, it is usually cardiac dysrhythmia (incorrect electrical-functioning of the heart muscle) that suddenly stops the heart. I would be remiss if I did not include an absolute recommendation that all facilities' hosting competitions and daily practices have ***at the ready*** an **A**utomated **E**xternal **D**efibrillator (AED) with ***trained personnel nearby.*** When used as quickly as possible, this particular devise can literally make the difference between life and death and is much more effective than CPR in restarting an arrested heart. (17, 18)

One particular brand claims it is the only one that can provide a 100% conversion to a viable beating heart with the use of appropriate shocking current. And it is virtually impossible to misuse these devices, since they are voice-activated and instruction-led to ensure, in the heat of an emergency, proper technique in resuscitation. With the advent of the "good Samaritan laws" in most states, concern over legal aspects should pale in comparison to the heroic task of doing all that can be done to preserve precious life.

In 490 B.C., the Athenian army turned back the armies of King Darius of Persia on the plains of Marathon in Greece. Afraid that the Persian fleet would retreat and attack Athens by sea, the Athenian general, Miltiades, sent his swiftest runner, Phydippedes, 25 miles to Athens with the news of victory. Weary from a previous 150-mile journey to Sparta, Phydippedes reached the city, gasped: "Rejoice, we conquer!" and fell to the ground, dead (probably due to the pooling of blood in his legs immediately after exertion and excess nor-*adrenaline* release).

Unless you want to end up like Phydippedes, remembered less for his deeds than for his death, be logical in your approach to exercise. Listen to your body. Seek out good medical advice and treatment, strive to convert to a healthier life-style, and above all, be thankful for the health you have… Never take it for granted.

REFERENCES:

1. American Medical Athletic Association (AMAA) Quarterly, April, 1994; Schulman, Charles, MD; p.10.
2. The Physician *and* Sports medicine, 1992, vol. 20, No 10; p.82.
3. Tsung, SH, Sudden death in young athletes. Arch Path Lab Med. 1982; 106: 168-170.
4. Maron, BJ, Sudden death in young athletes, Circulation,1980,62: 218-229.
5. AMAA Quarterly, Spring, 1998; Rowland, Thomas, MD; p.11. IBID p.10.
6. McCaffrey, FM, Sudden Cardiac Death in Young Athletes, AJDC, vol. 145, Feb. 1991, pp.178-180
7. Franklin, BA & Kahn, JK, Detecting the Individual Prone to Exercise-Related Sudden Cardiac Death,1995, Wayne State Univ Sc of Med, Detroit, MI, p.96.
8. Burke, Allen P, Farb, A, Am Heart Journal, Feb 1991, p. 571.
9. Wilmore, Jack & Costill, David, Physiology of Sport & Exercise,1994, p.485.
10. AMAA Quarterly. April, 1994; Schulman; p.10.
11. AMAA Quarterly, September, 1992;Jokl, Ernst, MD; p. 10.
12. Franklin, BA, Blair, SN, Exercise and Cardiac Complications, The Physician and Sports medicine, Feb,1994, vol. 22, No 2, pp.62-63.
13. Mittleman, MA,Triggering of Acute Myocardial Infarction by Heavy Physical Exertion, N Eng Jour Med,1993;329: 1677-1683.
14. AMAA Quarterly, April 1994; Ades, Philip, MD; p.11.
15. AMAA Quarterly, September, 1992;Cantwell, John, MD; p.10.
16. Cummins, RCS, Annals Emerg Med,1989, 18:1269-1275.
17. Textbook of Advanced Cardiac Life Support, Chap. 20, 1990, p.289.
18. Medtronic Physio-Control Corp., 1999, Redmond, WA 98073-9706.

CHAPTER 9

YOU MAKE ME BREATHLESS... EXERCISE-INDUCED ASTHMA (EIA), THE HIDDEN SYNDROME

OVERVIEW

Aside from the 1950's old rock-'n-roll tune by Jerry Lee Lewis, these words should be very familiar and ring true to every swimmer who honestly trains to go faster…

Rapid vigorous movement whether sudden or prepared is expected to bring about the body's compensating mechanisms which include the most visible and obvious: **increased depth and rapidity of breathing.** There have been many scientific experiments whereby normal athletes at sea-level were given pure oxygen to inhale before and after intense exercise in assumption of either delaying oxygen debt or enhancing recovery. Neither the arterial blood content of oxygen was increased nor the recovery time diminished. Since this proves that the body cannot store or accumulate oxygen to any great extent, the superficial interpretation of this intense breathing response would be that it is simply the body's way of bringing back its supply of usable oxygen. But this is only partially correct.

I submit that rather than simply developing an oxygen debt or deficit as a consequence of intense body movement, the **buildup of carbon dioxide (CO_2) from increased metabolism is the main cause of the sometimes nearly paralyzing symptoms of breathlessness.**

Even a benign situation like being tired (or bored) can cause the body to work at compensation by causing a *yawning sequence*. This happens more to cause the *blow off* (forced exhalation) of increased **CO_2 rather than to inhale more oxygen.**

One gets drowsy in a car (and begins to yawn) with several people as passengers and closed windows and vents more so because of the buildup of CO_2 in the air than any measured decrease in oxygen content. And this manifestation would be even more apparent and occur more quickly in aerobically conditioned athletes because of their ability to extract more oxygen from the ambient air per unit time and leave more CO_2 *to build up*.

There are two instances that come to mind, one relatively benign, and the other intensely desperate, where exposure to cold and its ability to cause the body to produce increased amounts of CO_2 have produced reactionary physiological responses. I have noticed on many occasions that simple *exposure to cold* would bring on the *yawning reflex*; here, due to the *increased metabolism* (shivering, etc.) necessary to raise body temperature, more CO_2 was produced which then needed to be blown off forcefully. The other much more serious situation is where we see many more victims dying of CO_2 asphyxiation than trauma when buried under snow as in an avalanche. CO_2 build-up about the face in the enclosed near-interment of snow and ice presents the fact that if the victim is not extracted within 15 to 20 minutes, the odds of finding him alive are greatly diminished.

Unlike plants and trees, which Nature has adapted to utilize carbon dioxide in a productive way (the manufacture of oxygen), human physiology has had to come up with metabolic pathways to neutralize or "detoxify" CO_2 since its production to excess has deleterious effects.

(Funny how Nature has adapted man's most annoying pest (the mosquito) to allow it to hone in on us for their blood feasts… They sense our presence by our release of carbon dioxide into the air and follow its trail back to us for meal time.)

This chapter will hopefully relate in part what happens to the body when it is asked to endure the vigorous activity of swimming fast. Depending upon the duration, intensity, and specific type of movement through water, and, of course, the physical condition and athletic aptitude of the participant, *breathlessness* is the endpoint for which to train.

This is not an easy thing to ask of an athlete, especially on a constant basis. It is one thing to become short of breath during vigorous *land-based* exercise… The body usually responds in its natural way of rapid respiration, in-and-out, without much thought given to controlling this process in any way other than the desire to recover as quickly as possible. But do the same in water, and we see a whole other story. No matter how athletic the participant, **if one cannot control the breathing part of swimming for as long as the race lasts, the whole technical aspect of the stroke usually breaks down,** and movement through water becomes, at first, less efficient, then downright counter-productive. AND, this negativity is magnified even more with the fact that as one moves faster through the water, the liquid medium holds the swimmer back with resistance that is either squared (under the surface) or cubed (at the surface). A land-based athlete with any logic might eventually analyze this and say: "why bother?" An experienced swimmer, on the other hand, comes to realize that, in the final analysis, it is **breath control that dictates speed throughout the race.** Miss-pace the race by taking it out too fast, or made the mistake of holding the breath too much in the beginning, and all too often the back end of the swim becomes more of a struggle than the swimmer bargained for… all because of the *sensation* that oxygen is in very short supply.

There are many complicated physiological processes that occur in cascade fashion when body movement becomes more demanding than staying in one's "comfort zone." There are dictums and theories about *oxygen deficit* versus *oxygen debt;* about *recovery oxygen uptake* or **Excess Post-Exercise Oxygen Consumption (EPOC).** I will discuss what I feel is the prime motivator to breathe, why we do this, and what happens if we do not.

SOME PHYSIOLOGY OF THE RESPIRATORY RESPONSE TO EXERCISE

Metabolically, to move fast in any fashion (for more than just a few seconds) creates biochemical demands that must be "caught up to" and dealt with by the body. The forced deep exhalations automatically proceeding right after vigorous movement is one way the body tries to bring back its overall pre-activity condition *(homeostasis)* **CO2 is one of the end products of metabolism; it cannot be prevented from forming, but it can be prevented or at least delayed from building up.** If there is muscular movement, CO2 is produced. If CO2 is produced in low enough amounts (light to moderate movement) it can be easily carried away by circulating blood through the muscles; there will be no buildup and no *sensation* to want to breathe vigorously. The typical breathing mechanism will allow for this transported CO2 to be adequately blown off at the lungs. The better the condition of the athlete, the more readily this process takes place.

Eventually, the more CO2 produced, however, the greater the responding respiration becomes. Any time **CO2 production rises to a greater extent than can be handled by the rate and depth of breathing, and blood will leave the lungs with some residual CO2 in it to be re-circulated through the heart and then on to the arterial blood supply and to the body's various tissues and organ systems.** If there is more CO2 in place in the circulating blood, there has to be less room for **O**xygen (O2) to be circulated. One of the typical end-result physical markers I look for in this case is seeing *a face with blue lips (cyanosis)* at the completion of an anaerobic (lack of oxygen) hard swim.

Since CO2 is being produced throughout the body with vigorous activity, adding more to the immediate tissue environment from the circulating blood only deepens its negative effects. One such effect is actually a *rescue mechanism* of sorts: there are *CO2-sensors in the arterial blood supply* which, when stimulated, produce the **sensation of "air hunger."** THIS, I feel, is the primary stimulus that causes the breathing center of the brain to want to engage in forced respiration, not what might be construed as a relative lack of oxygen.

With rapid inhalation and exhalation of ambient air, the oxygen exchange is really not that dramatic. As an example of quick inhalation-exhalation oxygen exchange, I submit the scenario of giving CPR to one who needs resuscitation. The ambient air contains 21% oxygen on average; forced air from a rescuer into the victim only contains about 16% oxygen; this shows that the body removes only about 5% of oxygen from quickly-inspired air. In addition, even with well-trained athletes, it takes time for all the respiratory trained mechanisms to kick in… Sometimes as much as three (3) minutes, so maximum oxygen consumption and oxygen exchange does not really come into play as quickly as the build-up of CO2.

PHYSIOLOGIC EFFECTS FROM EXPOSURE TO ALTERED OXYGEN IN AMBIENT AIR

To put this presentation in proper perspective, I must mention the importance of the amount of *available oxygen in the ambient air* where and when vigorous movement is initiated. Right from the start, the amount of oxygen in the air and its corresponding pressures do have an effect on athletic performance. Though this discussion is about work at sea-level, I want to show the powerful influence of available oxygen at different altitudes…

If one trains at *sea-level* where the relative oxygen content of the ambient air is 21%, and the barometric pressure is 760 mmHg (mercury), and the atmospheric oxygen pressure is 160mm Hg, the alveolar (air sacks in the lungs,) oxygen pressure averages about 110 mmHg, and the **arterial blood oxygen pressure rises to 96 mmHg.** The body gets used to this constant oxygen supply at this pressure while the adaptive enzymes become "trained" to extract what oxygen they have to work with from moment to moment.

Take the altitude up to *3000 feet*, and we see the barometric pressure drop to 687 mmHg, the atmospheric oxygen pressure drop to 142 mmHg, the alveolar oxygen pressure drop to 94 mmHg and finally the arterial blood oxygen pressure drop to 83 mm Hg… **an almost 14% drop in blood oxygen content from sea-level.**

Go to a *mile high* and the parameters drop to 631 mmHg barometric pressure, 132 mmHg atmospheric oxygen pressure, 85 mmHg alveolar oxygen pressure, and 75 mm Hg arterial blood oxygen pressure… **a 22% drop in blood oxygen content from sea-level.**

Go to *8000 feet* high, and the important parameters read thus: alveolar oxygen pressure drops to 69 mmHg, and the arterial blood oxygen pressure falls to 63 mmHg… **An almost 35% drop in blood content of oxygen from sea-level to 8000 feet.**

These physiologic numbers (lung and blood oxygen contents) are reduced by 10-15 mmHg in normal older athletes.

(No rocket scientist needed to see that if a poorly adapted athlete pushes hard at altitude, the reduced oxygen supply will manifest the sensation of breathlessness sooner and with more intensity; any CO_2 buildup will happen sooner into the exercise bout and will produce a prolonged effect of breathing distress. What usually presents is what is called "dragon-breathing." This is a type of involuntary adaptive reflex whereby the distressed athlete gasps for air with facial grimaces and neck muscle contractions.)

You can see from the above listings that absolute available oxygen is extremely important to the body's ability to extract it for metabolic use; have it (oxygen) compromised in content, and the ability to utilize it is diminished immediately. Here the breathing mechanism and corresponding oxygen metabolism are stressed such that not only is the probability of CO_2-build up a certainty, but any help from available oxygen to try and offset this will be hard to obtain. A physical manifestation that sometimes presents when respiration is compromised and the athlete is in distress is called "dragon-breathing." Mostly seen with asthmatics but not restricted to same, "dragon-breathing" immediately signifies intensely-labored respiration. Once started the body only attends to recovery from this state at the expense of all other movement.

Holding one's breath during training provides, in my opinion, only one benefit to the swimmer. It helps somewhat in the tolerance of CO_2 build-up… Something that could prove decisive with streamlining off the walls and into finishes. This having been stated; I am otherwise against breath-holding while swim racing most distances.

BREATHING PATTERNS WHILE SWIM RACING

There are **two types of distress that the body must be trained to withstand: physiological and psychological.** Correct physiologic adaptations are hoped for with appropriate training sets throughout the main racing season. But it is the **PERCEIVED** bodily response and adaptation to the swim training that will prove to be most important in producing fast swims. How you practice is how you race!

Cecil Colwin wrote an informative article on several aspects of breathing when swimming the four racing strokes (American Swimming, 2003, issue 5). I agree with his presentation that the **inhalation aspect of the breathing cycle is noticeably shorter than the exhalation aspect. But I disagree with Mr. Colwin that the "used air" should not be forced out with any great effort otherwise breathlessness will ensue more quickly. Exhalation must not be left to simple timing, in-and-out; as one approaches breathlessness during a race, concerted effort should be made to make sure the lungs have purged much of their stale air so more fresh air can be inhaled due to the natural negative pressure of the lungs.** Of course, the breathing and movement through each stroke cycle should by rhythmic, but this comes with practice and experience. Learning to pace an event and control the breathing cycle is just as important as knowing how to swim the required stroke… Maybe even more so. Many a good swimmer has taken a race out too hard and wished he hadn't; some are able to "feel" the mistake quickly and rely on their reserve of aerobic and anaerobic conditioning to hopefully salvage the effort, but most usually do irreparable damage physiologically (breathing-wise) and suffer the consequences.

I've seen this all too often with enthusiastic and energetic age-groupers. They get caught up in the immediate moment of competition and forgot the whole concept of *breath control for the whole race.* The 100 yard/meter freestyle is a strong example.

Usually thought of as short enough to allow breath-holding as in the 50 free, what proves out is the fact that *doubling the distance* (50 to100) *in water at full blast requires almost four times the energy (actual and perceived) since stressful metabolic alterations are occurring in an accelerated rate, so the back half of the race is happening in an already "unfriendly" physiologic environment.*

I suggest that the only breath-holding event be the 50 freestyle, and even here, some exhalations of CO_2 need to occur to assure a breath-holding strong finish. The 100 free should have the swimmer breathe every cycle going into the last 25 yards/meters where and when the athlete's ability to breath-hold during building discomfort will allow the quickest, strongest finish possible. Needless to say, this type of breath control needs to be practiced over and over for all freestyle events over a 50 so it becomes automatic during the "combat of racing."

I am against "double breathing" in backstroke only because of the negative influence on the smoothness of the stoke cycle; some gravitate to this breathing cycle because the head is out of the water, and no co-ordination of head movement with breathing is absolutely necessary. But the stroke should be trained with the same breath control as freestyle: of inhalation on one arm, exhalation on the other arm.

The correct breaststroke rhythm dictates one breath per cycle, and it is here that the inhalation is much shorter than the exhalation if one is to maximize the efficiency of the underwater glide… Good chance to blow out mounting CO2.

The butterfly, consuming the most energy per unit time of swimming, requires regular inhalation/exhalation. World records have now been swum with breathing every cycle… Just as much for controlling the breath and keeping the sense of breathlessness at bay longer into the race as for maintaining the rhythm of the stroke.

Everyone slows down towards the end of a hard race. But with proper breath control, I prefer to have my swimmers slow down *less* than their competition. Hopefully, this will mean a fast swim. *Breath control…* It keeps you in it to win it.

OVERVIEW

Though not in the same league as full-blown chronic asthma, Exercise-Induced Asthma **(EIA)** or *bronchospasm* is a special variant that has its own debilitating characteristics. Typically, EIA becomes manifest only after physical activity has begun or after its completion. This physical activity needs to be of at least of moderate duration and intensity to bring on EIA. Though it encompasses only a portion of the 26 million people *worldwide* who suffer from moderate to severe asthma, EIA affects athletes irrespective of gender and age. All too often, EIA is just a harbinger of an underlying condition which is **inflammatory in nature, mostly involving the small airways of the lung (bronchioles).** This should be of concern to both patient and medical practitioner. It should alert them to the fact that further investigation and appropriate treatment are a must. Were it not for vigorous and, or extended physical activity bringing on the hallmarks of asthma, this underlying inflammatory condition would go largely unnoticed and untreated, allowing the condition to worsen. Also with age comes the possibility of Gastro-Esophageal Reflux Disease (see my article on GERD in the Sept/Oct issue of Swim). This is a propensity to having gastric acid and related contents back up into the esophagus. And this can lead to a number of medical problems, one of which is asthma.

As mentioned above, EIA is usually brought on by vigorous activity lasting more than a few minutes, but symptoms can ensue rather quickly if the athlete has been emotionally and physically "pumped" for some time before vigorous movement and can persist for more than an hour after exercise completion.

Vigorous activity worsens symptoms in up to 80% to 90% of asthmatics, and EIA may appear in as many as 40% to 50% of patients with seasonal allergy symptoms. Additionally, 10% to 15% of the general population without any allergies, known asthma or any other medical problems can also exhibit EIA symptoms when challenged with vigorous exercise.

All asthmatic conditions are the result of an inflammatory process that causes narrowing of the airways and results in labored breathing. While not life-threatening in and of itself, an episode of EIA can affect performance in the water to the tune of a 50% drop in aerobic capacity and bring on an uncharacteristic bout of fatigue. There are several symptoms marking EIA, some obvious, some subtle.

SYMPTOMS OF EXERCISE-INDUCED ASTHMA

The most readily seen symptoms include cough during and, or after exertion, chest tightness or pain, wheezing (difficulty forcing air OUT of the lungs with "sounds"), fatigue, and general trouble breathing. More subtle symptoms include chest congestion, a feeling of being "out of shape," lack of energy, stomach pains, inconsistent or erratic physical performances, frequent colds, better performances during short exercise sessions, and poorer tolerance of running sports compared with swimming.

TRIGGERS OF EXERCISE-INDUCED ASTHMA

Specific triggers of EIA can vary from the obvious to the surprising. As mentioned above, high-intensity exercise (greater than 85% of maximal heart rate swims) tends to provoke attacks, theoretically because increased rapid breathing leads to increased circulation with its concomitant release of irritating endogenous (from within) bronchial chemicals, increased temperature, and resultant increased dryness in the airway. With age, comes the propensity of acid reflux, but this can be seen in anyone who uses poor discretion in ingesting food near to vigorous activity... Especially with a sport like swimming that puts the body in a prone position.

There are additional known environmental triggers for EIA: cold, dry, dusty, or Smokey air contaminated by automobile exhaust, smog components, cigarettes and other organic allergens. (In her book, *ASMTHMA and EXERCISE,* former Olympic gold medalist, Nancy Hogshead, documented the difficulty she had swimming in certain towns where the environmental conditions worsened her symptoms). Another almost "occupational hazard" for EIA sufferers is the chlorine content of various pools. Though not an allergen per say, since it has no organic components, chlorine is definitely an irritant. A high concentration of this oxidizing chemical and, or its breakdown products (hypo-chlorites and chloramines) measured in the air six to 12 inches above the pool surface has been shown to trigger more attacks in susceptible swimmers than any other cause. A feeling of a "wet lung" is usually the telltale symptom here.

For those experiencing frequent attacks of EIA, screening for occult (hidden) infection is indicated. While an upper respiratory infection such as the common cold or bronchitis would be an obvious trigger, sinusitis, otitis media or other systemic illnesses may flair asthma even though the athlete is unaware of their presence.

TREATMENT OF EXERCISE-INDUCED ASTHMA

There are several ways swimmers can try to control their EIA episodes. In an attempt to control their asthma condition and possibly avoid consuming excess medication, athletes should first try to take advantage of several natural factors that may help to keep EIA under control.

It is very important to take the time to warm up properly in order to prepare the respiratory system (as well as the heart) for the upcoming demands of vigorous exercise. A sufficient warm up of between 1000 and 1500 yards is needed to help lessen the amount of irritating chemicals that might naturally be present in asthmatics.

Other non-pharmaceutical methods include nasal breathing to warm the air before it enters the lungs, maintaining proper cardiovascular fitness, consuming sufficient amounts of non-irritating (to the GI tract) liquids to properly hydrate the mucous membranes of the airways, and to distance oneself from anything potentially irritating (perfume, cigarette smoke, exhausts).

The most reliable method of protection against EIA is the pharmacological. Here, obviously, an appropriate medical practitioner must be brought into the loop for proper diagnosis and treatment. And the athlete/patient must adhere to the appropriate dosing of medication prescribed for their particular condition. A caution here is for those swimmers competing in open competition… Some of the medications that work for this condition are banned by the various governing bodies in swimming. It would be wise to check first before taking *anything* that could possibly cause a positive drug test for a banned substance.

An athlete with EIA typically can be prescribed a quick-acting, but relatively short-lived bronchial inhaler like *albuterol* (e.g. Proventil) in a short a time as 15 minutes before needed. But with years of testing under race conditions, it has been shown that this type of inhaler actually works more thoroughly if taken *one hour* before needed. Effectiveness approaches 90% in most cases. Administration of *albuterol* is done with one or two measured inhalations as prescribed which affords the patient about two hours of maximum protection and up to six hours of moderate protection. Unfortunately, frequent or long term use will allow for a lessening of effect. And taking more than that which the prescriber has intended can produce negative effects on the body that, at the least, can interfere with rather than help performance. Therefore, it is best to use this type of medication on an "as needed" (for racing and, or training) basis. There are even extended-type medications and combination dosages that can provide relieve throughout the day and thru the night.

Another class of medication, called *leukotriene antagonists* (e.g. *Singulair*), may have an additive effect in controlling EIA. Taken once every 24 hours, *Singulair* gives more steady protection and is a Godsend to many sufferers. When added to the inhaler regimen, almost total control of breathing difficulty may be achieved.

Treating allergic athletes involves suppressing their allergic responses. Inhaled anti-inflammatory steroidal medications (e.g. *Flovent, Vanceril, Rynacort, Aerobid*, etc.) need to be taken daily from the start of the allergy season to keep both the allergenic and inflammatory components of asthma under control. These medications have their own cautions once of which to make sure the user rinses out the mouth after inhalation to prevent possible infections there.

Tighter control of asthma can be sought with the addition of two more types of medication: anti-allergen nasal sprays like *Nasalcrom, Nasonex, Vancenase*, etc., and non-sedating *antihistamines* like *Claritin, Clarinex, Zyrtec, Allegra*, etc. The nasal sprays act to help relieve congestion and stabilize the mucous membranes of the nasal passages against substances that can contribute to an asthma attack. The *antihistamines* present a synergistic effect by neutralizing potential asthma-causative agents that are all around us. These medications have been shown to increase airway function by at least 10% under vigorous activity. A new addition to this class is the promotion of Singulair (see above) to help control the body's response to allergens.

THINGS TO THINK ABOUT

A typical scenario for vigorous swimming would be for the athlete to re-medicate at least 20 to 30 minutes before practice warm-up, or about one hour before race time. The warm-up would be light aerobic exercise, at approximately 50% to 60% of maximal heart rate. Retaking medication is an individual circumstance and must be worked out beforehand to prevent any untoward effects on other vital systems. And, of course, the proper warm down is a must for many reasons including breath control. And let's not forget adequate hydration throughout the practice session or meet.

EXERCISE INDUCED ASTHMA. THE HIDDEN SYNDROME

The earliest known report of exercise as a cause of asthma dates back to the second century A.D. This syndrome (signs of the disease + symptoms) remained a mystery until 1864 when a physiologic researcher names H.H. Salter speculated that the rapid passage of fresh cold air over the bronchial mucous membranes might stimulate irritable airways. But it took all the way to the mid-1970's to confirm possible cause-and-effect and to elucidate further happenings in what has now come to be termed an "inflamed respiratory system." Since then, several researchers have clarified the complex pathophysiological mechanisms of EIA with the concomitant new anti-asthmatic drugs following suit. Because the stimuli for respiratory distress were shown to differ from some other causes of asthma, this condition more recently has also been termed **"Exercise-Induced *Bronchospasm*" (EIB.)**

There continues to be a vast amount of clinical research into the mechanisms and management of EIA, and knowledge in this field is deepening. The description, incidence, causes, and treatment of *exercise-induced asthma* will follow with their relationship to aquatic athletes.

DESCRIPTION AND INCIDENCE

Normally, when a person exercises intensely, the body adapts by allowing ventilation to increase to as much as 30 times greater than when at rest. Someone suffering EIA, however, is medically classified as having a 10 percent or greater reduction in stressed respiratory function under vigorous conditions. What is tested for physiologically is something called **F**orced **E**xpiratory **V**olume **(FEV)** in one second, or **P**eak **E**xpiratory **F**low **R**ate **(PEFR)** following a period of about six to eight minutes of strenuous exercise. The intensity of the exercise bout should be sufficient to increase the heart rate to at least 85 percent or more of the age-predicted maximum (Hrmax = 209 - 0.74x), where "x" is the age in years.

Airway obstruction becomes evident soon after, and in severe episodes, pulmonary function may take one hour or more to return to pre-exercise levels (milder cases remit within 15 to 20 minutes). In fact, this is a hallmark of EIA: spontaneous resolution of the attack 30 to 90 minutes after completion of exercise. There is an additional "late-phase" *bronchospasm* which occurs three to six hours after exercise in approximately **30 percent** of victims, **particularly children.**

Overt symptoms of EIA may vary with time among individuals and range from cough (during or after exertion), dyspnea (difficult breathing) with WHEEZING (trouble forcing air OUT of the lungs with "sounds"), and tightness or pain in the chest to generalized fatigue and stomach pain. Recognition of these transient symptoms as *bronchospasm* by the coach or athlete is important since they may be misinterpreted as signs of poor athletic condition.

EIB affects 80 to 90 percent of known asthmatics. However, it has been called the *"hidden syndrome"* because many victims have their first attack without a known history of asthma. Specific studies have shown that this situation can range from seven to 50 percent of previously normal children and adolescents. It can also occur in up to 50 percent of allergic patients. It has even been ascertained that accomplished athletes can suffer the debilitating **EIA syndrome** and not know for sure what is going on. A prime example is the former Olympian, Nancy Hogshead. In her book, *Asthma and Exercise,* Nancy describes a vague feeling of not being able to "get enough air" during demanding training sessions; at first she thought that she just was having a bad day, then a bad few days, then the feeling would make its presence felt on a regular basis. It progressed to the point that even if she competed in a city with polluted air, she would suffer the same air-deprived sensation.

How widespread is EIA? Studies at a few NCAA Division I colleges have revealed that just under three (3) percent of all athletes in all sports showed signs of diminished ventilation upon vigorous activity, yet two thirds (2/3) did not definitely know of their condition before matriculation.

For the 1984 Olympics, the U.S. Olympic Committee and the American Academy of Allergy and Immunology revealed that 67 out of 597 American athletes (11%) were suffering EIA when put through the rigor of training and competing. Yet, because they were treated properly, 41 won medals (including 15 gold) in 14 different sports.

Even 10-15% of the general population without any allergies, known asthma or any other medical problems can exhibit EIA symptoms when challenged with vigorous exercise.

PATHOPHYSIOLOGY OF EIA

When a person exercises strenuously, ventilation increases to about 30 times greater than when at rest. This stimulus and the subsequent cascade of biochemical events primarily differentiates EIA from typical allergic asthma. Current knowledge of the pathophysiology of EIA indicates that its *root cause* may be divided into **four components: (1) an irritating stimulus, (2) a translational event, (3) obstructive response, and (4) modulating factors.**

The main **IRRITATING STIMULUS** has been shown in several studies to be the stress imposed upon the airways by the need to **HEAT** and **HUMIDIFY** large volumes of air in a relatively short period of time. In other words, forced continuously-labored breathing is the primary culprit. Several studies over the years have proven that both cold and, or low-humidity air will bring on the effects of exercise-induced asthma due to the drying effect on the mucosal lining of the respiratory tract. But there is some controversy over which causes the greater negative effect.

There are several other substances that can help put someone over the EIA threshold: dusty or smoky air contaminated by automobile, bus, and truck exhausts, smog components including sulfur dioxide and ozone, cigarettes and various allergens (molds, dust mites, pollens, perfumes, etc.). One substance almost every swimmer knows all too well is chlorine… Needed to disinfect the water, but not the healthiest substance to breathe. Though not an allergen in the purest sense because it is not organic, its highly irritating character comes into play when it combines with ammonia to produce chloramines… this is what you "smell" of chlorine as you approach a poorly-regulated pool.

Another later approach to the etiology of the EIA condition has been investigated and shown to have a definite cause-and-effect relationship: EIA was also produced by RAPID and EXTENSIVE RE-WARMING of the airway AFTER vigorous exercise. This could explain the delayed *bronchospasm* seen sometimes as the swim training session pro

The TRANSLATION of this airway stress to produce *bronchospasm* is based on two subsequent events: (1) airway cooling and, or drying produces irritating bronchial receptors that in and of themselves can produce EIA, and (2) the excess drying effect causes certain cells of the airway lining to emit irritating chemicals which can, in and of themselves, cause EIA to happen… These chemicals include (*Histamine, Prostaglandins, Leukotrienes,*) and **N**eutrophil **C**hemotactic **F**actor (NCF)… All of which can produce EIA outright and produce an inflammatory cellular reaction.

The EIA OBSTRUCTIVE RESPONSE can be correlated to the release of the above irritating chemicals. Within 6 to 8 minutes, for the most part, the airway obstructive syndrome comes into play and breathing is, at best, labored; at worse, the athlete has to stop activity due to an overwhelming feeling of not being able to get enough air to continue… a sometimes frightening occurrence. After the initial *bronchospasm* or chest tightness, there can be a delayed physiologic clearance of these chemicals. They are depleted in amount, and their negative effects become diminished 30 to 90 minutes into the exercise bout; this can bring on a feeling of catching a "second wind" as one continues to exercise.

Then there is the truly delayed effect from the above-mentioned chemo tactic factors (NCF's); they take a longer time to produce inflammation in the area of release that can result in the delayed asthma that is seen in as many as one-third of EIA sufferers. Three to six hours post-exercise, these "late phase" EIA patients can present with great difficulty in breathing, which can be very perplexing to someone who is not presently exercising and has not done so in hours.

The final element in dealing with EIA is to MODULATE the body's response to all of the above. The better we can lessen all negative respiratory effects, the better the athlete/sufferer can deal with the rigors of intense training. The most obvious is to remove as many irritants from the ambient environment as possible. It would pay the afflicted athlete to get tested to find out what substances he or she is allergic to (molds, dust mites, etc.). Of course, correct diagnosis and pharmacologic treatment is a must, and this comes with a co-operative course of treatment from a knowledgeable health professional.

The objective here is to blunt the effects of irritating stimuli and, or deplete the troublesome mediators of *bronchospasm*... Not as easily attained as one might hope. The pharmacological treatment of EIA would have as its ideal objective, the complete eradication of EIA symptoms under all possible circumstances... Virtually impossible though medical science is making tremendous inroads to reach this goal.

The depletion of irritating endogenous (from within the body) chemicals entails both physical and pharmacological measures. The use of a PROPER WARM UP procedure to accustom the airways to impending strenuous exercise has shown to be of absolute benefit. The previously mentioned irritating molecules that are found in situ (right in the area) of the respiratory tract can be lessened in amount if they are forced to be released during a proper preparatory swim (warm up) or after a competitive race (warm down). These swims require enough time and the correct type of yardage if they are to work at all. When this happens in consort with the medications taken to help the athlete breathe, maximum benefit and effect can hopefully be produced.

Other physical measures to help in the battle against EIA include drinking enough liquids to help hydrate the mucous membranes of the respiratory tract to prevent the drying effect of vigorous breathing. Removing oneself from known irritating chemicals (perfumes, cigarette smoke, all sorts of fumes and exhausts) should be automatic ,and the controlled (relaxed) nasal breathing of the ambient air is something that needs to be practiced.

The most reliable method of protection against EIA is the pharmacological. An athlete with EIA typically can have his or her physician prescribe a quick-acting, but relatively short-lived bronchial dilator inhaler like *Albuterol* (*Proventil, Ventolin*, etc.) to be taken at least 20 minutes before needed. It has been found, though, that, for optimum protection, two inhalations of this type of inhaler needs to be taken about an hour before it is needed in the pool. It has a protective spectrum for up to six hours, but can be taken in as little as two hours after the initial dose if breathing becomes labored. Unfortunately, frequent or long term use will allow for a lessening of effect; therefore it is best to use this type of medication on an "as needed" (for training) basis.

Another class of medication, called "leukotriene antagonists," may have an additive effect on controlling EIA. A prime example of this class of medication is a product called *Singulair*. Taken once every 24 hours, this has proven to be a God-send to many sufferers. In fact, Singulair is now being touted as a prime protective against the allergic responses to pollens, molds, and the like. The combination of Singulair and the bronchiolar dilator has afforded many an EIA sufferer almost total control of his or her breathing.

The last element that needs to be mentioned is the ANTI-INFLAMMATORY class of medications that is designed to target allergic reactions in the nasal passages and the true etiology of all types of asthma: INFLAMMATION of the cells that line the bronchial tubes.

EIA is now officially classified as an inflammatory disease and needs to be treated vigorously to prevent chronic and progressively debilitating condition from ensuing.

The form of medication that can deliver the anti-inflammatory effect most efficiently and with the least amount of negative side effects is, again, the inhaler. Examples of oral inhalers include *Flovent*, *Rhinocort*, *Asthmacort* and several combinations of same with bronchiole dilators. Examples of NASAL inhalers include *Nasalcrom*, *Nasonex*, and *Flonase*. Oral medications for allergic susceptibility include the non-sedating *antihistamines*, *Clarinex, Claritin, Zyrtec,* and the **O**ver-**T**he-**C**ounter (OTC) possibly-sedating *Benadryl, Chlortrimeton*, and *Dimetane*.

Though it may seem that one has to go through an awful lot of trouble and become almost a "walking pharmacy" to keep asthma under control, those suffering repeatedly from an inability to catch one's breath while exercising vigorously, especially in the water, will do almost anything to be able to control what most take for granted… Letting the body get all the air it needs when it needs it.

THINGS TO THINK ABOUT

A typical scenario for swim practice would be for the athlete to pre-medicate 15 to 20 minutes before warm-up. Or approximately ONE HOUR before the main event on race day. The warm up would be light aerobic exercise, at approximately 50% to 60% of maximum heart rate, If necessary, the inhalers may be repeated before the competition begins if more than two hours have elapsed. If need be, another "hit" of a short-acting inhaler (e.g. *albuterol*) could be taken before the next race if the two-hour limit has expired. And, of course, the proper warm-down is a must for many reasons including breath control. And let's not forget proper hydration throughout the practice or meet.

CHAPTER 10

DEHYDRATION: YOU DON'T WANT TO GO THERE

If you find yourself in a state of *dehydration*, you made a mistake. Whether you are preparing for intense competition, trying to maintain a sustainable physiology during vigorous training, or partaking in the inevitable all-important recovery... If there simply is not enough liquid bathing the *internal* environment of the body, then impaired performance and delayed and, or poor recovery will mostly be what we see. And diminished physical performance is not the only possibility. Mental acuity can be compromised in a dehydrated state. Most "civilians" walk about day-to-day in a state of at least partial dehydration (and not able to be at their best) only to become aware that something is not right when challenged physically with intermittent vigorous exercise. A serious athlete in a state of dehydration, as stated above, made a mistake, and it should not be taken lightly. One of the "dictums" of physiology is to **"drink before you are thirsty and after you are not."** Relying on the body's thirst mechanism is fool's play at best. In fact, the older one gets; the less reliable the *thirst alert* becomes. In much of the population (almost 40%) the thirst mechanism is so weak that it is often mistaken for hunger.

There are several seemingly sophisticated preparations available to athletes today, either already in liquid form or in need of water to make the correct mix. Many serve the purpose, or at least claim to, of fueling the muscles, or providing a recovery environment for "spent" or damaged muscles, or replenishing what has been lost electrolyte-wise due to the body's heat-dissipation mechanism of sweating. **But the single most important element needed to make any of these preparations work is water.**

It may seem ironic that *swimmers*, literally "bathing" in water throughout their in-pool training, **can become dehydrated. Swimmers sweat like any other athlete** training vigorously; it just can't be noticed in the water. Ask any swimmer who forgets his/her drinking bottle to practice how the mouth soon feels like a bed of cotton. And this is made worse if the ambient air and water temp are allowed to rise to where heat is no longer able to be dissipated from the body moment-to-moment or with outdoor swimming in a cooler, but less humid atmosphere that only serves to hasten the drying effect of inhaled air.

Water is second only to oxygen in importance to life. A young healthy *male's total body weight is about 60% water*; that of a young *woman's is about 50%*. We can survive loses of up to 40% of our body weight in fat, carbohydrate, and protein, but a **water loss of only 9% to 12% of total body weight can be fatal.** *Approximately* two thirds of the water in our bodies is contained inside our cells (intracellular fluid) bathing necessary cellular elements with substances that sustain life. The remainder is outside the cells (extracellular fluid) performing tasks of transporting fuel and waste to and from metabolism-oriented structures.

WATER BALANCE DURING EXERCISE

Water plays several critical roles in exercise, mostly related to the blood's capacity to carry various elements (oxygen, *glucose*, fatty acids and amino acids, carbon dioxide and other metabolic wastes) to and from functioning cells of all the organs. **Water also plays a large role in heat dissipation from exercising muscles and the maintaining of blood pressure and cardiovascular functioning during physiologically stressful moments.**

An interesting relationship occurs when the body is forced to handle vigorous exercise. **Metabolic oxidation occurring during muscular contractions actually produces water as a physiologic by-product.** The more muscular contraction, the more water produced **but this is still only a fraction (maybe a tenth) of the water lost through other means:** evaporation through the skin, evaporation through the body's action of moisturizing inhaled and exhaled air, excretion from the kidneys and the large intestine. At rest, the kidneys excrete about two ounces (60 mls) of water per hour. You might think the kidneys would excrete more as the metabolic rate increases; well, they can for a while, but only to a point. Then **the production of urine goes way down when the body senses that fluid loss is occurring too rapidly to keep the body in a steady hydrated state. If not reversed.** How likely is the condition to occur?

HYPONATREMIA

There has come to light within the past few years the somewhat rare condition of *hyponatremia*. Though it should not occur in swimmers, in the spirit of complete presentation, this condition is discussed as a serious form of dehydration that potentially could arise in a swim-related event. In those competing in triathlons where the grueling distance run is saved for last, after the swim and then the bike legs, those who place themselves in the circumstance of potentially creating this condition can, at best, expect a poor finishing performance, and, at worst, place the body in physiologic peril. No argument that fluid replacement is desirable, but can too much of a good thing be bad? In the recent past, several cases of *hyponatremia* have been reported in endurance athletes, though *all land-based*. This condition is clinically defined as a blood-sodium concentration below the normal range of 136 to 143 mmoles/liter. *Symptoms* would logically appear in stages: **weakness, disorientation, seizures, and coma if the condition is not corrected quickly.**

The processes that regulate fluid volumes and electrolyte concentrations are normally highly effective, so consuming enough water to dilute plasma electrolytes to dangerously low levels is difficult under most circumstances. Distance runners who log between 15 and 25 miles per training session in warm weather and who do not salt their food excessively don't usually develop electrolyte deficiencies. Even those marathoners who lose three to five liters of sweat and drink two to three liters of water usually will maintain normal plasma concentrations of sodium, chloride, and potassium.

Tackling distances greater than a marathon (ultra-marathon, etc.) can obviously tax the physiology to extents that push all boundaries to their very thin limits. But a study done in 1991 by Barr and colleagues showed that when subjects consumed more than seven liters of plain water during six hours of exercise in the heat, their plasma sodium concentration decreased only negligibly by about 3.9mmmoles/liter.

The ideal solution to prevent hyponatremia would be to replace water at the exact rate that it is being lost or to add sodium to the ingested fluid to keep *homeostasis*. The problem with the latter approach is that sports drinks that have somewhat of a palatable taste contain only mild to moderate amounts of sodium concentration. So their consumption is more for energy and rehydration than pure sodium replacement. And taste is a very important element in the manufacture and marketing of sports drinks since palatability can change before, during, and after intense activity.

I would have to add the scenario that if an athlete, choosing to "push the physiologic envelop," happens to be on medication that can affect the immediate internal environment, for example, with diuretics, consequences not normally considered, are at risk of appearing.

DEHYDRATION AND EXERCISE PERFORMANCE

Even minimal changes in the body's water content can impair muscular contraction to the point where the swimmer feels "heavy" and slow in the water... As he or, she is moving through thick syrup rather than smooth-flowing water. The **muscle fibers** (*myofibrils*) will be rubbing against each other creating excess frictional heat in addition to the metabolic heat that is expected. Like a piston in an automobile engine that seizes due to lack of oil for lubrication, muscle fibers will go into spasm, and power production will be reduced noticeably. Many studies have shown that dehydrated athletes are intolerant to prolonged (greater than 60 minutes) vigorous exercise and heat stress. The heat stress factor is mollified somewhat by the immediate water environment of the swimmer, water having a much better heat-drawing capacity than air. But as the intensity of training increases, so do the effects of internal heat production, and **even an immersed vigorously-training swimmer will dehydrate and suffer during an intense practice session.**

The impact of dehydration on the cardiovascular and heat-regulatory systems is quite predictable. Fluid loss decreases plasma volume; this, in turn, decreases blood pressure, which then reduces blood flow to the muscles and skin. In an effort to deal with all this, heart rate increases. Because less blood reaches the skin overall, heat dissipation is hindered, and the body retains more heat in areas with a lot of muscle activity (we quite often see a flushing effect on the upper back of swimmers). As dehydration approaches 2% of total body weight, both heart rate and body temperature are elevated during exercise. If the water loss reaches 4% or 5% of body weight, say with land-based activity, the capacity for prolonged aerobic effort declines by 20% to 30%.

In athletic endeavors that require a mix of aerobic and anaerobic or more anaerobic activity (under 3 minutes… that covers most swimming events), the drop off in performance is not as dramatic but it is certainly there; especially if multiple events are swum over a relatively short period of time. Enough of a drop is seen such that the resultant effort can be diminished in close competition.

Below is a listing of physiologic parameters that show negative responses to dehydration; most are *not quickly improved*, if at all, when rehydration is attempted, which reinforces the dictum of prevention of dehydration is much better than trying to correct it…

Physiology	Dehydration	Rehydration
Cardiovascular		
Blood volume/plasma volume	diminished	delayed response
Cardiac output	diminished	delayed response
Stroke volume	diminished	delayed response
Heart rate	diminished	delayed response
Metabolic		
Aerobic Capacity (V02Max)	somewhat diminished	same
Anaerobic power	somewhat diminished	same
Anaerobic capacity	somewhat diminished	same
Blood lactate, peak value	diminished	diminished
Buffer capacity of blood	diminished	delayed response
Lactate threshold	diminished	delayed response
Muscle & liver glycogen	diminished	diminished

Thermoregulation & fluid balance		
Physiology	Dehydration	Rehydration
Electrolytes in muscle and blood	diminished	no change
Exercise core temperature	increased	delayed cool down
Sweat rate	diminished	delayed response
Skin blood flow	diminished	delayed response

74

Performance

Muscular strength	slightly diminished	slightly diminished
Muscular endurance	diminished	diminished
Muscular power	slightly diminished	slightly diminished
muscle movement to exhaustion	diminished	diminished
Total work performed	diminished	diminished

ELECTROLYTE LOSS DURING EXERCISE

In addition to body water lost during vigorous exercise, many nutrients, especially minerals, escape with sweat. We stated above; swimmers do not sweat as much as land-based athletes, but they do sweat, and they do lose body water. Sweat is a filtrate of blood plasma; it contains many substances found there including *sodium* (Na+), *chloride* (Cl-), *potassium* (K+), *magnesium* (Mg++), and *calcium* (Ca++). It is mostly water (99%) but contains enough lost electrolytes to produce altered physiologic responses in some athletes. What happens next is the body's sensing this loss and causing the kidneys to greatly shut down urine production; in effect, to hold on to body fluid. **An additional response also causes the kidneys to produce a powerful hormone called** *aldosterone*. This acts to make the kidneys retain sodium and chloride ions (Na Cl… salt). What follows is the amount of these ions rise and produces an increased concentration that signals the brain's *hypothalamus* to **produce the thirst alert** so we would increase our water intake. This dilutes them back to normal. Unfortunately, all this takes time… *It is not an immediate response*, which affords a delayed effect of recovery. Someone in the middle of vigorous training or competition that develops a healthy thirst has entered the **"zone of metabolic distress,"** and his or her **performance will most likely be compromised.** The damage is done, so to speak, though some effort can be salvaged if rehydration is done quickly and thoroughly.

If left to normal physiologic recovery, up to 48 hours may be needed for electrolyte and fluid rebalancing. This is an unacceptable time delay for those needing to partake in regularly-scheduled daily training regimens. This is where the commercial *"recovery drinks"* probably have a place. Though they do provide for moderate energy-replacement to the musculature (and are touted as such) due to the mild *glucose*-complex content, as mentioned above, they also have enough salt in them, among other things, to actually create a slight thirst, making the desire to drink more prominent which then helps to ensure adequate rehydration. *Gatorade* at 110mg of sodium per 8 fl. ounces has twice the content of PowerAde at 55mg per glass.

The author uses a 50-50 mix of red grape juice and PowerAde in his daily travails back and forth across the pool: grape juice to help with circulation (from resveratrol in the grapes) and PowerAde, with its better carbohydrate formulation, for energy and rehydration. A caution here is for those who have difficulty handling fructose which is in the grape juice.

TAKE HOME POINTS TO REMEMBER:

- *Our immediate need to replace lost body fluid is greater than our need to replace lost electrolytes or anything else consumed during vigorous exercise.*
- *Since our thirst mechanism does not exactly match our hydration state, we should* **"drink before we are thirsty, and after we are not."**
- *Adequate fluid and energy intake during vigorous training with appropriate timing for competition reduces the risk of dehydration and energy depletion and optimizes the body's cardiovascular and thermoregulatory functions which should eliminate two major causes of diminished performances.*

Step one. Pre and post run bodyweight. For the majority of weekend runners training for the general competitions, Saturday is usually their big running day. This is the morning they may cover 20-26km as their "big" run for the week. This is the best day to assess bodyweight loss. Weigh yourself before the run and after. Drink and hydrate as you would normally for that day (before and during). A loss of more than 3% bodyweight is a cause for concern as research demonstrates that a 3% weight loss corresponds to roughly a 10% drop in performance.

Step Two. Urine charts for a week. Standard urine color charts can be downloaded easily of the Internet. Print a couple of these off and tack one onto the bathroom wall at home and one at work. Unfortunately, you will have to frequently "collect" samples to compare your urine color to the chart. If you are in the "dehydration" zone then slowly increase fluid intake on a daily basis, until you are regularly in the "hydrated" zone. Drinking small amounts every 30 minutes is a better hydration practice than drinking large glasses 3 or 4 times per day. The gut is better able to absorb small amounts of fluid and not cause diarrhea that is a risk with large sudden water intake.

The Internet has a number of sites to download urin color charts for compairison. Please visit http://www.urinecolors.com/dehydration.php for an excellent chart and further information on dehydration.

Hydration in athletes is a science all in itself, as the sports performance staff employed to look after athletes and teams understand the detrimental effect that dehydration has on performance, incidence of cramping and also soft tissue injury. The weekend warrior does not the need the sophisticated interventions such as "glycerol loading," "IV fluids," and "controlled electrolyte drinks" that the sports people use.

Staying in the hydrated color zone and ensuring that you remain within 3% bodyweight loss range during exercise may be all that is required. Furthermore, replacing some of the fluid intake (water) with an electrolyte fluid drink (*diarolyte* or *gastrolyte*) may also be a worthwhile practice so that the "extra" water does not dilute the sodium content of the body (a condition called hyponatremia). Make up a liter of this in the morning (sachets can be purchased at all pharmacies) and slowly sip this throughout the day, as well as straight water.

SECTION II:

PUBLIC HEALTH TENETS AS THEY RELATE TO SPORTS... KEEPING THE ATHLETE HEALTHY

It is much wiser to prevent illness and injury and the subsequent inevitable downtime from training and participation than to deal with the sometimes long trek back to health or *homeostasis* by way of rehabilitation. Since it is almost a medical proverb that the "body never forgets," this section will illustrate instances where an ounce of prevention is worth much more than a pound of cure.

In this section, my graduate work in public health relating to sports will guide me in sharing what I know and have researched about intelligent choice that should be made by athletes of all ages as they commit to either intermittent or sustained training in various sports. Included will be very important nutritional guideline to prevent dehydration, allow for proper fueling and refueling protocols, and to bring to light many of the exotic energy-boosters that have recently shown to provide just what they claim. The appropriateness of adequate warm-ups, cool-downs, stretching, and rest and recovery will be illustrated as it pertains to athletes of all ages.

CHAPTER 1

STEALTH HEALTH

QUICK INFORMATION FOR ATHLETES

Information is presented in no specific order of importance. It is quick information that most people would not have given the importance to good public health. Of course, everything listed can be of vital importance to KEEPING THE ATHLETE HEALTHY.

- Environmental Issues

o Sun tan lotion **MUST** be applied at least 20 minutes before exposure to ensure adequate protection as expected; otherwise it just gets washed off if immersion in water happens before that; sunscreen must be re-applied after about 90 minutes in water no matter how long it is claimed to last on the skin.

o 15 minutes in today's sun equals about one hour's exposure 30 years ago; all sun-caused skin damage is cumulative, and we are susceptible from sun-up till sunset; UV-a & UV-b are the culprits.

o Sun rays bouncing off water or a shiny object like glass (rays of incidence) have more destructive power on the skin than direct sunlight.

o The sun is considered a major cause of cataracts as is cigarette smoke; using polycarbonate swim goggles when in the pool will greatly protect the eyes from forming cataracts; wear polarized and UV-coated sunglasses if there is sun up in any amount.

o In strong sunlight, an outdoor pool has its chlorine content heavily vaporized off the top 12 inches of surface; this provides for an irritating mixture of fine water mist and chlorine which can aggravate breathing problems.

o The prescription cream, *Efudex*, is being used on those people who are pre-disposed to developing skin cancer. Fair complexion, blue eyes, red hair and who spend lots of time in the sun; Yet the skin may seem normal, but hidden cell changes are brought out within days to be treated before more serious skin damage can ensue. Once these pre-skin cancers are discovered they can be burned away chemically.

o People who are bombarded with excess electronic media information diminish their ability to exercise sufficient critical thinking.

o It is safer for general health to live on the **WEST** side of a major highway than the east side because the prevailing westerly winds will blow traffic exhaust **AWAY** from you on the west side and **TOWARD** you on the east side.

o If ever exposed to poisonous plants like ivy or sumac, you usually have around 2 hours to remove the toxic irritant before it penetrates too deeply into the skin; rubbing alcohol is the best and most easily available to remove these toxins.

o It is a wise move to disinfect A/C ducts in homes and cars at least once every 2 weeks throughout most of the year but once weekly during cold and flu season; this stems from studies regarding Legionnaire's Disease in hospitals where the offending bacteria grew in air ducts.

o During colder months the relative humidity in ambient air when heated to room temp dries out to less than 50%; this can bring on dryness and irritation in the respiratory tract rendering people susceptible to respiratory infections and asthma.

o A hot-steam vaporizer in the bedrooms at night and, or spending several minutes in a steam shower can help moisturize the bronchial tree, raise the air humidity and provide soothing relief.

o **NEVER** dive head first into cold water; the cold contracts the blood vessels and keeps blood away from the heart and lungs allowing for potential fainting or cardiac arrhythmia; always enter feet first to squeeze the blood **TOWARD** the heart and lungs.

o Closing the toilet seat cover or spraying a Lysol type product above the toilet when flushing prevents bacteria from being spread up to 10 feet away.

o Ethyl rubbing alcohol instilled in each ear after swimming will draw out residual moisture to prevent Swimmer's Ear.

o If there is a fire that is burning old trees, be aware that stored methyl mercury in the old wood will be released into the air; spilled mercury from a broken thermometer, for example, must be vacuumed up to prevent it from sublimating into toxic mercury fumes.

o Chlorine by itself is **NOT** allergenic; it must be combined with body fluids or something organic in order for the compound to bring about an irritating allergic-producing reaction.

o Mosquitoes are drawn to their blood meals by their ability to sense carbon dioxide; we exhale, they find us to bite and feed. They do not like the hot sun and begin their marauding as the sun sets.

• Physical Body Issues

o A major rule of public health is to hydrate before your are thirsty and after you are not; do NOT rely on the thirst reflex to ensure adequate hydration especially as we age; this reflex presents as hunger rather than thirst in the elderly with dehydration becoming more pronounced; when the temp/humid index is over 75, liquids should always be brought along and consumed throughout the day; most kidney stones are formed during hot months with inadequate liquid intake.

o   Newly established methods for CPR now have the one administering it NOT use mouth-to-mouth; instead, removing the hands from the chest after finishing each compression allows the lungs to fill by negative vacuum as Nature intended for their use.

o   Warm-up and cool-down procedures are a must before and after strenuous exercise to prevent pooling of blood in the legs and the creation of a blood volume void in the heart, both of which can lead to fainting or cardiac arrhythmias.

o   Skeletal muscle stretching need to be done in a static mode (no bouncing or ballistic movement) and held for about 30 seconds to stop the inhibiting stretch release mechanism; the more muscle, the more need for stretching; the older the athlete, the more need for stretching; if kept warm, the athlete's stretch will last for about 2 hours; new research has shown that stretching less than an hour before need will weaken the muscles by as much as 30%; stretching should be attempted only when the muscles have been warmed sufficiently.

o   Hydration is very important to maintain adequate blood volume not only for performance but for prevention of blood pressure irregularities; red grape juice has a special property (*resveratrol*) to prevent blood platelets from sticking, allowing blood to flow more easily and quickly to where it is needed: the muscles, but since it has fructose, the gut may have difficulty digesting it; diluting with an electrolyte liquid (*Gatorade*), or plain water could help. Now the Welch's Company has combined red grape juice with the benefits of a strong antioxidant and anti-inflammatory (cherry juice) to make what I feel is the ideal training liquid.

o   Studies have now shown that strenuous exercise in the early morning can place extra stress on the body may present with an extra danger since the anti-stress hormone, cortisol, is at low titer in the blood until around 11 AM; most will show greater strength, power, and speed after 6 PM, when cortisol is at its highest level in the circulation due to *circadian rhythm*.

o   When engaging in progressive-resistive training (the weight room), the legs should be worked first thing to prevent blood pressure spiking; **NEVER** engage in breath-holding (*Valsalva maneuver*) when moving heavy weight because the build-up of pressure on internal organs can produce a dangerous situation with their circulation; try to change the weight-lifting protocol each session to "keep the body guessing" and prevent it from plateauing; ideal order of activity: go from legs to core to arms and chest, rotating the cycle in different ways each lifting session.

o   Tropical fruits, mainly pineapples, have an ingredient, the enzyme, **BROMELAIN**, which helps digest food in nervous stomachs, and also helps the body heal throughout from strenuous exercise. By breaking down and removing the by-products of muscle activity.

o   Whenever learning new neuro-muscular movements, it can take up to 48 hours for the brain to have it imprinted because our highest center of the brain, the cortex, is relatively slow in digesting new information; this lag time is necessary for it to get down to the cerebellum, a more primitive area of the brain. If new physical movements are experienced, say, with another sport, what was just learned from the first sport can be wiped out or at least diminished enough to delay its implementation.

o It has been stated that 10,000 quality repetitions under guidance is necessary to master a particular movement under the stress of competition, and 10,000 hours of same to become elite at it.

o Strong *antihistamines* are an important medical treatment for trauma and must be taken almost immediately since the chemical, *histamine*, is released quickly. This medication acts to lessen swelling and tissue damage and helps the body heal more quickly.

o There are two main physical rules of hydrodynamics for swimmers: laminar flow and hull design; the longer the hull in a streamlined fashion, the faster it goes for the same effort since resistance is greatly reduced; keeping the body flat and in line with the spine as much as possible even when fatigued will allow the swimmer to hold pace longer stronger through the water.

o **D**elayed **O**nset **O**f **M**uscle Soreness (**DOMS**) occurs usually within a few hours of intense physical movement and mostly due to elongation (eccentric), or the recovery phase, of that movement.

o The United States and Japan have shown that their citizens average the **LEAST** amount of sleep on work day nights (6 hours, 30 minutes) while Mexican citizens and Canadian citizens get the most sleep (averaging around 7 hours 10 minutes).

o Eating gummy bears candy can protect your stomach lining from the damaging effects of alcohol and can reduce ulcer size by up to 50%.

o If you are lacking sleep over an extended period of time, or are stressed in any number of other ways, the body reacts by producing the hormones *Ghrelin* and *Cortisol*; the former increases your overall appetite while the latter increases your desire to eat sweets and other calorie-laden food and inhibits the action of insulin receptors... all to produce increased body weight, *glucose* intolerance over time and generalized increase in all the bad blood markers for handling fats in the diet.

o The number one cause of kidney failure in the United States, today is the over-prescribing by doctors and the overuse by patients of the class of drugs known as NSAIDS (non-steroidal anti-inflammatories); some over-the-counter examples are Advil, Motrin, Aleve and their generic equivalents; a safe protocol for this class of drug is 5 days on, 2 days off as a drug holiday to spare both the kidneys and stomach; always take these meds with food, NEVER on an empty stomach.

- Athletic Training Issues

o Drink before you are thirsty and after you are not; a dehydrated athlete puts his muscle fibers at extra stress since they are not lubricated with proper amounts of fluid.
o Sprinters' muscles produce much more lactic acid than distance athletes, and this is magnified by the fact that fast-twitch muscle fibers do **NOT** have a blood supply to carry away the built up lactate as does the slow-twitch fibers.
o Re-fueling the body is optimized within one hour of exercise, but can still have a dramatic effect within two hours.
o *Mitochondria*, the actual energy segments of cells, are optimally induced by intense exercise; there are lactate receptors on *mitochondria* that stimulate their growth as lactic acid builds up from intense exercise; *mitochondria* protectors are needed here because intense activity can also bring about oxidative damage to the *mitochondria* because of their poor cell membrane structure.
o Swimmers who utilize the kick board for various kick training sets should place their face in the water every few seconds and align the head, neck, and spine; this prevents calcium deposits and inflammation (arthritis) from starting even at an early age.
o Swim practices should be started with a kick board and the swimmer leaning on the board kicking and kicking on his side; he should be looking back toward the starting wall; this puts the swimmer in perfect position to stretch the muscles of the shoulder girdle, upper back and neck along with attendant tendons and ligaments to prevent swimmer's shoulder and help relax the muscles groups that perceive stress the most.
o Do not do the same training routine day to day; whether, in the pool, the weight room, on a bicycle, or the ground, the body must have variety and different intensities to bring about the greatest adaptations the quickest; otherwise, the body just trains to train. We want to keep the body off balance and always challenged; as the athlete ages, bringing the legs into the workout protocols becomes more and more important.
o Certain elements and procedures bring about greater abilities to focus... what I call the **POWER OF THE MOMENT**; amber goggles and peppermint scent and flavor act on the brain's **R**eticular **A**ctivating **S**ystem (**RAS**) to bring the athlete into the moment to do his best; also, breathing exercises to enhance the air-exchange and help focus are extremely important; most athletes breath improperly... rapid, shallow breaths and even breath-holding when they spot a threat to their efforts.
o The most important part of dedicated and intense training is the rest and recovery; the body needs time to recover aided by appropriate supplements to offer up its best for continued intense training.

ISSUES FOR LAND-BASED AND AQUATIC ATHLETES

- Physical Body Issues

o Stretching needs to be done in a static mode and held for about 30 seconds; two 15 second stretching bouts will work if they are done consecutively within 15 seconds of each other; the more muscle and the older the athlete is, the more stretching is needed; the colder the ambient temperature, the more stretching is needed but only after the muscles have warmed sufficiently (a hot shower or heating pad works fine); stretching lasts for about two hours; latest research shows that stretching less than an hour before you engage in vigorous exercise may have a weakening effect on muscle groups by as much as 30%; I have found that stretching about 60 minutes before training or competition works well; a moderate stretching effect can occur from an appropriate warm up and cool down.

o Proper warm-ups and cool downs of the specific muscle groups brought to bear during training or competition must be undertaken; the warm-up procedure must be no less than 15 minutes long, with the cool down lasting about half that; this is not only for the musculature but for the cardio-respiratory systems; these protocols help bring the athlete back "down to earth" safely and help ready them for the next bout of intense movement.

o Hydration is vital to maintain adequate blood volume not only for muscle performance but for prevention of blood pressure and cardiac irregularities; RED GRAPE JUICE has special properties to prevent blood platelets from sticking thus allowing more blood to flow more quickly to where it is needed: the muscles, but since grape juice has fructose as its main source of energy, the gut may have difficulty digesting it at first; diluting with PowerAde could help.

o It is safer to engage in strenuous exercise after 5 PM than before 9 AM; the body is more powerful in the late afternoon as a result of circadian (24 hour cycle) rhythm.

o When engaging in progressive-resistance training, the legs should be worked first to prevent blood pressure spiking; NEVER engage in breath-holding when moving heavy weights...what is produced is called the *Valsalva maneuver* where the athlete vigorously holds his breath building up pressure in the chest cavity (this can prevent adequate venous blood return to the heart); don't repeat the same routine resistance-training repeatedly since the body will adapt and begin to train to train, not train to get better; we want to keep the body off balance with different routines each time; you work the legs, then the core, then the arms and back and chest and return to the cycle.

o Whenever learning new neuromuscular movements, it can take up to 48 hours for the brain to have it imprinted, but if the body is exposed to completely different intricate physical movements (a different sport), what was just learned can be diminished or totally wiped out.

- o *Antihistamines* are an immediate recommendation to take after sustaining physical trauma; *histamine* is always released upon trauma which causes swelling and delays healing; an *antihistamine* lessens swelling and helps speed healing;
- o Muscle tears and consequent pain due to (DOMS) usually occur due to eccentric movement (forced elongation) of muscle groups; this is in contrast to concentric movement (forced contraction) of muscle that is the normal function of this tissue.
- o Enhanced day-to-day recovery is achieved chemically by use of supplements such as glucosamine & chondroitin to protect and help heal the joints, the enzyme bromelain which reduces inflammation throughout the body, a near-perfect food source: skimmed chocolate milk; ribose, muscle-friendly whey protein, and creatine, all used to provide for muscle repair and building and a quality energy source.
- o It seems the USA is the country with the most sleep-deprived populace. More than two million fall asleep while driving per week. We average about 6.4 hours of sleep per 24, where the optimum should be around 8.2 hours daily. Athletes need even more @ 8.4 hours per 24.
- o Symptoms of sleep deficit include: slower reaction time, poor balance and coordination, missed signals in your visual field, increased tendency to illness, greater inflammation which lingers to hinder healing from injuries, dulled memory, burnout, exhaustion and depression.
- o We drink the most coffee in the world, 587 million cups per day to try and combat this lack of sleep.

- • Athletic Training Issues

- o Drink before you are thirsty and after you are not.
- o Sprinters make much more lactic acid (lactate) than distance athletes; buffers need to be induced with the proper training to handle this lactate build-up.
- o The greatest gains from intense practice are during (R & R).
- o As with physical body issues above, re-fueling is most beneficial within two hours of a training session or a competition, preferably within one (1) hour; *Endurox*, *Accelerade*, *Accel Gel*, chocolate milk, creatine, ribose, high quality whey protein, and adequate hydration are all important "refuelers."
- o *Mitochondria*, the actual energy-producing segments of each cell, are induced to form only during intense exercise; new studies show that lactate receptors on *mitochondria* stimulate their growth as lactic acid builds up; when vigorous training is coupled with *mitochondrial energy boosters*, the amount of these energy-inducing segments can double more easily.
- o Do not repeat the exact same routine on land, on the bike, in the weight room or in the water; we want to always keep the body "guessing" as to what you throw at it each training session; as one ages, the legs become more important to train well; the best, most thoroughly-trained athletes are worked from the legs up; aging usually brings about losing a step on land but it does not have to occur in the water.

- o Certain elements enhance focus for imminent effort, what I call "**The Power of the Moment;**" peppermint dissolved in the mouth brings the parts of the brain into play that help focus; amber goggles or glasses do the same thing; enhanced breathing exercises do the same thing; when athletes begin to "lose it" and become self-doubting or distracted, they start to breathe shallow and rapidly; many even hold their breath when they perceive a "threat;" what needs to be done is to control inhalation and exhalation almost every minute before intense effort; breathing in deeply with mouth open causes the belly to expand and lower the diaphragm, enabling the lungs to fill more completely with fresh air; if inhalation occurs through the nose, nitric oxide is released from back of the throat that opens up blood vessels for enhanced circulation; blowing out through the mouth (exhaling) in a concerted but controlled manner reduces or eliminates the build-up of carbon dioxide; knowing that you can control your breathing capacity is very important to feeling confident.
- o Any muscle cramping must be attended to quickly; always rub the muscle *in one direction, downward toward the length of the muscle*; never rub it up and down to prevent rubbing the cramp back into the muscle; if no physical damage is the cause, it is most likely from dehydration, build-up of lactic acid, or lack of fuel.

CHAPTER 2

KEEPING THE ATHLETE HEALTHY

When lecturing on public health, I often start out with the statement: "If you all knew what was out there waiting to get you, you would all go hide in a cave… Until I told you what was in the cave." This succinctly means that there is really no place to hide against sickness, injury, or worse. They are waiting to get you, especially if you put yourself in their path. When, by choice, we venture out of our caves and place ourselves in positions of challenge it becomes our responsibility to be constantly vigilant regarding our own welfare and health, and what we do as young people all too often can present itself years later as cause and effect. A mature (Masters) athlete who has remained intact with little, if any, permanent damage to any major organ system and who trains intelligently can remain in the arena of choice for many years. An injured or ill athlete is good to no one and having the realization that whatever put him on the sideline could have been prevented or greatly lessened only adds to the frustration.

A lot of public health is the "shining light of logic." People need to be exposed to this light in such a way as to convince them to incorporate it intelligently into their lives. A coach-and-athlete combination who abides by the rules of good public health will most probably have a training advantage over those who don't. To quote an oldie from my pharmacy days: "A dram (5 mls.) of prevention is worth a liter (1000 mls.) of cure," every time.

Lesson #1 is to try and put balance in one's life. To give vigorous athletic training equal billing with the rigors of today's demands in the classroom, the workplace, the home, and society, the successful athlete has to be aware of all that can tear at him, both physically and emotionally. Just as a successful competitive swimmer must learn to "make friends with the water" and move through it with an economy of effort that belies the ease spectators see, so must the athlete move through life. Those athletes engaged in long-term training toward a specific goal must be aware of and try to avoid all possible roadblocks to their efforts to improve. Every day should be looked at as a chance to get better in some way. The ability to exercise hard every day might be a genetic gift or the result of extreme focus on a specific goal. In fact, it has been proven many times that the body can "train to train;" adaptation is a remarkable hallmark of the human condition, but good physiologic sense suggests that easier training bouts inserted into the mix and appropriate rest and recovery are all required to properly climb the mountain of condition and solidify possession of those four magical words: "being in great shape." It is then incumbent upon all who seek to be in shape to make the right choices every day… Not an easy task for most young (and, sometimes, not so young) healthy people.

Most of us take good health for granted… Until it leaves us. Many people carry the notion that they are "bulletproof" and that they can expect their bodies to respond to every demand quickly and successfully. The thought of getting sick or injured just isn't as tangible as it should be. My goal and experience have burnished this in my mind, is to educated all my athletes to the point just shy of being obsessive. However, as important as it is to know when to push yourself, it is equally important to know the difference between working correctly toward physiologic goals and putting yourself in harm's way.

There are many subtopics that would easily fit into the title of this work: (1) the importance of adequate warm ups and cool downs, (2) the when, why, and how to stretch, (3) the proper way to fuel the machine for training, and (4) the psychology for competition. For this writing I have chosen to explore more esoteric thoughts that can have great influences, both positive and negative, if acknowledged or ignored.

OVER-REACHING VERSUS OVER-TRAINING

Those who know physiological adaptation to training know that the most important part is the **R**est and **R**ecovery (R&R) between exercise or competition bouts. What goes on here can make all the difference in performance, both in day-to-day training and at the big competitions. *Over-reaching* and *over-training* describe the syndromes (signs and symptoms) of pushing too hard and, or too often. The main difference between the two is the length of time and the degree to which performance is hindered. This is an important distinction. It is not the overt symptoms the athlete exhibits that define the condition; it is more the degree to which performance is diminished. The same symptoms can be experienced with both conditions, but it may take only a few days to a few weeks to recover to full performance after over-reaching, whereas it can take weeks or even months to come back from over-training.

In addition, different athletes react to the stresses of vigorous training differently. Some athletes exhibit some of the symptoms of overtraining, yet are able to race fairly well. Some exhibit few or no symptoms during practice sessions but race poorly. It takes a wise athlete and an understanding coach to spot problems that relate to performance upon demand.

Clues that an athlete may be over doing it are several: the overt physical signs of excessive stress can manifest as irritability, difficulty sleeping (often being too tired to sleep properly through the night), walking around with constant body aches, decreased ability to concentrate, susceptibility to colds and other illnesses, and a change in eating habits. According to the **I**nternational **C**enter of **A**quatic **R**esearch (ICAR) at the **O**lympic **T**raining **C**enter (OTC) in Colorado Springs, Colorado, to be considered "subjectively stale," as the condition is described, an athlete has to present with at least three of the above.

There are also internal physiological parameters that mark an unrelenting stressful condition. Analysis of the athlete's blood would show muscle damage, including a rise in enzymes that would otherwise be contained within the muscle cells proper (two of these markers being *creatinine phosphokinase* and *lactic dehydrogenase*) and an increase in urea. An elevated concentration of the hormone *cortisol* is a classic stress marker, along with a rise in white blood cell concentration, which can signal that the body is fighting off an infection or dealing with inflammation.

In addition, the effects of over-training whether in the pool or on land with the "bad intentions" of hard intervals or racing produce a reduction in aerobic capacity. This can manifest itself as an out of air feeling too early into a practice or during a race. We see a shift to anaerobic physiology rather than a reliance on the aerobic physiology built up during training.

We must not forget the mental and emotional consequences. As over-training takes control of our physiology, the mental energy seems to wane. This is a result of two things: (a) absolute brain energy depletion (diminished *glucose* supply for the energy needs of the brain due to it being in such high demand by the muscles), and (b) the **knowledge** that the body is going to make energy demands that cannot be met. A dedicated athlete does not suffer from short-term memory loss; what hurt yesterday and the day before will most assuredly hurt today, maybe even more so with a cumulative effect. Fish are prisoners of their environment; they have to swim to survive. We, on the other hand, are all prisoners of our minds; we choose to swim, or run, or bike, or…

One of my heroes from the swimming world, former Olympic Coach Jack Nelson, esteemed now-retired head coach of the nationally known and respected Fort Lauderdale Swim Team, is justly famous for his motivating slogan: "Access to Success is Through the Mind."

Student athletes: "note bene" (note well): since *glucose* is by far the most important source of energy to adequately fuel the brain, it becomes a matter of necessity to replenish *glucose* supplies right after practice. In fact, it is now mostly well-appreciated that there is about a two-hour window where (depending upon how one replenishes with the correct food choices) eating can measurably affect the re-supply of *glucose* and glycogen to meet the energy requirements of a demanding life. Since carbohydrates, utilizing the compound tryptophan in a biochemical process, forms serotonin in the brain, we see a tranquilizing effect, they need to be balanced with some protein and fat, which produce *epinephrine* (*adrenaline*) and *nor-epinephrine* (nor-*adrenaline*) as stimulants to help counteract the drowsy feeling one may get from an intense carbohydrate load. And all athletes who choose to take part in vigorous exercise and constant training must ingest a sufficient and appropriate energy supply to adequately nourish the brain, the muscles, the immune system, and all vital organs, all of which must work overtime to prevent over-training.

If symptoms of "too much" begin to cloud the days, then immediate rest from all vigorous specific training is a must. What works for the older athlete is usually a week off from everything and a change of schedule to allow for mental healing. After a week, some easy cross-training can be instituted in different venues: leisure bike-riding or relaxed walking in pleasant sensory surroundings that would get the swimmer away from the pool or some easy pool time to get the runner away from the track or biker off the road. No guilt should be felt for missing practice; an imbalance in the athlete's schedule brought this about in the first place, so some short-term rehab is in order.

INFECTIOUS DISEASES

In addition to the mental and physical effect of over-reaching and over-training, vigorous exercise also involves the risk of immunologic breakdown, which leave the athlete open to infectious diseases. When the athlete is exhausted from training hard and working in close physical proximity to others of similar ilk, it is easy to become sick and to suffer from it.

There is a 3-foot rule in public health: if you can separate yourself from someone who is sick with a cold or other Upper Respiratory Infection (URI) by at least three feet for the short time that you may share proximity, your chances of coming down with the infection are reduced. I want to emphasize the fact that a short time of exposure means just a few minutes at best. Double the distance, and you cut the risk to at least a quarter (providing you do not get drenched with infected saliva from a direct "hit" of a wet sneeze or cough. If you are walking behind someone who is sneezing or coughing during cold season, take a detour off to the side so as not to inhale the trailing effluence of spreading germs. If forced to share space with someone exhibiting symptoms of a cold or URI for longer than an hour, try to get as far away as practical and have as many people fill in the space between you and "germ central," and, if at possible, open windows to circulate fresh air. If able and appropriate, spraying a Lysol-type product through the air and onto fabrics in the confines of a contaminated space will help to reduce virus and bacteria load. The air ducts and accompanying filters in the home and car should be sprayed at least once a week. Years ago, it was discovered that the infecting bacteria for Legionnaires' Disease in hospitals found a "home" in the hot water pipes and air ducts heating the rooms. A cough or sneeze in your car can cause several thousand infecting organisms to find the same type of resting place (A/C-heating ducts) for many hours… A major vector for infection and re-infection without most people even being aware.

In terms of the viruses and bacteria that cause the vast majority of URIs, there are three main components to consequential infection: (1) the infecting load or total amount of initial exposure, (2) the length of time exposed, and (3) the condition of the body and its defense mechanisms at the time of exposure. The absolute simplest yet most important procedure to keep the spread of infection down is to prevent potentially contaminated hands from coming in contact with mucous membranes (eyes, nose, mouth) since this type of tissue is much more permeable to things that land on it than the outer covering of our bodies. Good public health procedures dictate a lessening of the amount of exposure. Removing contaminants from the hands should be of concern to the extent that maybe a gel-type hand wipe would be useful before eating out if no restroom is available or, if it can be accomplished tactfully, after shaking hands.

A major dictum in public health is to "drink before you are thirsty and after you are not." This will be presented a few more times throughout the book to ensure the reader comes away with the importance of a reliable effort to hydrate throughout the day. This adequate, consistent hydration is very important as the seasons change from humid summers to the cooler, drier fall and winter months. This becomes even more important in extreme climates, both hot and cold, since they can each dry out the body's portholes to its surroundings rendering them less effective in keeping out infecting organisms. If the relative humidity in your home is less than 50% during the dry, colder winter months, then the air is lacking sufficient moisture.

Dehydration, a major cause of muscle fatigue and cramping and sometimes progressing into more troublesome blood pressure consequences can even negatively affect the body's ability to fight off invading organisms by way of the respiratory tract. Everybody sweats even swimmers in the water, when pushing through vigorous exercise, and when hydration becomes compromised the upper respiratory tract has its ability to capture and expel invading organisms diminished. Motility of cilia is reduced, mucus is thickened with less motility, and the lining of the upper respiratory tract can become raw and irritated adding to the inflammatory response that occurs with infection.

Another simple but very important procedure is to blow the nose after exposure to airborne infectants or at least at the end of every day, to help eliminate many of the infecting organisms caught in the nasal passages and the upper respiratory tract before they can "dig in," since it takes up to several hours for most infecting organisms to penetrate the mucous linings of the body. Doing this in a hot steamy shower aids, in removal by thoroughly liquefying the mucous membranes and thinning secretions which can thicken in cold climates.

Swimmers are at risk if the pool water's chemical balance is not maintained. Chlorinated water in pools is very drying and irritating to all mucous membranes. The water may be wet, but if the chemicals in the pool are not correctly adjusted when hosting swimmers, upper respiratory involvement progressing all the way to bronchitis and asthma is not uncommon. If you can smell chlorine in the pool area, it is broken down with a very irritating pH of 11 or so. The same caveat holds for land-based athletes: don't exercise to where air-exchange becomes prolonged and intense when the ambient air is contaminated with any of a number of air-born irritants.

With swimmers and every other athlete pushing through vigorous activity in challenging environments, respiratory function can be helped with soothing hot steam. A shower is good but ephemeral; better yet is a hot steam vaporizer through the night. Cool mist units have been in vogue for quite a while, but they can spread contaminated moisture and are not as soothing. Hot steam is sterile and provides a sense of comfort. Public health logic suggests that the bedroom be aired out in the morning and sprayed with a disinfectant to prevent mold build up by the windows and their coverings. It is worth all this extra effort? Ever try to be physical and can't breathe easily due to infection or inflammation? I rest my case.

PAIN VERSUS DISCOMFORT

It is important for a swimmer to do everything possible to prevent over-training, over-reaching, injury, and illness, and a major element in this prevention litany are the ability to differentiate between pain and discomfort. This might seem to be a trivial distinction; in reality, it is what makes successful participation in athletics long-standing. There is obviously a difference between pain and discomfort, usually a question of duration and degree. It is up to the individual athlete (and his coach, if applicable) to know where the boundaries lie and what the consequences are if they are crossed. We must also add the concepts of present-time and delayed-onset pain or discomfort to the mix to provide a more complete and accurate picture of what is happening as an event progresses.

Every athlete worth his sweat gets better only by forcing his body through the rigors of sport-specific training and any appropriate and beneficial cross-training. This will guarantee discomfort both immediate and delayed. Sometimes an athlete will be in all-over pain, and it can last for quite a while. While many athletes need to have this feeling to be sure they are training at a level that will produce results, the discomfort may cause others to drop down in intensity and stay within their relative "comfort zones." Experience in a particular sport will usually help the athlete learn to deal with this reaction in an adaptive and positive way. An athlete *should* move in and out of the comfort zone; this is sound physiological practice and creates the adaptability necessary for continual improvement.

The mental and emotional aspects of this reaction to training is centered around the perception of the progression from discomfort into pain, and this is something that must be successfully dealt with if the athlete is to progress. Swimming fast manifests the feeling of being "out of air" more than on land since humans evolved as land-based beings, and any resistance to movement is felt and perceived to be at least four times as great in the water as on land. But struggling to breathe anywhere is daunting.

Pain, on the other hand, is where good medical and physiologic sense take over and respect what the mind and body are signaling. Pain is Nature's way of protecting the body from imminent damage or greater injury later on. There is nothing wrong with backing down from pain, especially if it becomes localized, intense, and unremitting. Training past this kind of sensation can be strongly negative and derail the training schedule. If the pain is skeletal-muscular, conditioning and, or rehabilitation may bring the athlete back. If pain is repeatedly sensed to come from an internal source, medical attention is absolutely required. If the perception of pain in an otherwise sound athlete keeps interfering with performance, then the mental or emotional aspect must be addressed, and a cause sought out and corrected. Often it takes a sports psychologist or other expert to get to the root problems and place things in proper perspective.

As it is with just about anyone who has lots to do and much to share, I have been sick, and I have been well… I like well better.

CHAPTER 3

CAN YOU COOK TO SAVE YOUR LIFE?

OVERVIEW

We've all heard this many times: people either eat to live or live to eat. From the way the present-day "plump" US population is presenting itself, the latter seems to have more weight (pun intended). But there is another very important aspect to cuisine and how we fuel ourselves day-to-day, and that comes in the form of how we actually have our meals prepared.

More and more studies are showing the importance of **how** food is cooked as it relates to whether it is harmless, prevents or causes disease. The American people, for the most part, have always enjoyed their meals, and our society has traditionally been more centered around how food preparation affects tastes and textures than its concerns about totally healthy eating. A prime ready example is fish. We know that those who primarily eat ocean fish have fewer heart attacks, but if one eats only **fried** fish, risk of heart disease increases. Depending upon the cooking method, and the ingredients added, the same food can either accelerate obesity, inflame internal tissues, or aid in weight loss. And much less is understood about how most food is prepared and how **that** can convert foods into deadly **toxins.**

A large study published in 2002 in the *Proceedings of the National Academy of Sciences* produced a dramatic finding that cooking food, especially animal protein, at *very high temperatures with minimal moisture* **increased** the rate at which the aging process progressed. The study emphasized the fact that **high-temperature-cooked foods** resulted in **increased generalized inflammation throughout the body** and **accelerated glycation (sugar-combined denaturing of functional proteins).** And several more studies have concluded the same difficulties where it has been shown that *breast* and *prostate cancers* are sharply **increased** in those who regularly eat strongly-cooked meats like steak and hamburgers. The emphasis in this research article is to enlighten the reader as to how and why to choose safely cooked foods and methods to protect the body against the lethal impact of eating what we now know can be dangerous to our overall health.

When any food is heated to high temperature **(over 300 degrees)** chemical changes occur that inflict damage to human cells after that heated food is eaten. Whether fat, carbohydrate, or protein, when exposed to high temperatures, toxic compounds form that you really don't want in your body. The type of food most indicted in this "heated" revelation is meat.

As one of the top three cancers (and growing) in men, researchers have been seeking cause and effect for prostate cancer for years. Diet has proven contributory. Statistical analysis shows that those who eat **1.5 servings**, on average, of pan-fried red meat per week **increased** their risk of **advanced prostate cancer** by **30%**. Those who consumed **more than 2.5 servings** showed **increased incidence** by **40%**. This is seen as a cumulative effect over many years, and since many aging men consume well-cooked red meat almost daily, no wonder prostate cancer has risen to epidemic proportions. But now many have become aware of their risky eating habits and, rather than totally give up their favorite foods, have started taking what they hope are neutralizing supplements to hold in check this advancing incidence of prostate tumors.

THE BODY'S RESPONSES TO HIGHER-AND LOWER-TEMPERATURE COOKED FOODS

There was a breakthrough study in 2002 that brought to light where diabetics who consumed a **low-temperature cooked diet lost weight** compared to a group that consumed the same number of total calories through the same carbohydrates, fats, and proteins that were cooked at **higher temperatures.**

Not only the loss in weight but a *reduction in blood glucose* with **reduced cooking heat** were highlighted in the study. This six-week study also showed that eating the same food cooked at lower temperatures **reduced glycated** Low-Density Lipoproteins (LDL) **by 33%** whereas diabetics consuming the same higher-temperature-prepared food **increased glycated LD by 32%.**

Moving forward to 2012 with a team of researchers at Mount Sinai School of Medicine (NYC), a compound, **methyl-glyoxal**, was shown to play a major role in the development of abdominal obesity and its related diseases. Experimenting with pre-clinical specimens (mice and rats), the scientists saw the development of significant abdominal weight gain, early insulin resistance, immune changes consistent with inflammation/oxidation and type II diabetes. *Methyl-glyoxal* is one type of dangerous chemical species to the physiology called **A**dvanced **G**lycation **E**nd Products **(AGEs)** which are produced to excess with high temperatures and *dry heat.*

As mentioned, **glycation is a deadly mechanism of aging that destroys functioning proteins** in the body and **induces chronic inflammation** that can promote weight gain. Nutrients like *carnosine*, *Benfotiamine*, and *pyridoxal-5-phosphate* are potent anti-glycation agents and are now being included in various advanced vitamin/mineral formations that expound an additional anti-inflammatory activity.

In the Mount Sinai study, two groups of mice over a four-generation time period were fed equivalent amounts of similar food, the only difference being the forced ingestion of *methyl-glyoxal* for one group and the total exclusion of this *glycation end product* in the other. The generations of AGE-fed mice all developed early insulin resistance and increased body fat, whereas the control group had neither of these conditions. Reinforcement of this dramatic biochemical demonstration has brought to the fore the importance of how dangerous *glycation-inducing compounds* can be. Further study has revealed this same pattern of disturbed metabolism is reproducible in humans. What was also discerned from this study was that the induced abdominal fat produced ***pro-inflammatory cytokines***... a *major causes of disease and weight gain in humans.*

The research team that conducted this study recommends that clinical guidelines be revised to eliminate foods cooked using dry heat and replace them with methods that use lower heat and, or lots of moisture (water) as in stewing, poaching, stir-frying, utilizing a slow-cooker, or steaming. Examples given were for consuming stewed beef, chicken, and fish instead of grilled meats.

ADVANCED GLYCATION END PRODUCTS (AGES) AND FOOD PREPARATION

AGEs are also called *glycotoxins*. Overwhelmingly found in foods that are overheated or cooked at very high dry temperatures, their production predominates in the various dishes that are prepared by frying, barbecuing, broiling or cooking in the microwave. While the worst culprits are animal products since they contain a higher amount of "bad" fats that speed up the formation of *glycotoxins*, any food exposed to extreme high heat can scorch the natural sugars present and create this dangerous chemical. This is also true of many pre-packed foods that have been preserved, pasteurized, homogenized, or refined, such as white flour, cake mixes, canned milk, dried milk, dried eggs, dairy products including pasteurized milk and canned or frozen precooked meals. It should become obvious that we cannot totally avoid *glycotoxins* in our diets, but we can reduced exposure by changing at least some of our food preparation as mentioned above. Not only is the heat reduced with these methods, but moisture is introduced in the cooking process. The more moisture allowed to mingle in the process the greater the delay in the reactions that lead to *glycotoxins*. Marinating foods in olive oil, cider vinegar, garlic, mustard, lemon juice, and dry wines can also help in reducing glycotoxin content. And finally, the researchers have been convinced that even small changes in the general diet can remove dangerous amounts of this damaging agent by adding more fresh fruits and raw and steamed vegetables to almost every meal.

EXTINGUISHING INFLAMMATORY FIRES WITHIN

Unfortunately, *as humans age*, there is a systemic *increase in inflammatory cytokines* (destructive cell-signaling chemicals) that contribute to **virtually every degenerative disease.** While these *inflammatory cytokines* can cause *agonizing pain* as in arthritis, they also *disrupt* the *linings* of our *arteries, mutate DNA*, and *degrade brain cells.* **Chronic inflammation is directly involved in diseases as diverse as cancer, atherosclerosis, diabetes, aortic valve stenosis, congestive heart failure, Alzheimer's disease,** and **kidney failure.**

In our aging population, the "silent signs" of increasing inflammation begin to show as elevated blood levels of **C-R**eactive **P**rotein **(CRP).** This is a marker for generalized inflammation due to excess circulating levels of one or more of the ***pro-inflammatory cytokines*** occurring somewhere, anywhere, everywhere in the body. There is also a refined specific CRP test for cardiac inflammation.

For those desirous of either preventing or reducing inflammation or eliminating what has already taken hold in the body, there are now several active anti-inflammatory substances that specifically target the inflammatory response. Several of my research articles on PQQ, Rhodiola, Ribose, the healing enzyme, Bromelain, and *Mitochondria* Energy Boosters have detailed their anti-inflammatory and energizing activity within the human physiology. And now an increasing body of evidence is revealing that the simple physical activity of **avoiding foods cooked at very high dry-heat temperatures** can also reduce the production of these troublesome inflammatory cytokines.

HOW GLYCATION "COOKS" US TO DEATH

The glycation process that turns a chicken brown in the oven closely resembles what happens to the proteins in our body as we age. When body proteins react with sugars, they turn brown and fluorescent, lose elasticity and cross-link to form insoluble masses that generate free radicals. The resulting *glycotoxins* or **A**dvanced **G**lycation **E**nd products (AGEs) accumulate in our collagen and skin, corneas, brain and nervous system, arteries, and vital organs as we age. Unfortunately, *glycotoxins* are highly resistant to the normal processes of protein turnover and renewal that maintain the healthy tone of youthful body tissues and organs.

How does the body try and cope with these chronic assaults on proteins? Long-lived cells such as neurons and muscle tissue cells build to contain high levels of a salvage dipeptide called *carnosine* that is composed of *histidine* and *beta-alanine*. Unlike ordinary antioxidants, carnosine blocks numerous pathways involved in the actual *glycation* process.

As mentioned above and simply put for clarification, *glycation* is the binding of a sugar (*glucose*) molecule to a protein molecule resulting in the production of a damaged protein. Many age-related diseases such as arterial stiffening, cataracts, and neurological impairment are at least partially attributable to *glycation*. Once formed, these glycation end products are barely functional. As these degraded proteins accumulate, they cause cells to emit signals that induce the production of other damaging inflammatory cytokines. And we know that virtually all diseases are rooted in inflammation whether it be chronic, sub-acute or recurrently acute. The simple ingestion of **fish oil** can suppress inflammatory cytokine production as can *curcumin, Boswellia, DHEA,* and *vitamin K.* Taking steps to *shed abdominal fat* and *reduce blood glucose* is also of enormous benefit in lowering production of *pro-inflammatory cytokines* in the body.

What one eats plays a major role in the chronic inflammatory process. Consuming low-glycemic foods reduces the insulin surge that also contributes to the chronic inflammatory process.

Several studies have shown that consuming foods high in *glycotoxins* can be responsible for the induction of a low-grade, but chronic state in inflammation. The *glycotoxins* produced in food cooked at high temperatures also promote the formation of *glycotoxins* in our functioning tissues. Thus, when we eat foods altered by high temperature cooking, they inflict inflammatory damage to many living proteins in our body.

PROTECTING YOUR GENES AGAINST OVERCOOKED FOODS

Studies going back to the 1990's have shown that heavily-cooked foods have the potential to inflict massive damage to the very essence of living cells, the genes. A group at the University of Minnesota reported in 1998 that women who repeatedly ate overcooked hamburgers had a **50% greater risk of breast cancer** than women who ate rare or medium-cooked burgers. The famous Iowa Women's Health Study found that women who *consistently* ate well-done steak, hamburgers, and bacon had a **4.62-fold increased risk of breast cancer.**

Cooking foods at high temperature causes the formation of gene-mutating **heterocyclic amines,** which is the root problem for the danger from deep-fried foods. Heterocyclic amines have pervasively been linked to cancers of most of the vital organs and tissue groups such as prostate, breast, colorectal, esophageal, lung, liver and others. While health-conscious people try to avoid foods that are known carcinogens, even grilled salmon contains a potent dose of gene-mutating heterocyclic amines.

Even if one works diligently to reduce overt exposure to cancer-causing heterocyclic amines, it may be impossible to totally keep these dangerous compounds from forming within the body. Enzymatic activities that naturally occur in the liver can inadvertently manufacture heterocyclic amines from otherwise harmless organic compounds.

The first lines of defense against carcinogens consumed in the diet are agents that prevent gene mutations. Many anti-mutagenic agents have been identified in fruits and vegetables, the most potent being **indole-3-carbinol** and *chlorophyllin.*

An eye-opening study presented in the journal *Mutation Research,* in the late 1980's showed that the plant extract *chlorophyllin* was the most effective anti-mutagenic discovered up to that time. It suppressed the mutagenicity of substantiated carcinogens such as fried pork, diesel emissions, and coal dust by more than 90%. No other supplement came close to *chlorophyllin's* ability to inhibit deadly gene mutations. It acts at the cellular level to "trap" heterocyclic hydrocarbon carcinogens by reacting with their structural "backbone," making it impossible for them to form deadly compounds within vital cellular DNA.

Additional protection against carcinogens is found in the activity of **I**ndole-3-Carbinol (I3C) which is found in anti-cancer vegetables such as cabbage, cauliflower, and broccoli. In pre-clinical trials, rodents given strong doses of known carcinogens had 96% fewer tumors when pre-treated with I3C, and the length of time between exposure to deadly chemicals and the development of tumors was extended by over 200%.

The main activity of I3C at the cellular level is to prevent DNA mutations. It has shown benefit in protecting breast tissue by 92%, white blood cells by 82%, liver cells by 69%, and colon tissue by 67%. Other studies have confirmed this strong benefit with 90% protective activity in the liver, lung and trachea and other tissues by 55%. Clinical trials have shown that, when eating strongly over-cooked food, a dose of 100mg chlorophyllin and, or 80-240mg of indole-3-carbinol and other cruciferous vegetable extracts have proven definitely protective.

SUMMARY

There is compelling evidence that eating too much over-cooked food causes a physical reaction that can increase inflammatory products mainly of which are called *cytokines*. And inflammation is directly associated with disease. The longer it exists, the greater the amount of disease it can create. Since many of our favorite fast ("junk") foods are cooked at very high temperatures, it makes good health sense to avoid the choice of eating the likes of French fries, hamburgers, hot dogs, potato chips, most fried foods and many cooked snacks and desserts whenever possible. These foods not only contain the potentially dangerous *glycotoxins*, but they also create other metabolic disorders that can induce degenerative diseases. Supplements such as carnosine along with Benfotiamine and *pyridoxal-5-phosphate* act to neutralize these dietary dangers by actually inhibiting the formation of the root cause: glycation reactions.

Avoiding foods cooked with mostly dry heat to high temperature not only reduces *pathological glycation processes*, but also prevents the formation of gene-mutating toxins that are known *carcinogens*. When food is chronically over-cooked without added moisture, toxins invariably form that can *mutate cell regulatory* genes. What results is *increased cancer risk to several organ tissues.* Research has shown this for several years, and it is now getting to the general population which is becoming more and more conscience of eating healthy from properly prepared food. Though occasional dalliances with high-temp foods should not bring about total metabolic destruction, if we see no change to safer eating over time, or one chooses not to consume neutralizing supplements with their meals, we will be literally seeing people playing with metabolic fire as they age and cook themselves to death.

CHAPTER 4

COACH NESSEL'S ENHANCED ACTIVITY SUPPLEMENTS

The following list presents the suggested supplement; its strength/dosage, where to purchase, and know the use as of this time. Everything listed is determined to be SAFE, EFFECTIVE, and LEGAL for all means and purposes regarding competition in United States Swimming, NCAA swimming, and YMCA swimming. At this time, my suggested dosages should be observed since no adverse side effects have been reported over the last several years. In some instances, at this time, we truly do not know the optimum amount of a beneficial effect that can be elicited. Continued testing and observation with my "lab rats" of various ages and abilities keep this most exciting topic at the forefront of my interest. I am personally included in my "lab rat" population and can definitely feel the difference.

Though I consider all the substances on this listing to be beneficial with many overlapping in effect to enhance positive outcomes, I fully recognize the effect on the all-important family budget. Therefore, I have listed the following in descending order of importance (greatest to least) as to my considered opinion for all-around enhanced well-being.

- **RIBOSE**; in my opinion, is the single most important substance ANYONE engaging in vigorous activity can take. It is a 5-carbon sugar (pentose) that is the limiting factor in the body's producing the energy molecule ATP. It is of specific benefit in protecting the body from depleting its deep energy reserves thus keeping the heart from dangerously-low amounts of ATP that could lead to heart failure under extreme circumstances and severe disablement and even death. Dosage is two scoops (comes in a container) per day, in the morning for those 15 and under (or under 150 pounds) or three scoops daily for those over 150 pounds. Nutrabio.com is the place to order it. Best pricing is when several containers (500 grams each) are purchased together.
- **PQQ** (Pyroloquiniline Quinone); this is a relatively new substance discovered in Japan that has proven to be the ONLY substance known to actually produce *mitochondria*, the energy segments of each cell. When *mitochondria* die, the cell dies. When enough cells die, the body sustains serious energy loss and even debilitation. It has been classified as the first new vitamin in 55 years and is listed as a B-vitamin. Original discoveries of PQQ's worth came from its remarkable ability to stop early to moderate Alzheimer's Disease in its tracts and even reverse early stages of this insidious and terrible disease. Research is actively progressing as to

how much *mitochondria* can actually be "stuffed" into important muscle groups, and PQQ is the main thrust of this work. Dosage is one 10mg capsule twice daily with meals. Vitacost.com provides the best pricing.

- **Mitochondrial Energy Booster**; this supplement has all three of the necessary ingredients that act to protect the actual *mitochondria* from self-destruction as they produce the thermal activity that affords us the vital energy to move; the ingredients are co-enzyme Q10, alpha lipoic acid, and l-carnitine; these ingredients can be purchased separately, but this particular combination product obviates the need for that. I get mine from Vitacost.com and take two capsules twice daily with breakfast and dinner.

- **Rhodiola Rosea:** this product came to the attention of American physiologists only relatively recently since The Soviet Union, during the Cold War era, kept this under wraps. They gave it to their military, Olympic athletes, and astronauts. While the best of our best space explorers could only stay in space for relatively short periods, the Russian astronaut crews could withstand the rigors of gravity-free much longer and in better condition over the long hall. The product works to enhance the immune system and provide the body with deep energy reserves from which the vigorous athlete can draw to sustain efforts and repeated demanding training sessions and multiple-day competitions.

- **Resveratrol:** this is one of the potent anti-inflammatory substances we can add to our diets; it enhances our immune system, allows for increased recovery from intense training and competitions and also lessens the tendency of the platelets in our blood to stick together; this allows for more blood to flow more easily to the muscles needed to produce quality movement. I get mine from Vitacost.com in a product called LONGEVATROL in 200 mg capsules; one twice daily with food. RESVERATROL is also found in purple grape juice. The Welches company has combined purple grape juice and cherry juice (which adds more anti-inflammatory activity) into a great tasting healthy juice mix that I and my swimmers consume before practice and at meets.

- **Omega-3:** I get the very important antioxidant and anti-inflammatory from FISH OIL capsules containing 300mg OMEGA-3 each; this is another antioxidant/anti-inflammatory that protects the body from free-radical damage that ensues from intense training. I take one capsule twice daily. It also allows for better blood flow throughout the body and especially to the muscles when needed for vigorous exercise.

- **Green Coffee Bean Extract:** the active ingredient here is CHLOROGENIC ACID that also enhances the immune system, has anti-inflammatory activity, controls blood sugar and cholesterol amounts and acts to enhance the total body system to withstand the rigors of vigorous exercise.

- **HA JOINT FORMULA:** this is a specific product that helps coat the joints of the body and protect and heal them from trauma and constant over-use. The body normally makes this substance (*Hyaluronic Acid*) but as we age, it cannot produce enough to keep up with intense demands placed upon body parts day after day. It has proven effective even in younger athletes in need of repair from trauma. I get my supply from Purity Products.com and take three capsules at one time in the morning to protect me throughout the day.

- My "famous" **FLORIDA COCKTAIL:** this I take almost every day in some form; by this I mean that the three main ingredients (watermelon, fresh pineapple, and fresh cherries) are consumed by me almost daily. I mixed these fruits in a blender, add lime juice to taste, pit the cherries, and enjoy all the benefits of what I feel are the very best fruits for energy, recovery, and to build enhanced energy reserves. Tropical fruits, of which pineapples have the most, contain a healing enzyme called BROMELAIN. This absolutely helps the body heal and recover from intense training, trauma, and demanding competitions. It only attacks and remove dead or damaged tissue and also settles the stomach to help digest food.

- Watermelon is the absolute choice for the perfect food to take to help the body throughout intense activity. It contains three natural sugars, three physiologic stimulants, 93% to 95% water and L-citrulline, an amino acid that can hasten the removal of lactic acid from muscle tissue for faster recovery. Taking this before and after vigorous activity is the what I recommend.

- For added energy and sustained sustenance I take either *Accelerade* powder or *Endurox* powder and mix with water just before I leave for training sessions. I also have a bottle mixed for swim meets. This is well-tested and has shown absolute positive results with extended time in the water or training other sports. It is made by Pacific Health Labs and can be purchased from their website or at GNC or the Vitamin Shoppe.

- For those wanting to increase muscular mass and increase instant and extended muscular power, CREATINE powder is the way to go. It is safe, effective, and legal in all sports, but the user MUST keep well hydrated to prevent muscular cramping. The dose is 5 grams per day.

- Purple grape juice and cherry juice combination from Welch's. This provides antioxidant and anti-inflammatory activity all over the body from its resveratrol activity and the benefit of the healthiest berry in our diet: cherries.

Always keep well hydrated.. "drink before you are thirsty and after you're not." Once you sense thirst, you made a physiologic mistake that an athlete should never make.

The overall take-home points from this listing is to keep the body energized and well-supplied with substances that reduce both inflammation and the damaging oxidation that results from physiologic reactions elicited during vigorous training. The body needs to undergo appropriate physiologic stress to improve, yet we need to remove the inevitable oxidative damage that ensues. Since every disease in the human body is most probably caused by the inflammation process... the obvious reason for all the anti-inflammatories and anti-oxidants.

RECIPES

This very tasty drink is a formula concocted of many things that I feel are not only healthy, but will aid in the recovery of the muscles and connective tissue after they have been put to the test either from vigorous training or intense competition... the closer to the finish of the physical exertion, the better for recovery...

All items are placed in a large blender to make approximately 5-6 servings; ideally, the athlete should take at least two servings (12 oz. each)15-30 minutes apart and as close to the end of training or racing as possible...

- At least 12 oz. of sweetened frozen strawberries in syrup.
- At least 12 oz. RED grape juice or 30 RED grapes.
- Two large fresh bananas.
- Six ounces of EGG BEATERS.
- 12 oz. of SILK vanilla low-fat soy milk
- 8 oz. of flavored-to-taste yogurt with active cultures.
- 6 ice cubes to cool and dilute the mixture.

Blend thoroughly for at least 30 seconds or until all the ice has been mixed. Repeat blending if the mix stays for any length of time...

The ingredients in this delicious drink provide natural energy boosters, muscle-friendly casein and soy protein, natural anti-oxidants (including resveratrol from red grapes), and many vitamins and minerals necessary to catalyze energy reactions that all aid in repair and recovery.

If taken on a regular basis, recovery for the next training session or day of competition will be enhanced with corresponding increases in the ability to put forth greater effort toward fast swimming.

The use of either pure whey protein or a product like *Endurox* as an added ingredient is to ensure that "hungry" muscles are fed before vigorous exercise; of course this type of breakfast is also quite suitable for recovery from vigorous exercise. In addition, I list Canadian bacon and individual side servings of Egg Beaters to balance out the meal with their quality protein offerings. These work with the various fruit toppings to give the mixed flavors we have all come to enjoy, but with the additional advantage of not spiking blood sugar too quickly. Since variety is the spice of life, the more choices of fruit toppings, the better to keep interest high and the taste flavorful in this type of meal.

"MUSCLE TOAST" INGREDIENTS LIST

- 2 scoops either pure whey protein powder or vanilla *Endurox*
- 1/2 teaspoonful cinnamon spice
- 4-egg equivalent of Egg Beaters
- 1 cup fat-free (skim) milk
- 4 slices whole-wheat bread

FRUIT TOPPING

- 1 ripe banana, mashed
- 1 tablespoonful strawberry, blueberry, apricot, or cherry preserves
- 1 tablespoonful water
- 1 tablespoonful fruit-flavored syrup or confectionary sugar to taste

SLICED CANADIAN BACON & EGG BEATERS

In a large bowl, mix the protein powder or vanilla *Endurox*, cinnamon, egg beaters, and milk. Whisk until blended smoothly. Next, soak each slice of bread in the mixture for at least 30 seconds. Coat a non-stick pan with no-calorie cooking spray; cook each slice (both sides) on medium-high heat until bread is slightly firm.

As the toast cooks, mash the banana and mix it with the choice of fruit preserves and water. Top the toast with the fruit mixture while still in the heating pan. A little extra fruit-flavored syrup or confectionary sugar can be added to taste; makes two servings. While the toast is cooking also heat up enough egg-beaters to serve two to three eggs equivalent per person. Finally, heat two slices of Canadian bacon per person that balances the meal by adding the meat protein with lots of minerals but with very little fat.

Strong muscle benefits are derived from this meal by way of dairy protein, egg protein, meat protein and pure whey protein... all muscle friendly and which provide needed refueling that lasts over many hours.

QUICK NUTRITION FACTS FOR ATHLETES

Most swimmers, and most people for that matter have no idea how many calories they can and should eat in a day.

DAILY CALORIC ESTIMATE

- Figure out your **R**esting **M**etabolic **R**ate (RMR) by multiplying your body weight by 10... this is the number of calories you need to stay alive.

- Figure out how many calories you need to get through the day apart from when you are swimming and otherwise training. If you are pretty sedentary (desk-bound),

- Take 30% of your RMR. If you are moderately active (on your feet a lot, say as a teacher or walking mailperson) during the day, take 50% of the RMR. And if you are quite active (construction worker, military, athlete-in-training), take 70% of your RMR.

- Finally, figure out how many calories you burn working out: a 150-lb man uses 10.6 calories per minute swimming fast freestyle with fairly efficient technique; a 170-lb man burns 12 calories per minute, while a 190-lb man consumes about 14 calories/min. Men usually have more lean body weight (muscle mass) than women consequently burn more calories per unit time doing ANYTHING.

- *Working example: a 190-lb man swimming mixed strokes with a push to a fast pace in a relatively quick interval for an average of 90 minutes (swimming and recovery time) will consume about 1100 calories during the practice session.*

- Of course, calorie-burning will continue to be above normal for at least two extra hours after practice, since the **B**asic **M**etabolic Rate (BMR) has been raised by the training effect. This aids in total calorie consumption for the whole day and also provides a heads-up as to when to re-fuel (eat) and not have all the calories add to body weight.

- Add up each answer to get your day's total caloric need. Example: for a 190-lb Man who trains for a 90-minute session and is moderately active throughout the rest of the day, he would be able to consume over 3900 calories without gaining any weight. Keep in mind that these calories should be easily handled by the body... mostly complex carbohydrates (65%+), some protein (20%+) and only a maximum of 15% fat, preferably mono-saturated (e.g. olive oil). This scenario is strongly influenced by the athlete's individual metabolism, his general health, and his age and degree of full-body muscularity. As people age, physical activity throughout the day tends to lessen, the metabolic rates are not elevated as easily nor as high in response to vigorous exercise, and most will tend to put on weight. What has come to light during the aging process that greatly helps keep body fat lower, is the fact of adding lean muscle. The more muscle, the more calories burned throughout the day, plain and simple.

QUALITY CALORIES

It is not just a matter of getting several thousand calories down the hatch; rather, they need to be quality calories that deliver the kind of fuel an athlete needs, when he needs it. As stated above, about 2/3 of the caloric intake should be composed of quality carbs; swimmers tremendous carb cravings which should be satisfied to ensure adequate energy intake. Examples would include *whole grain cereals, whole wheat breads and bagels, quality energy bars* (*Promax*), fruits, juices, and mixed pastas.

A small bag of potato chips delivers nearly the same number of carbs as a slice of whole-wheat bread, but with 10 times the fat. In addition, the bread has more fiber and protein and a little iron and calcium to boot. That's the deal with most healthy foods... you get something extra with your energy... nutrients. Not just empty calories!

MAKING THE RIGHT CHOICES

To calculate how many quality carbs you need as an athlete, multiply your body weight by three (3). This gives you a number you can use when reading food labels. But you also need to learn to eat with your eyes... always be open to trying something new; do not settle for the usual fast (and often tasty) food. If the taste or texture seems to reek of fat, you are making a poor choice. Once in a while is okay, but eating this on a regular basis is, again, making a poor choice in quality fuel selection.

We see a lot of young athletes not only make poor food choices, they mostly eat a very small variety of food. Blame it on convenience, on laziness, or just ignorance. Ironically, even those wanting to eat healthy many times have narrow diets as well. These people become fat-phobic and reliant on food supplements at the expense of a rich, varied selection of nutrient-dense foods. Athletes need to eat more than the average person; it would behoove them to make quality choices in selecting a lot of different foods.

There is a significant segment of student/swimmers that tend to under-eat due to foolish reasons like claiming to not have enough time or simply wanting to look trim and strong in a bathing suit. We all know this is counter-productive. Not eating when energy demands are strong only make for poor training and competition experiences and puts the athlete at risk for illness and injury. But with a little imagination, proper nutrition can be instituted throughout the day: a midmorning snack when a break in class allows; a pre-practice snack can make all the difference in the workout that follows. Having high-quality appropriate carbs to re-fuel after practice is also very important to refuel the muscles and the brain. The body is extremely receptive during this time to replenish the carbs burned during practice and for some time after. Re-fueling within an hour if possible allows for the greatest amount of glycogen replenishment in both muscle and liver. Since the brain uses only *glucose* to fuel its demanding needs, ingesting various sources of this is the smart thing to do especially if studying demands must follow training demands.

Plan to eat six to eight small, fast meals, rather than one or two huge meals per day. I call this "grazing?" It keeps the body fueled and energized appropriately throughout the day. Each mini-meal should have the proper balance of carbs, protein, and fats along with adequate hydration. If protein is eaten in to a greater extent in one small meal, then other food stuffs must be consumed in correct proportion at other meals to keep the day's food intake in balance. One final thought here: the newer formulated energy bars that contain balanced nutrition are almost always in order, and they taste pretty good, too. They should be kept in swim bags, lockers, cars, wherever you go.

EXAMPLE DAILY MEAL (NUTRITIONAL ANALYSIS FOR 3500 HEALTHY CALORIES)

BREAKFAST: 1 /2 cups orange juice; 1 cup strawberries, 1 '/2 cups fiber cereal or oatmeal; 12 to 16 oz. 1% or skim milk, 1 roll, 1 teaspoonful butter substitute (e.g. *Smart Balance Light*), 1 tablespoonful strawberry jam.

651 calories (19% of daily total), 127 grams carbs, 19 grams protein, 10 grams fat.

MID-MORNING SNACK: 1 plain bagel, 1 teaspoonful butter substitute, 1 tablespoonful jam, 16 oz. *PowerAde* or the like.

388 calories (11% of daily total), 80 grams carbs, 7 grams protein, 6 grams fat.

LUNCH: I lean roast beef sandwich, 1 cup cranberry/grape juice, 1 medium apple, 2/3 cup potato salad, 1 peach.

898 calories (25% of daily total), 144 grams carbs, 25 grams protein, 26 grams fat.

MID-AFTERNOON SNACK: 3 pretzels, 16 oz. *PowerAde* or the like, 1 cup grapes.

345 calories (10% of daily total), 80 grams carbs, 5 grams protein, 2 grams fat.

DINNER: 1 '/2 cups chicken chow mein, 1 cup of rice, 6 oz. green tea (calorie-free sweetener), I orange, **1** cup 1% or skim milk.

762 calories (21% of daily total), 90 grains carbs, 60 grams protein, 18 grams fat.

EVENING SNACK: 1 banana, 1 cup 1% or skim milk, 3 graham crackers, 16 oz. *PowerAde* or the like.

470 calories (13% of daily total), 98 grams carbs, 12 grams protein, 7 grams fat.

Grand Total: 3517 calories, 620 grams carbs (68% of caloric total), 129 grams protein (14.2% of caloric total), 70 grams fat (17.4% of caloric total).

The first order of business for someone who participates in continuous vigorous exercise is to keep the body's immune system intact. To strengthen the body's ability to ward off illness is a strong step toward proper training. To be sick is to be unable to train up to one's potential.

My choice of vitamin/mineral supplement is ***MASTER GREEN MULTI***. Four capsules a day (two twice daily with food) supplies not only the correct selection and amount of vitamins and minerals but many beneficial phytochemicals. These are substances that come from a natural source (e.g. plants) which act to prevent oxidative damage to various organs and tissues. Phytochemicals help the body repair itself more quickly than if none had been ingested… something of importance if the athlete is to train vigorously on a regular basis. This product can be obtained by either calling the company, Great American Products, from Destin, Florida @1-800-466-8615 or online @ www.greatamericanproducts.com.

My next recommendation ensures intake of worthy ergogenic (work-enhancing) substances. The product called ***ATP EVOLUTION*** (www.nutrabio.com) has what I feel are synergistic (greater than the sum of the total) components that work to greatly enhance muscle force.

The two main ingredients in this product are *RIBOSE,* a natural 5-carbon sugar, and *CREATINE*, an energy substance composed of amino acids, which is naturally found in and around muscle tissue. RIBOSE is a vital component of the energy molecule ATP. It is not found in its 5-carbon state in the body but has to be biochemically built from other sugars. This takes time, and when instant energy is demanded, there is no time for biochemical delay. Having a ready supply in reserve of this limiting vital element can make a noticeable difference in many sprint athletes. It has also been shown that having large doses of ribose can actually protect the heart from beating to exhaustion.

Much has been written about CREATINE in the past few years. It has been put to the test at the highest athletic levels since 1992 and proven itself to be of great benefit to those who need POWER to succeed in their sport. CREATINE acts as a first-line (immediate) supplier of **C**reatinine **P**hosphate **(CP).** CP, in turn, can immediately supply more ATP to the muscles upon demand. The body is able, on average, to deliver about a 10 second supply of ATP for immediate sprint usage. Ingestion of CREATINE can usually double this. Any reports of dangerous side effects have mostly been overstated. Improper and inappropriate usage is usually the cause of adverse results that include possible muscle cramping if dehydration is present. One MUST prevent dehydration to allow the body to utilize CREATINE correctly.

Two relatively new products in the sports nutrition market that have proven themselves efficacious to many different types of athletes come from Pacific Health Labs in New Jersey. What makes their patented nutritional formulas work is the fact that it has been shown that ingesting an energy source with a 4:1 ratio of carbohydrates-to-protein allows for a greater absorption of muscle-friendly substances for both energy-supply and recovery. *ACCELERADE* is the pre-activity supplement that provides the correct energy source to the musculature, while *ENDUROX* R-4 is the all-important recovery formula… This has the *ACCELERADE* ingredients plus tissue-sparing antioxidants that prevent or heal muscle damage from intense training. Both are in powder form to be *MIXED WITH WATER ONLY… NO CARBOHYDRATE-CONTAINING LIQUIDS (will throw the ratio's off).*

Another energy alternative is found in ***PROMAX BARS.*** Each bar has a good amount of muscle-friendly ***WHEY protein (20 grams),*** along with the proper carbohydrates for athletic energy demands. All the flavors are delicious. ***PROMAX*** can be used as acceptable energy snacks throughout the day if under physical stress.

If one can tolerate the fructose content, I strongly recommend the ingestion of ***RED GRAPE JUICE*** either before a workout or race or during same. *This has the phytochemical RESVERATROL which not only acts as a powerful anti-oxidant, but also inhibits the platelets in the blood from sticking. This allows for better blood flow to exercising muscles, lungs, heart, and kidneys.* Better blood flow means better ability of the body to handle the physical stresses of vigorous training. I bring this mix to the pool when training: *half GRAPE JUICE, half either Gatorade or PowerAde. NEVER COME TO THE POOL WITHOUT A HYDRATING DRINK OF SOME KIND. WATER IS BETTER THAN NOTHING, BUT NOT MUCH. IF THE WORKOUT IS LONGER THAN 60 MINUTES, AN ELECTROLYTE SOLUTION IS REQUIRED FOR PROPER HYDRATION.*

As far as *fruits* are concerned, the magnificent *BANANA is one of the best choices. It provides natural sugars, natural stimulants, a great source for potassium and 80% to 90%*

water. When in season, WATERMELON is the best source for potassium, has natural sugars and stimulants and is up to 96% water.

STIMULENTS can come from either natural sources as in the BANANA and watermelon or from a produced source. The main point here is to do no harm, to keep it legal, and to use something that works. We all know of caffeine. In fact, it is the most used drug in the world. So much so that the international swimming governing body (FINA) has allowed its use but within finite measurable limits. One of the "drugs" that are tested for at international competitions is caffeine. This can actually make an effort in the water seem less taxing. It is both a psychic stimulant and a physiologic stimulant. It makes the muscles fire more intensely during "power swimming." It also utilizes free fatty acids as energy sources to spare glycogen (carbohydrates) for use to sprint home a mid-distance or distance race. There are side effects that can be disturbing to some athletes: shaking, increase in nervousness, and an increased desire to urinate causing a mild dehydrating effect… All not the best effects for a competitor. But this mostly goes away in time and with continued regular use. Early on there was concern that the possible dehydrating effect of caffeine would negatively affect the musculature with cramping and possible muscle tares if consumed with creatine but over the years there has not been seen this negative interaction to any great extent as was originally feared. Caffeine, it turns out, is not the all-powerful dehydrating chemical in actuality as originally thought… A case of text-book information not being realized under the conditions of actual physical duress.

A "stimulating" drug that is allowed by some swimming governing bodies and not others is the oral nasal decongestant, *SUDAFED, or its generic equivalent, pseudoephedrine.* It is much safer than ephedrine all around, but it can stimulate the heart to beat faster and stronger and open up the nasal passages for better breathing, especially if one is suffering from allergies or a cold. It is allowed by high school, YMCA, and NCAA swimming. For all intents and purposes it is NOT allowed in United States Swimming since only very small amounts are permitted to be found in the urine.

What has recently been found in psychological studies with competitive athletes is that either the **smell of PEPPERMINT or the taste of it will stimulate the brain to increase its ability to concentrate and focus on the task at hand.** We can see the benefit this implies with pre-race concentration and visualization.

With all this exercise and training that the body has to go through, it would be helpful to find substances that help it recover. There is an *enzyme* found in tropical fruits, mostly in pineapples, called *BROMELAIN. It aids digestion that would help calm "nervous" stomachs and attacks only damaged or dead tissue. Bromelain also helps to reduce inflammation. It is a definite help in allowing the body to recover after a demanding workout. BROMELAIN can also be found in capsule form in shops that sell health food items. Along with bromelain, fish oil containing sufficient amounts of omega-3 oils (EPA and DHA) can act as an antioxidant and anti-inflammatory.*

GLUCOSAMINE (*a lubricating substance) either with or without CHONDROITIN (an enzyme) is a natural substance found in the joints of the body. As one ages or if the joints are damaged due to trauma or overtraining, GLUCOSAMINE and CHONDROITIN can re-*

supply what is needed to "bathe" the area in nature's lubricant to allow for easier movement through the complete range of motion of the affected joint and reduce inflammation and pain.

The newest product to show physiologic promise is MITOCHONDRIAL ENERGY BOOSTER. It is composed of co-enzyme Q-10, alpha lipoic acid, and actyl L-carnitine. This protects the mitochondria (the only segments of a cell that can produce energy in the form of ATP) throughout the body and allows it to rise to a higher level of condition and energy production more quickly.

The last item for this listing is the *antacid, TUMS.* Though not a nutritional supplement, it comes under this category only because more and more testing has shown that to prevent *lactic acid* from building up the use of a body-friendly antacid can provide for greater effort in a vigorous athletic situation. There are substances that work better, but the side effects (gastrointestinal distress) are not worth the potential benefit. There is a specific dosing regimen which is still being refined (depending upon body weight and size) than can actually delay the buildup of lactic acid until later in the race. Anywhere from three (3) to Five (5) tablets are chewed at a time every five (5) minutes starting from 20 minutes away from the race right up until almost time to go to the blocks. Water or the like is drunk each time to wash down the chewed tablets and help in the antacid's absorption. It is NOT recommended that this regimen be repeated back-to-back for races. But it CAN be used for a specific race and for prelims and finals of same.

There are many products touted to help the athlete achieve every goal sought. Most fall short of what is promised. What I have suggested above is a strong list of products that have proven themselves worthy with hundreds of athletes over many years. Some of the newer products have produced positive effects immediately. All are safe, effective, and legal according to the various governing bodies of the swimming world.

CHAPTER 5

THE MANY BENEFITS OF RESISTANCE TRAINING

INTRODUCTION

It is common knowledge that regular participation in vigorous physical activity, especially of an aerobic nature (e.g. swimming, running, biking) will most likely contribute to a decrease in the risk, or at least prevent the progression, of several chronic negative conditions (high blood pressure, stroke, coronary heart disease, *osteoporosis*, diabetes, obesity) that produce the greatest amount of morbidity in present-day America. In fact the **A**merican **H**eart **A**ssociation (AHA) has identified physical inactivity as a prime risk factor, along with high cholesterol, cigarette smoking and uncontrolled hypertension (high blood pressure), contributing to the number one health problem in the USA today: **C**oronary **H**eart **D**isease (CHD). As a positive alternative and intervention the **A**merican **C**ollege of **S**ports **M**edicine (ACSM) and the Surgeon General's Report on Physical Activity and Health have established a list of benefits due to aerobic exercise programs designed to positively affect health status; these are based on a preponderance of evidence on disease prevention.

Up until recently the effects of resistive exercise (strength training) on health status have been largely overlooked. Traditionally, strength training has been seen as a means of improving muscular strength and endurance (muscle mass) and power, but not as a means for improving general health. But there is increasing evidence that strength training plays a significant role in many health factors. The ACSM (1990, 1995), AHA (1995) and the Surgeon General's Report of Physical Activity and Health (1996) all have recognized strength training as an important component of health.

Improving muscular strength and power has been traditionally viewed as important for athletes, competitive weightlifters, and bodybuilders, but not for improving general health status. Much recent evidence indicates that this conception is no longer true.

Though every benefit listed in this chapter can pertain to most sports and athletic endeavors, no matter the age, understand that I related all the positives specifically to masters swimming since that is what I have dedicated my daily training to and from which I have reaped the most benefits. Since swimming is what I know best both from participation and instruction, it only seemed logical to bring it into the presentation.

IMPROVEMENTS IN STRENGTH AND FUNCTION

Aging is normally seen with an associative decrease in muscle mass and strength, which is linked to decreased mobility, decreased functionality and an increased risk of falling in older people. Falls, in and of themselves, have been identified as the single most frequent cause of injury related mortality in the elderly, and it has been statistically verified that 90% of all hip fractures in the elderly occur as a result of a fall. A logical approach to lessen this statistic would include exercises to strengthen all the muscles of the legs, the hips, and the torso. This would then provide the foundations for better body positioning and awareness throughout all kinds of movement. Taking this a step further (no pun intended), strengthening the upper body would also help protect the victim if a fall should happen by allowing better positioning of the body to handle a collision with either the ground or any object in the way.

Though utilizing a small statistical population, a most dramatic study was performed in San Francisco with elderly residents in old age homes, in the mid-1990's. Average age of the subjects was 87 years; both genders were studied. A 10-week program of a few simple but important resistance exercises allowed for some startling results. Granted the subjects came to the study relatively inactive and subject to the advanced aging process concurrent with their years. But an average increase in general muscle strength of 113%, gait velocity (12%), stair climbing power (28%) and a specific quadriceps (front leg muscles) strength improvement of 174% all seem astounding. But they really shouldn't be. A lifelong involvement with resistance training has shown that increased strength can be achieved and maintained at a relatively high level into the sixth decade of life.

Isolating another area that has pronounced negative effects if kept in a weakened condition, low back pain and spinal disorders become the predominant reason for disability in the workforce. It is estimated that chronic low back pain accounts for nearly 80% of the annual cost of low back disorders even though this classification represents only 10% of all spinal disorders. The state of chronic poor lumbar strength has been associated with the development of chronic low back pain and dysfunction and contributes negatively to an already too sedentary population.

APPLICATION TO MASTERS SWIMMING

Applying this resistance training philosophy to Masters Swimmers of all ages can (and most often does) produce remarkable results in the water. Whether one uses latex tubing, free weights, universals (or other mechanical devices) or simple body-weight calisthenics, the ability to move water is directly related to the ability to generate POWER. The concept of strength forced to occur over a period of time (power) is the pivotal element that seems to produce the remarkable results we now see in all age groups, in the world of competitive swimming. An additional benefit of consistent weight training allows for increased endurance and articular (joint) strength which seem to translate a great deal into injury prevention, which at any age can spell the difference between a washout or a successful season.

A different concept altogether that has proven itself repeatedly to increase strength in the largest target set of muscles (the legs) has been the use of flexible swim fins. The forceful working of all the muscle groups of the lower extremities in a concerted continuous fashion has produced remarkable results leading to some very fast swimming. The Soviet Union of the late 1970's into the mid-1980's utilized this type of training aid to great advantage. Then more and more USA Swimming programs came to see the light as to the fins' potential and began utilizing the same concepts to increase leg power and flexibility.

BONE MINERAL DENSITY

Osteoporosis is a degenerative disease that is characterized by a decrease in **B**one **M**ineral **D**ensity (BMD). This loss produces a fragile framework of bone quite susceptible to fractures, which, in turn, can lead to decreased physical activity and possibly increased susceptibility to further health problems and mortality. Research has clearly indicated that bone formation can be stimulated by placing a strain on it as is seen during resistive and aerobic exercise. Although both forms of exercise can increase BMD, the increase is site-specific to the joints exercised. It is a common finding that, in people who weight-lift, for instance, their arms have greater BMD than those seen in runners. But the legs of both have about equal BMD. It is also seen in active and retired weightlifters a greater BMD in the hip, spine, tibia, and forearm than in those who never exercised as such. Several studies with varied populations of relatively advanced age have proven the obvious: stress the body with weight or resistance against the constant force of gravity, and you increase BMD in the site-specific areas stressed. Those who have lost BMD through disuse have been able to regain it at times to near baseline levels of their youth. Or they could maintain an increased BMD compared to those not engaging in resistive or other activities. Thus, a meta-analysis (an analysis of several studies on the subject) of the body's reaction to movement against force, be it mechanical or gravitational, indicates that resistance and aerobic exercise can both positively affect BMD but that this influence is absolutely site-specific to the mode of exercise.

APPLICATION TO MASTERS SWIMMING

Swimming occurs in a gravity-free environment, yet movement is guided by a medium (water) 1000 times as dense as air. It is the resistance to movement in this dense medium that contributes to the retention of BMD in those Masters Swimmers who train vigorously and consistently, regardless of age. This added to the very popular tendency to cross-train with weights, affords the aquatic athlete the resultant effect of maintaining solid bones throughout the body into much later in life.

Another theory put forth in this class of athlete brings out the rule of muscular stress against bone. Even though the swimmer is in a gravity-free environment, intense muscle contraction is still pulling (by way of tendons) on the various bones involved in joint movement; this causes them to keep a need for increased BMD over their non-physical counterparts in the population.

AEROBIC CAPACITY

Exercise programs that emphasize endurance usually elicit a 15-30% increase in maximum oxygen uptake (VO2Max). Available evidence indicates that traditional weight training (greater than 1-2 minutes rest between exercises) does not increase VO2Max. But it has been shown that performing circuit training regimens can increase VO2Max 5-8%. These regimens consist of a circuit of approximately 10 exercises. A resistive force (amount of weight) is then chosen that can be moved quickly (in one second) for 15 repetitions of that particular exercise. The rest period for each exercise is between 15-30 seconds.

Though resistive training is obviously not a grounded method of aerobic training, it can aid in the body's ability to engage in same.

APPLICATION TO MASTERS SWIMMING

To swim faster longer, and rise to a higher level of aerobic condition, the body's musculature must be trained to have enough strength, power and endurance to allow for both longer swim sets and increased numbers of repetitions and intense intervals. Weight and dry-land training are the established forms of cross-training that allow for the muscles' adaptive behavior to move more water with each stroke cycle.

BODY COMPOSITION

Obesity is a risk factor for several health problems including diabetes mellitus, arthritis, Cardio Vascular Disease (CVD), and kidney dysfunction. In addition, several new arterial and venous pathways, forced to travel through the increased fatty tissue, have to be fed and lead by the heart placing a correspondingly excessive stress on it. Though it is a given that dedicated aerobic activity has been prescribed successfully to control body weight and reduce fatty tissue, there is also increasing evidence indicating that strength exercise is an effective means of influencing body composition.

Muscle tissue is denser than fatty tissue. Since muscle is classified as part of the Lean Body Mass (LBM), as we add it to the skeletal structure and reduce body fat content, we may see only a slight reduction in total body weight changes unless large amounts of fat are eliminated. (The logical combination of aerobic and resistive training is the most efficient way to eliminate the fat and put on the muscle. The more muscle on the body, the greater the calorie expenditure with any movement). Then a noticeable metamorphosis occurs. What is produced is the presentation of an appropriate athletic body composition: the average non-professional nor elite athletic male under 25 years of age--10-12% body fat. Average athletic male 25-35 years of age: 12%-15% body fat. Average athletic male over 40 years of age: 15-

20% body fat. Women who classify as an average moderately-dedicated athlete need to just add 5% to the above listing.

The aging process lends itself to a cascade of physiological and biochemical events that result in a reduced resting metabolic rate in the general population. A reduction in muscle mass, growth hormone, and testosterone all act to produce a diminished resting metabolic rate which allows for increased fatty tissue buildup. To counteract this decline in metabolic activity, participation in an aerobic exercise program that includes consistent resistive weight training is the most logical, the most practical and the most successful path to take to push back Father Time and produce a more youthful and healthful body type.

Even with a genetic tendency to expand the waistline and soften all around, dedicated participation in the above combined type of physical activity will belie the chronological age and hold in check any deleterious effects that could arise over time.

APPLICATION TO MASTERS SWIMMING

Consistent, vigorous swim training positively stresses the body by bringing into play most of the appropriate musculature for movement through water. The resultant physiology, to a greater or lesser extent, depending upon the athlete's genetics, will adapt such that a more completely toned body will be produced. Seeking this, a growing number of competitive Masters Swimmers have found that time spent in the weight room or with dry-land activities is time well spent. Though swimming itself is not the ideal activity for weight reduction as compared to running, for example, due to the reduced need to move against gravity, the addition of moving a land-based resistance in a structured effort against gravity (weight room activity) will add the desired increased muscle size and strength.

Masters swimmers are in a perfect situation to add valuable physiologic information to the study of aging in comparison to the relatively sedentary general population. It has been well documented (and readily seen) that body composition in a Masters swimmer presents quite well as to a leaner, more toned generalized musculature, regardless of gender; this leads to a greater strength-to-weight ratio and a reduced body/mass (weight-to-height) index.

EFFECT ON CARDIOVASCULAR RISK FACTORS

There is growing evidence to indicate that strength training may also be important to risk intervention. Strength training exercise has been shown to increase insulin sensitivity, decrease *glucose* intolerance, and has a modest effect on decreasing diastolic blood pressure and may positively alter serum lipids.

Several studies have been designed and conducted to show the positive effect strength training has on the physiology related to insulin regulation. As lean body mass, increased so did the insulin response to ingested *glucose*. Studies comparing aerobic and strength training regimens have proved that both modalities positively controlled insulin physiology on a day-to-day basis.

Problems arise when insulin regulation is not tightly controlled, and uncontrolled insulin leads to diabetes, and diabetes very often has as its side effect vascular problems. It is from these vascular problems that circulatory disturbances to the heart and other vital organs and the extremities produce the debilitating and deadly sequelae we so often see.

Aerobic endurance exercise is a well-established method for raising high-density ("good") cholesterol (HDL-C) in many people. The HDL-C works its "magic" by scouring the inside lining of blood vessels to draw out the type of cholesterol (Low-Density--LDL) that can clog the arteries. If this cholesterol is allowed to react with oxygen and then harden, potentially deadly clots can form. These produce the most morbidity and mortality in the United States.

Several studies have given conflicting results as to how efficient resistance training is in raising HDL-C. Some researchers have found that heavy strength training over a period of several months can produce the positive results we seek (as much as a 13% increase in HDL-C). Others have derived results that show no real positive influence of the cholesterol picture. What has come from several analyses of resistance programs is the fact that one would have to do several exercises quickly and sequentially with very little time to rest between exercise bouts to produce any positive results; in effect, the resistance training becomes somewhat of an aerobic exercise.

APPLICATION TO MASTERS SWIMMING

As a group, Master's Swimmers are relatively knowledgeable about health matters. Most choose to take the "high road" as regards to what constitutes overall good general health and well-being. They eat relatively healthily, or at least know they should. They know or at least surmise the benefits of regular vigorous exercise. And they are mostly aware of what precautions should be taken as they approach the various markers of aging.

Though whether by genetic default or advancing age, even Masters Swimmers may find themselves prisoners of their own metabolic defects. The very popular (and now common) addition of strength training to their in-pool time affords them this additional method of controlling *glucose* metabolism, keeping any aberrant cholesterol readings under control, and bringing blood pressure into line.

If, in fact, any of the above physical means is not adequate to keep either blood sugar or serum lipids (fats) under control, Masters Swimmers as a group are well-monitored by the appropriate health professionals, and chemical intervention with any number of medicinal choices will most likely occur. It is out of the norm for a long time masters swimmer to ignore any biochemical or physiological warnings that may arise as aging takes place. Though they rely heavily on the continuous and dedicated aquatic training Masters swimming offers, and the dry-land exercise they seek out to augment their strength, power, and endurance, very few are foolish enough to go through life not being monitored adequately so as to evaluate the total benefits of both aerobic and strength training.

SAFETY AND PRACTICAL APPLICATION

Data regarding the safety of strength training and testing shows that it is safe if properly administered and performed. No adverse cardiovascular events should occur if appropriate steps are taken to account for relative strength at the time of participation and the effects of aging.

There is one precaution that should be addressed: there could be a problem in some people if they hold their breath when performing strength training. This puts extra pressure on the internal organs and causes blood pressure spiking and vascular difficulty. It is called the *"Valsalva maneuver."* To prevent this buildup of pressure on the internal organs, one should blow out as the strength movement is made and should breathe in as the recovery takes place.

Muscle soreness is a common resultant especially as one ages or for beginners into the regimen. Special care must be taken to prevent injuries at this point by not moving too much resistance too quickly. No more than a 10% increase in resistance per week is a usually safe modality.

Also, as one ages, there develops a need for an exogenous source (outside the body) of substances that normally protect the joints. *Glucosamine* and *chondroitin,* taken as a dietary supplement, act to replace what naturally becomes diminished, reduce pain and discomfort, and allow more complete functionality of all the stress-bearing joints.

An important reason why strength training is beneficial in daily life and may cause less risk in doing various lifting tasks is related to the training effect of simply getting stronger. The spine is protected by stronger supportive muscles of the trunk and all the joints enjoy the same protective condition throughout most movements.

We also see that blood pressure measured during sub-maximal lifting decreases following the training period. Thus, strength training can decrease the stress placed on the heart during lifting tasks and any other demanding activity that requires vigorous effort. Heart attacks that are a risk factor with such activities as shoveling snow, lifting heavy objects and executing vigorous movements whether by choice or need can be lessened by the overall beneficial adaptive effects of strength training.

APPLICATION TO MASTERS SWIMMERS

It is a wise choice to include strength training on a regular basis through the training week along with the regular swim bouts that Masters Swimmers endure. The number one over-use injury with aquatic training is "swimmer's shoulder." What this most often turns out to be is that the four muscles of the *rotator cuff* (*supraspinatus, infraspinitus, Teres major*, and *subscapularus*) are not strong enough to handle the repetitive movements through the various planes the shoulders must move to execute the four main competitive strokes. Educated and experienced Masters Swimmers wisely spend time keeping the *rotator cuff* strong enough to balance the work of the major shoulder and upper arm muscles like the deltoids, biceps, triceps, trapeziums, pectorals and rhomboids.

Swimming places the body in a horizontal position in a medium that produces a gravity-free ambiance. This usually keeps the blood pressure and heart rate at a lower number than would be seen in an upright athlete dealing with body weight, resistive elements of a chosen sport, and the all-encompassing presence of gravity.

Making the muscles of the trunk as strong as practical is key to moving through the water in a powerful manner. Whether swimming the long-axis strokes (free and back) or the short-axis strokes (breast and fly), the true power is basically generated from the hips and includes the whole torso. Strength training with free weights, latex tubing, and, or mechanical devices is as important to fast swimming as in-water training.

On average, it takes a land-based athlete about three years to fully acclimate to the gravity-free environs of the pool. The reverse is true but with a caution: as one ages, gravity and ground of land based sports can take their toll on joints that have not had to endure the pounding and weight-bearing that non-swimmers do. Overall strength can only act to help the body deal with whatever we put it through.

CONCLUSION

The effects of resistance/strength training on muscular strength and endurance (muscle mass) and rehabilitation from musculoskeletal injury is well known. As a result, most of the major health organizations have included it as an important component of a well-rounded exercise program along with aerobic endurance and flexibility exercise. More recently, strength training has been shown to be beneficial in improving many factors associated with good health. These factors include increased function and prevention of falls, decreased pain in chronic low back pain patients, improved *glucose* tolerance and insulin sensitivity, increased BMD, increased basal metabolic rate (weight control), and improved quality of life. It appears that most of the above findings can be attained in strength training programs that include 8-10 exercises that are performed 2-3 days per week, using one set of 8-15 repetitions to fatigue.

CHAPTER 6

WHY YOUR SPORTS DRINK SHOULD CONTAIN PROTEIN

Carbohydrate is usually considered to be the most important nutrient for endurance athletes. Protein, on the other hand, is associated with strength and power sports such as football and weightlifting.

It's true that endurance athletes do not require especially large amounts of protein in their regular meals. However, exciting new research from leading sports science laboratories is reshaping our conception of the ideal sports drink. This research has shown that, when consumed during aerobic exercise, a sports drink containing carbohydrate and protein in a 4:1 ratio provides four benefits compared to a conventional carbohydrate-only sports drink: 1) better hydration, 2) greater endurance, 3) less muscle damage, and 4) faster muscle recovery.

1. BETTER HYDRATION

In a study conducted at St. Cloud State University and published in the *International Journal of Sports Nutrition and Exercise Metabolism*, researchers compared the rehydration effects of a sports drink containing carbohydrate and protein in a 4:1 ratio (*Accelerade*), a conventional carbohydrate sports drink (*Gatorade*), and water. The carb-protein sports drink was found to rehydrate athletes 15 percent better than the conventional carbohydrate sports drink and 46 percent better than water.

2. GREATER ENDURANCE

In a study conducted at the University of Texas and published in the *International Journal of Sports Nutrition and Exercise Metabolism*, researchers found that a carbohydrate-protein sports drink increased endurance by 29% in cyclists compared to a conventional, carbohydrate-only sports drink. Consuming protein during exercise may increase endurance by providing an additional energy source to the muscles and by improving the efficiency of carbohydrate usage during exercise.

3. LESS MUSCLE DAMAGE

A study published in *Medicine and Science in Sports and Exercise* found that a carbohydrate-protein sports drink reduced muscle damage in an exhaustive workout by 83% compared to a conventional sports drink. Consuming protein during exercise may reduce muscle damage by reducing cortisol levels. During hard workouts, cortisol, a stress hormone, is normally released in large amounts and subsequently breaks down muscle proteins, causing muscle damage.

4. FASTER RECOVERY

When athletes experience less muscle damage during a workout, they recover faster and perform better in the next workout. This was demonstrated in the above-mentioned study in which a carb-protein sports drink was found to reduce muscle damage compared to a conventional sports drink. As part of this study, athletes returned to the testing site the next day for a follow-up workout. On average, the athletes had 40% greater endurance in the follow-up workout when they consumed a carb-protein drink in the first workout than they did when they drank a conventional carbohydrate sports drink.

RESEARCH YOU CAN USE

All of the latest research on the benefits of consuming protein during aerobic exercise adds up to one conclusion: If you are serious about your performance, you should consume a sports drink containing a 4:1 ratio of carbohydrate and protein in every workout.

CHAPTER 7

THE BATTLE OF THE BULGE

It may be that most Americans are obsessed with being thin, but if you look around you'll see that most are overweight. In fact, at least one-third of the adult American population is approaching obesity (depending upon height, at least 20 to 30 pounds overweight), and nearly one-half are considered overweight. This is more than a 10% increase from the 1980's, and the number continues to climb.

We also know that several potentially catastrophic diseases can arise from being overweight. For example, **C**oronary **H**eart **D**isease (CHD) and diabetes are now both definitely linked to an expanded waistline. We also know that those wanting to partake in athletics will definitely be at a disadvantage carting around more non-muscular body weight than they should.

So how do we reduce our nation's fat and your waistline? Consistently inserting moderate to vigorous exercise in the daily/weekly schedule is a proven way to fight the bulge. But if you do not follow a low-fat diet, in conjunction with your regular exercise program, you may be waging a losing "battle of the bulge."

There has arisen of late a major dietary controversy over what type of foods (or that type of diet) actually causes the most harm in regards to increasing body fat. Aitkin's Diet followers believe that it is mainly *carbohydrates* (simple and, or complex) which produce the unwanted fat, while consuming fatty dishes and protein at will is the way to body leanness. There have been weight-loss situations on the Aitkin's Diet; enough so as to make many stop and consider is this a possible avenue to permanent weight loss. They should also ask the big question: is this the *safest* way to a *permanent* ideal body weight?

To lose weight, the obvious should be clear: take in less calories than you burn up with activity, or to put it in a more logical way: burn up more calories than you take in throughout the day, the week, the year. By this, I mean *consistency.* Going on a diet should not be the goal of the weight-loss seeker; entering into a life-style change in eating describes what should be the intended objective.

Many health professionals say you have to go on a low-calorie diet to lose weight; true but too simplistic. They say "A calorie… is a calorie… is a calorie" and "All excess calories will be stored as fat." Be cautious of these warnings. They are only half-truths, and are not the main issue when dealing with weight control. You do not eat calories, per say; you eat carbohydrates, fat, and protein. And each of these food groups are utilized and stored differently by the body.

WHAT IS A CALORIE?

A kilocalorie (*Kcal... 1000 calories*) or what we conveniently refer to as a ***calorie***, is a measure of heat energy. Scientifically, it represents the amount of heat needed to raise the temperature of one kilogram of water (slightly more than a quart) by one degree Celsius. For example, a can of chicken noodle soup with 90 calories per serving has the chemical energy in one serving to raise the temperature of 90 quarts of water by one degree Celsius, or 1 quart of water 90 degrees. But if the can of soup is actually chemical energy that produces heat, what happens when you eat it?

WHERE DOES IT ALL GO?

The protein in the soup (coming mostly from the chicken), which equals four calories per gram, is broken down and then reassembled to replace protein in your body lost by routine cell turnover, especially in the muscles. Some of the protein is also used to make enzymes and other key chemicals needed to make your metabolism work

Suppose you add up all the protein in your daily diet, and it comes to more than your body needs. What happens then? The calorie counters say it is all turned into fat. But this would call for some monumental biochemical processes to occur, and the scientific literature does not support this type of metabolism. What happens is that the excess protein is oxidized, which means it is burned off and converted to compounds that are eliminated from the body (assuming the kidneys are up to the task).

What happens to the fat in your soup, and from the other foods you eat? Some replace lost tissues such as cell membranes and certain cells in your nervous system. The rest is first utilized as energy for body function and movement. But since fat is the highest food energy source (providing nine calories per gram), it is quite easily stored as such by the body for later use. Nature has always provided this biochemical energy pathway. The trouble with all this is that the body's ability to store fat is seemingly limitless. People who consistently eat more fat than they can burn up keep storing it day after day… Getting fatter and fatter.

The fate of the carbohydrate in the chicken soup (coming from vegetables and pasta), and from the rest of the daily food intake is more interesting. A little Carbohydrate (CHO) is utilized in cell turnover, but the majority is consumed for muscular energy. Although it only produces four calories per gram, carbohydrates provide the "high-octane" readily-usable fuel the body needs to move though all the demands we choose to put it through. Thus, a diet consisting predominately of carbohydrates will provide plenty of energy upon demand.

What if you eat too much carbohydrate? The calorie counters say it is simply turned into fat. However, the scientific literature tells a different story. Some extra carbohydrate can be stored as *glycogen,* which is the breakdown product of carbohydrates and the storage component of *glucose; glucose* is the prime energy source the body seeks to move muscle and everything else attached to same. This glycogen is stored somewhat in the muscles proper for an increased ready supply of energy and stored to a greater extent in the liver, which is the second line of defense against energy drain.

If one eats more carbohydrates than the body can store, the rate of oxidation increases. The body "turns up the heat" and the **B**asic **M**etabolic **R**ate **(BMR)** is raised burning carbohydrate faster. Only when the body has filled all possible stores and turned up the burners full blast can it begin converting some of the extra carbohydrates into fat. And by this time, very large amounts of food would have had to be consumed.

Results from clinical nutrition studies show that the conversion of carbohydrate to fat in healthy physically active people is minor, compared to storage of dietary fat. The body only readily converts carbohydrate to fat if the body is deprived of fat, or it needs more fat as in the third trimester of pregnancy, or it has **MUCH** more caloric intake than it needs on a daily basis.

What has come to be of tremendous benefit to those who train intensely on a regular schedule is the scientific discovery that a certain proportion (4:1) of carbohydrate to muscle-friendly protein (whey) can have a synergistic effect in powering the muscles and allow them to recover faster and more completely than they would otherwise be able with carbohydrates alone.

WHAT SHOULD YOU DO?

The evidence that counting grams of fat is the key to weight control is well documented. The mechanism for the process is logical and true, and the scientific literature supports it. The evidence that simply counting calories is the way to go is inconsistent, seldom corrected for the known influence of fat, often flawed, and there is no mechanism to explain how those excess calories contribute to weight (except for those from fat), that is consistent with human biochemistry.

It is very hard to overeat on pure carbohydrate foods because they are bulky and often contain a lot of water. A good rule of thumb is if you are in good health, have a normal metabolism, and exercise regularly, consuming one gram of fat for each kilogram (2.2 lbs.) of body weight (or target body weight) will not add on the pounds Americans seem to be so attached to.

It is never a pleasant situation to cut out your favorite foods to lose weight; that is why so many diets fail. The best way to lose weight and keep it off is to remove as much fat from the diet as possible. Always select the low-fat alternatives; your taste buds will become accustomed sooner than you think. Choose several servings a day of fresh fruits, vegetables, breads and pastas (minus the high-fat spreads or sauces) with a complimentary amount of quality protein and as little fat as you can get away with. There will always be too many opportunities to consume fats; work at dodging them as you would anything that would jeopardize your working out.

MORE ON FOOD INTAKE FOR BUILDING MUSCLE AND ENERGY THROUGHOUT THE DAY

There are three main seasonally-influenced diets that I recommend to my athletes for building endurance into strength and then into power. The most obvious physical alteration is the building of muscle with the attendant athletic "thickening" of the body. Put simply, the body cannot perform up to its potential under the challenge of vigorous exercise unless it has the muscular force from which to draw. I build a meal as I would build one of my model radio-controlled boats; I add the correct things to give it balance and make it work up to my expectations and needs.

The diets are broken up into the **fall-into-winter segment,** the **winter-into-spring segment,** and the **summer segment.** Each is correlated with the ambient weather conditions which in Florida are not nearly as diverse throughout the year as in the more northern latitudes. I tweak my diets (though they are much more complicated) as the various petroleum companies do with their gasoline mixtures when specifically formulated for time of year and locale. My diet recommendations try to ensure the nutritional/energy demands of the athlete as he chooses to train appropriately for his athletic needs.

The most basic concept for weight gain is to take in more calories than one would consume in a day; for weight loss to burn more calories than consumed in a day. But we do not want to simply put on weight that most easily would wind up as fat stores in the body, or lose weight at the expense of muscle tissue. We want muscle with enhanced formation of all the appropriate enzymes needed to produce energy. Energy is produced only by certain molecules within muscle tissue. These energy powerhouses are called *mitochondria.* They are the energy centers of the body. Appropriate vigorous training will produce more *mitochondria* but they can only work to efficiency if supplied with sufficient nutrients throughout the day. Though suffering a bad reputation in modern nutritional circles when taken to excess, a small percentage of fat intake is absolutely necessary to ensure adequate production of very important regulatory hormones, cell membranes, and the covering of nerve fibers (*myelin*).

I highly recommend the consumption of food at least five to six times per day, and the intake of adequate liquid as often. Most people walk around in at least a semi-dehydrated state which won't usually manifest itself unless put under physical duress. What is seen is a "heaviness" or sluggish feeling throughout the day, waning in concentration, small aches and pains that should never be a bother become more noticeable, and any sense of endurance or strength becomes dissipated.

If one sweats, one needs to drink; if one breathes, one needs to drink. If one thinks, one needs to drink... get the picture. If you are alive, you need to drink. You must never wait until you are thirsty... then it is already too late to prevent sluggishness. This holds true whether you are in a hot climate, a moderate climate or a cold climate. Just because you are not ostensibly sweating, you can still become dehydrated in a very cold dry climate due to simple respiratory and skin evaporation. You must also drink past when you feel you have had enough. In a few words: "drink before you are thirsty and after you are not." Have fluid replacements around you most of the time. I like diet green tea the best. Green teas have many phytochemicals that simply act to protect the body's "innerds." The diet form of this provides no extra sugar and calories.

Another important concept that must be considered for athletes is not only to fuel-up before activity but to re-fuel after workouts or competition. Depending upon what foods and, or supplements are taken, fueling up can require different lead times. Some foods require at least an hour to get properly absorbed; some as long as two to three hours. Some energy supplements are ready to go within 15 to 30 minutes. The optimum time to re-fuel is within two hours of the exercise bout, with the first hour after exercise presenting the greatest window for energy uptake.

Some easy biochemistry: 3,500 calories to equal the energy to make (or lose) a pound of weight. Protein and carbohydrate provide four kilocalories of energy per gram of weight; fat provides nine kilocalories per gram of weight. Obviously, fat provides more than twice the caloric content per unit weight than other food stuffs. We want to add "athletic" weight, mostly muscle, with a little with fluid, and a little with fat.

Since the season is now winter, we will present the fall-into-winter diet. No matter what time of year we are in, it is best for the general physiology to consume foodstuffs five to six times per day. I call this "grazing." No real gigantic meals where you come away stuffed and ready for a dozing session (except for special holiday or celebratory occasions.) Breakfast, smart snack, lunch, smart snack, dinner, smart snack. This is the template throughout most of the days of the week. The relatively constant intake throughout the day keeps the metabolism stoked allows for a continuous stream of nutrients to bathe the internal tissues, and provides the necessary energy for an active lifestyle. Right along with this numerous intake of food is the above-mentioned required consumption of various types of liquid; hydration is a must in an athlete... throughout the day!

BREAKFAST

No question, the most important time of the day for food intake. The name itself breakfast says it all. We need to break the fast of the night with good food choices and to stoke the furnace of metabolism. You must take the time to allow breakfast to become a strong part of your daily food intake. A quick pastry and cup of coffee (or anything similar) is no way to fuel an athlete and is the path to an unhealthy internal physiology. By eating, the body's metabolism is raised. By eating smart, the physiology is allowed to proceed in a relatively healthy state as it fuels the body's needs for the day. Many well-conditioned athletes feel a sense of warmth come over them immediately after eating... metabolism has increased due to the intake of calories. Consume the correct type of calories in the correct proportions, and fueling becomes an efficient process.

SOME MENU SUGGESTIONS:

- This is a relatively light meal and easy to digest. For ease of preparation there are variously-flavored instant hot oatmeal cereals (*GREAT VALUE* brand name from Walmart) that are a wise choice. I add a bit of water and at least a cup of milk to wet down the cereal. (All milk intake, whether on cereal, in coffee or other beverages, or in cooking should be skim or no more than 1% milk fat. We want to add solid body weight (mostly muscle) not fat stores.) Add either fruit placed on the cereal directly or eaten alongside to vary flavor and nutritional content; the best fruit-in-cereal choices are bananas, blueberries, blackberries, strawberries, cherries. The best side-dish fruit selections are cantaloupe, pineapple, orange and grapefruit slices. (Oatmeal provides long-lasting energy with water-soluble fiber to help control cholesterol and *triglycerides*; the suggested berries are loaded with phytochemicals that are natural substances that provide natural metabolic protection for the body. I like pineapples whenever I can eat them because of their bromelain content. If no pineapples, then I take a bromelain supplement in tablet form. This enzyme helps in general digestion and to help the body rid itself of damaged and dead tissue whether from trauma or vigorous exercise). You want to make sure you consume at least 5 servings of fruit and, or vegetables every day. A glass of orange juice is equivalent to one serving, for example. A typical day for me includes my eating at least one apple, a banana, some mixed fruit cocktail, mandarin orange slices, and anything else in season. I buy the Dole prepared fruit in plastic containers for ease of administration throughout the day. I also try and squeeze fresh juice a few times a week; not just for the great taste of wholesome fresh, but also to consume the PECTIN that makes up the body of the fruit, This pectin helps to capture excess fats that might be ingested and binds with them to prevent deposition into the arteries.

- If no cholesterol or other blood-fat problems exist, the equivalent of two eggs plus three slices of Canadian bacon plus hash brown potatoes is a hearty way to start the day; I usually choose egg-beaters or something similar to get all the nutritious elements of eggs but not the cholesterol. Canadian bacon is a good source of protein and minerals but with much less fat than regular bacon. Caffeinated coffee does not bother me if taken early enough in the day, but if consumed after 6 PM or so, I can suffer acid-reflux from caffeine's effect of producing more stomach acid and also relaxing the esophageal sphincter, allowing acid to reflux back up and cause the heartburn sensation. Keep in mind that chocolate, citrus fruits, acid and spicy condiments, mints and nasal decongestants all can act to relax the esophageal sphincter to bring on an attack of acid reflux. If you do not stiffer this condition (yet), then caution with these foods is not necessary, but if you do, then heed my advice.

- A third choice can be the quickest, but not the poorest in nutritional content: either solid or liquid yogurts with various fruits provides an easy method for a mixed intake of various important food elements. This dairy class of food provides casein, a specific type of muscle-friendly protein that is usually easy to digest and is readily incorporated into the body's physiology. Many tasty varieties exist which prevents meal-boredom. Along with this choice, I suggest some other fruit source like a glass of orange juice, cut melons, or fruit cocktail. The healthiest choices to pick from the fruit source are blackberries, blueberries, raspberries, strawberries, and cherries. I add these to my yogurts and cereals whenever I can. They taste good, and know that they are the highest sources of anti-oxidants you can easily find. Make them a strong part of your daily diet.

- If you have the time and means to splurge and treat yourself, or are able to patronize an eatery that can provide, an American favorite of a mixed egg-omelet is a good choice for the weekly variety. I usually do this on Saturdays after an intense workout. I look at this as a nutritional reward for enduring the "combat" or intense training at my age. Onions and mushrooms are a mainstay in my omelets because they provide valuable antioxidants and minerals yet cause no harm to the cholesterol and *triglyceride* picture. Green and red peppers, if able to be tolerated, are also a good choice for the omelet, as well as spinach, which has a strong amount of leutin in it which can prevent bad things happening to the back of the eye... a condition called macular degeneration is a devastating condition that can come with age and excessive exposure to the sun. The antioxidant, lutein, protects the back of the eye-grounds and keeps the eye healthier longer. If cheese is a favorite, you certainly can partake but try for "light" varieties with at least half the fat content. Mozzarella light cheese is always a good choice if you want to add cheese to an omelet or just to any meal. As a rule, the darker the cheese, the more the calcium content but also, the more the fat. Dark cheddar and American have normally more fat content than lighter varieties. If shopping for this type of foodstuff check the labels for content. Try to always choose the low-fat varieties... nowadays the taste is the same but the healthy choice is greater.

MORNING SNACK

If you have had breakfast by 9 AM, a late-morning snack (past 11 AM) is in order. This is really not to stave off hunger or even to quench that somewhat "empty feeling" in the gut that may arise, but rather to re-fuel and re-energize the metabolism to keep stoking the body's ability to make energy. Since hydration is a must throughout the day, part of this snack must include at least 16 oz. of liquid. A good choice with very little calories and minimal carbohydrate is the new product, POWERADE OPTION. This comes in a 32 oz. bottle in various flavors. I utilize this to hydrate throughout the day, but it does not provide the optimum amount of caloric energy to sustain a vigorous workout lasting more than 60 minutes. If you are trying to put on solid weight, this product is only good for hydration during down time, but not to energize a serious workout. This would also be a good time to consume a few pieces of fruit, some *Wheat Thin Harvest Grain crackers* with strawberry-flavored Philadelphia light cream cheese, or some flavored yogurt. The beauty of the many varieties of flavored yogurt is that you can have several a day and not become "food-bored." I also recommend the consumption, if possible, of pure red grape juice at least twice daily. I save my daily doses for snack time, and while I work out. I have recently added another nutritious drink to my menu: *V8 brand V-FUSION*. This is a very tasty mixture of various fruits and vegetables in liquid form; absolutely no fat, and with 170 calories in the 12 oz. container, it really hit's the spot when an energy/hydration mix is called for. It comes in a variety of flavors. It is so loaded with the good "stuff" that it qualifies as a complete serving of a vegetable and a fruit.

LUNCH

Many times a busy business, personal, or social schedule obviates the ability to sit and consume a decent amount of energy replenishment. This is not a good thing. Eating on the run is just that... The excessive movement interferes with proper food ingestions and digestion, and a constant schedule of this will only allow for inappropriate food intake and the consequent poor digestible processes that will follow. If the body cannot properly assimilate its energy intake, how do you expect it to turn it into the energy you demand and the re-building of tissue needed for an active lifestyle?

Though this is a very important time for refueling, it can take a step back from a strong breakfast. But if the breakfast was suspect, then the lunch needs to be a bit more hearty... not stuffing the body, but containing sustainable foods that the body can handle while it is asked to perform the tasks of the day. Recommended options:

- A lean roast beef sandwich on grain breads, which include any whole grain, rye, wheat, or pumpernickel is a solid nucleus from which to build. Pickles, Cole slaw, sauerkraut, tomatoes are all good add-ons. I especially try to consume several tomatoes per week because of the lycopene content. This anti-oxidant helps to protect the body from oxidative damage and is especially helpful for keeping the prostate gland in a healthy condition. Along with this good protein choice, some quality complex carbohydrates besides the bread should be consumed. Here is where mixed fruit, yogurt, or a side of vegetables come in. You want to end up absolutely not hungry but also not stuffed to the point of feeling bloated. Keep it clean, lean, keep it mean. I strongly suggest that while you eat, you rest. You should eat in peace and have the time to help the body handle the digestion process by not moving around too vigorously right after eating. This is where a little quality "down time" comes in.

- If possible, a baked fish sandwich or platter is a wise choice for a strong lunch. Notice I suggested *baked, not fried.* Try not to eat fried anything if possible... not a good choice due to *trans fats* and extra calories of the wrong kind. Soup should be a mainstay in the weekly diet. If the weather is cooler, warm soup with hearty ingredients are just the thing to help stoke the metabolism with quality nutrition. I like the Italian Wedding Soup, beef noodle, chicken, noodle, tomato rice, and a host of others so long as the taste is as hearty as the ingredients. For those trying to put on muscular weight, eating breads during the lunch and dinner menu is appropriate. A few slices will add substantial carbohydrates to help fuel the following hours' energy needs helping to spare any breakdown of muscle tissue to do the same. We

126

want to build muscle, not tear it down just to do daily tasks; to fuel our daily needs for basic energy, it is best to get them from carbohydrates and fats. To build the muscle tissue that we desire at the end of the day, we need the quality muscle-friendly choices of protein: whey, soy, casein. A mix of the three would be ideal and approach a near-perfect meal, but that does not have to be the case all at the same time. If consumed, one-at-a-time, throughout the day, that would work sufficiently well to build and rebuild quality muscle tissue throughout the body.

- Having made the above statements, I would also suggest a new product that I found which has good taste, no fat, quality protein, ample calcium, and aids in the daily hydration: the product is called SKINNY COW FAT-FREE CHOCOLATE MILK. I go through about two quarts a week as a supplement to my regular intake of fluids. I sort of look at this as almost a dessert. It truly tastes rich and creamy, but is absolutely healthful in every respect.

- There are many times when the Italian craving comes over me; I handle the call by heating up a can of 99% fat-free *Chef Boyardee* beef ravioli. Though the can says it contains two servings, I suggest you eat the whole container's worth that only provides about 300 calories with 3 grams of fat. The taste is quite good, and it sustains me for many hours. This would make up the mainstay of the lunch along with some fruit and, or vegetable juices to wash it down.

- Sometimes when I am really hungry, and the clock says, "after lunch hour" I take one of a select menu listing from the *Marie Callender* line of frozen dinners. Of course, this only works if you have access to a microwave that may or may not be the case for many lunch times. There are several delicious choices that have surprising less calories (fat included) for the taste. Suggestions include Sweet & sour chicken, slow-roasted beef, herb-roasted chicken, and beef tips in mushroom sauce. Calories are in the 400 to 800 range, which is good, but you will probably need to supplement this when you choose it for dinner.

AFTERNOON SNACK

I take my creatine and ribose mixture that I concoct before I train. I take this about two hours before I need to draw on my energy reserves since it takes about that long for this to get to the muscles to produce any positive effect. This can also be taken right after a workout to help in recovery for the rest of the day or the next exercise bout. My creatine comes in the form of *CREATINE SURGE* from Jarrow Labs in California, and my ribose comes from *NUTRA BIO* Labs in New Jersey. (www.Nutrabio.com). The two substances (creatine and ribose) together is a case where $1+1 = 3$... they produce a synergistic effect to produce long lasting energy.

An energy supplement is also taken at this time to help balance my fuel supply for the *mitochondria*. Since I am on the Board of Consultants of Pacific Health Labs in NJ, the makers of *Endurox* and *Accelerade*, I am one of their spokesman as to the efficacy of their products. They do work, and they present no side effects worth mentioning. The products are tasty especially the vanilla and chocolate flavors. It is almost the perfect energy supplement physiologically, and something I strongly recommend to my serious athletes. I also take, since it has been proven to provide a moderate amount of oxidative protection to the heart, some DARK CHOCOLATE around this time of day. The chocolate usually contains a decent amount of caffeine, which stimulates the body into activity and helps it focus mentally. My choices are those with at least 60% cocoa in the formula... usually in the 70% concentration... not too sweet, but with that great chocolate taste and the fact that something great-tasting is actually doing me some good.

Any other choices previously mentioned can be consumed at this time, especially from the fruit list; I would not suggest an energy bar or carbohydrate replacement at this time unless you are about to engage in vigorous activity. What can happen to many is an energy spike (sugar rise in the blood) followed by the release of insulin that then super-lowers the sugar level bringing on a precipitous drop in energized feeling. And once you begin taking an energy bar supplement, you must keep up the intake with at least an energy drink or the like to keep the sugar in the blood elevated long enough to last through the exercise bout.

DINNER

Though traditionally thought of as the most wholesome and hearty meal of the day, it does not have to be. In fact, dinners should be tasty, well rounded with nutrition and substantial enough to satiate hunger, but not to the point of over-stuffing the digestive tract. There are many ramifications, mostly negative, that arise out of over-eating at night, including acid-reflux syndrome, dyspepsia (difficult digestion), and difficulty in falling asleep.

It is still sort of an "unwritten law" that you shouldn't eat no heavy foods after 8 PM if you want to enjoy a good night's sleep. Not such a stupid statement. Many foods taken after that time can have a deleterious effect on trying to hit the sack at a decent time to get up early the next day. My dinner choices center around a strong protein content to help my body repair itself from the day's "combat." At night is when most of the body's healing and growing occurs. Those who constantly deprive themselves of adequate sleep deprive their bodies of vital recovery time. It is also incumbent upon the athlete to ensure adequate hydration for the night's sleep. I also try and re-fuel with *Endurox*, ribose sugar, and creatine to help prepare me for the next day's physical demands. Recommended options:

- Any of the above-mentioned *Marie Callender* (or similar) frozen food entries. But for dinner supplementation is needed with choices like applesauce (that I eat almost with every dinner... also a fruit choice for the day); hearty soup, salad with tomatoes. A choice that I enjoy is the tomato-mozzarella, artichoke salad made at my local *Wal-Mart*. I also try to eat Cole Slaw several times a week.
- Lean chicken cutlets with Marinara sauce and low-fat mozzarella cheese melted over. For a typical male athlete looking to put on muscle, four pieces should comprise this hearty entry. Right along with this should be a vegetable dish like Green Giant creamed spinach, vegetable medley, Brussels sprouts, asparagus, cauliflower, and broccoli.

- The only Chinese selections that are not overly fat-laden are their chicken dishes other than General Tao's. Most of their vegetables present a healthy choice especially if sautéed or heated in the right oils (peanut, canola, soy, corn, etc.). When I eat out Chinese, I will take their baked or roasted dishes (chicken, fish, beef and broccoli, etc.)

- Protein from the sea is the best for keeping a lean but muscular body; this is when I make sure I have my two servings (at least) per week of baked fish. Tilapia is an excellent choice for its omega-3 fatty acids and good protein content. Sea scallops, sole, flounder, and mackerel all make for good fish choices. Scallops are the healthiest of all the shellfish choices, though eating shrimp no more than once a week will not harm the blood-fat picture and yet still provide a good source of protein from the sea.

- Dinner can be an excellent time for making a thick, loaded omelet with good side dishes. Having baked apple for dinner is not only a tasty treat, but it provides a nutritious filling food choice. When eating out simply, say at the Cracker Barrel, they provide several tasty and filling side dishes... their chicken-and-dumplings really hit the spot on all accounts.

- Pizza can be eaten for lunch or dinner; there is good and bad with this. The healthiest toppings to add to a pizza are mushrooms, onions, spinach, and anchovies. The fatty beef and pork choices should be avoided. Pizza is a treat and should be treated as such. No more than once a week do we do "street Italian."

There are a myriad of food choices that I left out. Mine is only a guide. If you have questions, just ask.

CHAPTER 8

THE IMPORTANCE OF PHYTOCHEMICALS IN YOUR DIET

There are many sophisticated methods for calculating daily caloric needs for weight control, be it for maintenance, gain, or loss. Besides the obvious about lessening caloric intake by reducing portion size and making wiser (healthier) choices of foods, the true key to weight control is the amount, the intensity, and the frequency of exercise one chooses to implement into his/her weekly schedule. I chose **weekly** instead of **daily** because if you truly want to become immersed in a healthy lifestyle, the overall schedule of events over a period of days must follow a pattern that allows for recovery from vigorous exercise yet exposes the body to certain strengthening bouts to increase muscle content. In a short sentence… This is about your **personal energy equation.**

It is a physiologic given that the more body size you have, the more calories you burn doing *anything.* Since muscle is more dense than fat, adding muscle will cause the body to burn the most calories per unit effort.

I present four levels of daily caloric expenditure: sedentary, light, moderate, and strenuous. When you know approximately how much energy your body burns in a day, you can estimate how many calories you need to maintain, lose or gain weight. Here is an easy formula to help get you going on balancing your personal energy equation.

A. To find the **base (minimum) number of calories** needed to "run" your heart, lungs and all your internal systems, simply **multiply your weight by 11.**

Write the number here; BASE = _____.

B. Determine your *level of activity* from the list below and **multiply your basal metabolic rate by both the low and high percentages listed. This gives you a range of the additional calories you require for the day.**

Write the numbers here; low_____ high_____

Activity Level	Percent
Sedentary (no sports or exercise at all)	30-50
Light (an easy stroll)	55-65
Moderate (moderate swimming or walking at a brisk pace	65-70
Strenuous (regular heart-pounding exercise such as vigorous Swimming or serious running)	75-100

C. Add the base number to the "low" activity number to determine your minimum daily calorie needs. Add the base number to the "high" activity number for your maximum daily calorie needs.

Example: if you are a 190 pound man whose daily activity level is in the moderate range, you will need 3,449 to 3,553 calories per day. Here is the math:

Step 1. 190 x 11 = 2,090 calories
Step 2. Low: 2,090 x 0.65 = 1,359
    High: 2,090 x 0.70 = 1,463
Step 3. 2,090 + 1,359 = 3,449
    2,090 + 1,463 = 3,553
Calorie needs for this 190-pound man: 3,449 to 3,553 per day.

CHAPTER 9

STAYING HEALTHY

PART I.

The time spent training, and competing must not be wasted or undermined by issues and events that can, for the most part, be prevented. If the athlete is to be true to his or her sport and the ideal of being the very best he or she can be, then what is done outside the athletic venue is just as important (in the grand scheme of things) as what is done in it.

THE HUMAN BODY'S RESPONSE TO ITS AMBIENT ENVIRONMENT

As I see it, going through life is analogous to walking over a very high-arching bridge in the deep black of night with just a few pale lights interspaced here and there for weak illumination. Surmising there is a very deep body of dark water under the bridge, we come across randomly-spaced large open trap doors along the roadway that become more numerous as we travel. Logic would dictate that as we move along the bridge, we better look down and watch where we are stepping lest we fall through and disappear into the black deep. Sound like a bad nightmare? Well, life is a lot like that bridge walk. There are many "trap doors" out there waiting to have us fall through them. How we watch ourselves as we travel along can make a great difference in whether we get far on the bridge or fall through much too early.

When lecturing on Public Health I often start out with the statement: "If you all knew what was out there waiting to get you, you would all go hide in a cave... Until I told you what was in the cave" ...meaning that there is really no place to hide against that which could make us sick, injured or worse. It is incumbent upon ourselves to be ever vigilant as to our welfare and health, and what we do as *young* people all too often can present years later as cause and effect.

A lot of Public Health *is* logic. People need to be exposed to this logic in such a way as to incorporate it into their planned existence. A coach and athlete combination who abides by the rules of good Public Health will most probably have a training advantage over those who don't. An ounce of prevention is worth MORE than a pound of cure, every time.

Public Health lesson number one is to try and put a balance in one's life. But to make *vigorous* athletic training on a par with the rigors of today's demands in the classroom and with modern socialization in general, the successful athlete has to be made aware of all that

132

can tear at him, both physically and emotionally. Just as a successful competitive swimmer must learn to "make friends with the water" and move through it with an economy of effort that belies the ease spectators see, so must the athlete "move through life." Those athletes engaged in long-term training toward a specific goal must heed and avoid all possible roadblocks to continued efforts to improve. The ability to train hard (day-to-day) requires devotion to making the right choices (day-to-day)… not an easy task for most young *healthy* people. Most take good health for granted (don't we all). They seem to think they are "bullet-proof" and that they can expect their bodies to respond to all demands quickly and successfully. The thought of getting sick or injured just doesn't seem to be an important possibility. The ideal is to educate the athlete to the point just shy of being obsessive.

INFECTIOUS DISEASES, THE CAUSE OF MOST ILLNESSES

The biological dictum of "cause-and-effect" is what steers us through the day-to-day activities that comprise our existence. There is a cascading series of events that usually rule how we react to our surroundings. How the body is prepared to deal with its ambient environment is what drives Public Health to its importance in our everyday lives. Though previously presented, this topic is covered in greater detail in Section III, Chapter 16.

VIGOROUS TRAINING AND TRYING TO KEEP THE BODY HYDRATED

Though one would think no sweating goes on in a liquid environment, it does. In fact, it is quite common to lose up to two pints of fluid per practice. One pint equals about one pound in weight. Weighing oneself before and after practice (if no liquids are consumed during workout) would show a weight drop of up to two pounds.

It is not adequate to just drink water, though that is better than nothing. The modern sports drinks have electrolytes (various salts) which not only add the correct elements to the body's natural fluids, but also make you somewhat thirsty so you will want to drink throughout the training session. I recommend taking in 32 ounces of this type of liquid, half before practice, half throughout the practice.

There are now even more sophisticated hydrating and energy re-supplying supplements on the market, but that will be discussed under a different topic.

The muscle fibers need moisture to bathe them in their contractile activity. If there is not enough hydration, the fibers can "seize" just like an automobile engine with insufficient motor oil. A major cause of muscle cramping is the simple fact of being dehydrated. A relatively pale yellow urine signifies adequate hydration during physical exercise. Once you are thirsty, it is actually too late to get properly hydrated for a race that will occur shortly or to work a training session intensely. Proper hydration takes time to occur… at least a half hour depending upon the type of liquid imbibed. The Public Health dictum with regards to fluids is: **"drink before you are thirsty and after you are not."**

PART II.

Keeping athletes in good physical and emotional health is key to training harder and longer. Training with intelligence (as to rest and recovery) is paramount to keeping the athlete in proper tune, allowing for optimum performance upon demand. Attaining the proper **balance in life** is a paradigm for staying physically healthy and emotionally strong. These last two states sometimes seem like "lucky gifts" from the gods. But working within proper Public Health guidelines and with some healthful common sense, the training sessions can produce what they were intended to do without excessive negativity tearing at the athlete. Yes, it pays to be lucky (not to get sick or injured), but luck is something that cannot be counted on as a planned result. Most of the time being "lucky" is being **prepared** when **opportunity** presents itself.

THE "POWER" TO MOVE

My approach to teaching and coaching **swim racing** requires what I feel are the three most important elements needed to swim fast (in order of importance), (1) **technique**, (2) **strength (power)**, and (3) **condition.** It used to be that I would list *"condition"* second, behind *"technique."* But as I developed my own philosophy of coaching over the years…that of a "power-swimming" or sprint coach, I have come to realize the importance in the ability to "move water" upon demand. I use the word, *"power"*, instead of *"strength"* because what is most needed to move the body through water (a medium 1000 times more dense than air) is the ability to grab hold and pull the body through it *QUICKLY.* The added strength and power gained with an appropriately-instituted resistance training program will also go a long way to preventing injuries.

Power, for purposes in this discussion, is the concept of **strength over time.** Just being strong is not enough, though that is good as a foundation. We must add **quickness** into the formula for success, and we must also incorporate the concept that moving through water requires **muscular endurance.** Even race-swimming a 100 yards or meters demands that the musculature hold on for about as long as it would take to run 400 yards or meters. Add to this the fact that the faster one moves through water, the more the water resists movement through it, and one can see the special type of muscular training needed to swim fast.

A logical approach to strength gain is best undertaken by ensuring that the body is generally prepared to handle the rigors of progressive resistance training. The medical dictum: "Do no harm," is key to preventing injury. At first, **lighter resistance** with **more repetitions** allow the body to adapt to weight training in a safe manner; this also enhances the effect of creating **endurance.** Once a stronger foundation is developed, then increased resistance can safely be added with **power-lifting** the objective. In fact, the best plan to produce a balanced effect is to cycle the two approaches in weekly segments. *Circadian rhythm* (what goes on physiologically in our bodies at different times in the 24 hour cycle) has a definite effect in how the body reacts to resistance training. There are several physiologic parameters related to strength that peak at certain times during the 24 hour cycle… all of which allow the body to perform better as it adapts to gaining strength.

Body temperature peaks between 5PM and 6PM. One of the parameters in Public Health that can be used in a crossover fashion to weight training is that if a patient is suffering a systemic infection that produces fever, said fever will peak around 5PM. This same general peaking in body temperature while healthy allows the muscles to warm more so they can handle physical movement more efficiently. If resistance training is to be performed at various times, it is very important to make sure the musculature is sufficiently warmed so as not to tear. It also appears that, in the average athlete, **skeletal muscles become about 10 percent stronger around 6PM.** The other parameter that becomes very important in strength training is that **perceived exertion of energy expended** with resistance training **seems less between 6PM and 7PM**; since the workout seems easier, one is able to push harder to gain more strength.

It was mentioned earlier in the series that **stretching is very important to protect the muscles from tearing.** It is good Public Health to ensure the elongation of the various muscles to be stressed (while they are in a warmed state) before dry land and, or weight room exercise bouts. It is also good Public Health to have older athletes and those that are heavily muscled to take extra time to stretch especially if the weather is cold. Nature provides that muscle tissue is more easily stretched for increased range of motion and efficient movement than the connecting tissue surrounding it. If the muscle is not elongated sufficiently, then the connective tissue will tear, and this usually involves much greater medical intervention and recovery time. The body's adaptation to resistance training actually starts with the connective tissue (tendons, ligaments, fascia…all called *integument)* that attaches the muscles around joints (*articular* areas) and other areas where muscle influences muscle and muscle influences bone movement. This connective tissue becomes thicker and stronger, which, in turn, forces the bones to which they are attached to become thicker and stronger to support their attachments. What this produces for improved Public Health is a bone structure that will resist *osteoporosis* (hollowing out of the dense bone structure, allowing for possible breakage, and usually seen in the sedentary elderly population) and possible hairline and other fractures seen in overuse syndromes, no matter what the age of the athlete.

The ideal way (in a Public Health sense) to allow the body to adapt to progressive resistance training is to use *latex* (rubber or surgical) *tubing*. The benefit here comes from the fact that there is no actual weight-lifting per say to possibly hurt the spine or other supportive structures. Also, the instant adaptability of moving either closer or farther away from the area where the tubing is attached allows for appropriate resistance at that instance (more or less) depending upon how one feels at the time. Fighting gravity plays a minor part when using latex tubing compared to free weights and some resistive machines, and that is good since it is more closely related to the gravity-free environment of movement through water.

Once the supporting connective tissue is made stronger with *gradual increases* in resistance training (no more than 10% in resistance amount and, or frequency per week), then safe increases in muscular adaptation can be sought. This "go-slowly-but-carefully" approach ensures less chance of injury in the weight room. It is good Public Health and wise athletic training to take more time and build gradual strength with a carefully-planned regimen of weight training than to try and seek quick strength and risk serious orthopedic injury.

If there is muscular and related tissue injury of an acute nature, good first aid and sports medicine procedures would and should prevail. *Immediate trauma* means swelling, inflammation, and pain will follow in the next few minutes. Various treatments to lessen these markers should be in position ASAP as time is of the essence in reducing the sequalae of taking a "hit." Ascertaining the degree of damage to the athlete and getting him or her to a stable safe position with immobilization should be the prime effort; ice packs come next in quick order. Following this   procedure brings in pharmacology. Taking an *antihistamine* will help keep swelling down by preventing the body's release of *histamine*, a substance usually released with most trauma and injury. When the damage is from an over-or chronic use injury, after immediate icing to control pain and potential swelling, *applied heat* is the procedure of choice. This causes blood to rush to the affected area bringing the body's own (*endogenous)* healing enzymes and also allowing *exogenous* sources (from outside the body) like the enzyme, *bromelain,* from pineapples to provide a healing environment. Heat also provides the obvious: a soothing feeling of warmth, especially appreciated when the weather turns cold.

PART III

In the simplest of terms: it is SO much easier to prevent injury and illness than to cure or heal them. But if we are faced with the necessity of recovery, rehabilitation, or renewal of strength (in body and mind) and vitality, then what I present should aid the athlete in quest of maximum performance.

SPECIFICITY OF TRAINING

Unfortunately, nowadays it takes an all-year-round commitment to be competitive in a particular sport, and the sport of swimming is as guilty as any in requiring total immersion. There are a few exceptions where extraordinary athletes can excel in more than one specific sport, but that situation is rare. To reach the maximum of one's ability (and then possibly a little more) takes a total "student of the game." What is done out of the pool is as important as in it. **Stroke-specific** dry-land muscular exercises are what need to be worked. For events of 200 yards or meters on down, doing stroke-specific exercises for the **length of time it takes to swim the target event** is a very logical approach to muscular adaptation for early to mid-season training. As training continues, more **power lifting** with quick, sharp muscular recruitment needs to be instituted replacing some of the many-repetition lifting bouts.

Since **swim training** is done in a **gravity-free environment**, making the swimmer run (against gravity) is just asking for articular (joint) trouble. Many coaches require **running** as part of the early conditioning regimen each year, even doing steps. Some aquatic athletes can handle this pounding; many cannot. This can be **poison** for *breaststrokers*, who produce tremendous tension on the inner aspects of their knees, and other swimmers who live and die by their legs. It is a wise coach who heeds his athletes complaints about joint pain after an extended dry-land running and jumping session. A better **cross-training** choice would be **bicycle and, or stationary bike riding**… better to let the rubber tires and, or the mechanical set-up take the pounding than the knees, ankles, and hips, since most trauma can have a negative cumulative effect over the long haul in a swimmer's career.

ASTHMA AND THE ATHLETE

There are two main types of asthma, though they affect the respiratory system similarly. Chronic asthma affects the sufferer continuously, sometimes made worse by infection, being in the presence of irritating and, or allergenic substances, or for seemingly no reason at all. The asthma that occurs **only upon vigorous exercise** is classified as Exercise-Induced *Bronchospasm* **(EIB). EIB can affect swim performance as much as 50%.** It is found in chronic asthmatics, highly-allergic individuals, and in about 15% of the healthy general population. EIB is treatable with oral inhalants, oral medication and nasal sprays which need to be coordinated with a physician. Unfortunately, irritating pool chemicals can aggravate the condition as can cold, dusty, smoky air, cigarettes and noxious exhaust fumes. This last category brings in a major dictate, in Public Health: **do not reside on the EAST side of a major highway unless you are near the ocean.**

(Since we are under the influence of prevailing Westerly winds, all who reside on the EAST side of a major thorough-fair get vehicular exhaust blown in their path day-in and day-out. At least one mile of separation (with hopefully much greenery in between) is needed to afford some protection unless near very influential on-shore ocean breezes.)

A hallmark of EIB is the fact that *symptoms* usually **develop between six and 12 minutes into the exercise bout and can resolve itself up to 90 minutes after exercise stops.** Wheezing, cough, feelings of fatigue and not getting enough air, chest tightness and even stomach pain are all hallmarks of EIB.

Proper hydration is a must to keep the airways moist and non-irritated (maybe a reason many asthmatics take up swimming), and an appropriate warm-up period before vigorous exercise is strongly suggested to help rid the body of chemicals that are irritating to the upper respiratory tract. Along with all this is the correct timing and administration of appropriate medication.

CHAPTER 10

SWIMMER'S EAR

ANATOMY OF THE EAR CANAL

Your ear has several sections. The eardrum separates the outer ear (slightly S shaped canal in most people) from the inner ear. The outer ear canal contains hair follicles and glands that produce earwax for normal protection, but it is this area that is most susceptible to the condition called Swimmer's Ear. This outer ear is normally relatively free of organisms. However, there are times you can develop a bacterial infection of the outer ear. Swimmer's ear is one such infection. It occurs when your ear is exposed to moisture for a prolonged period. Activities such as scuba diving, underwater swimming, synchronized swimming, or the daily grind of competitive swim training can lead to swimmer's ear.

PREVENTION OF SWIMMER'S EAR

Prevention is always easier than treatment; with this in mind… one should never attempt to remove earwax by methods that utilize rigid or semi-rigid apparatus. To remove wax to excess will only serve to sensitize the ear canal and make it vulnerable to infection. Wax has a natural lubricant function that protects the lining of the canal.

When you bathe or shower, you should only cleanse the outer ear by using a washcloth. You should not insert cotton swabs in the ear canal. They only seem to work by taking out a small portion of wax, whereas they actually push wax further in toward the ear drum where it can cause a plug known as an impaction.

Water should only be removed gently from the ear either by head movement to dislodge the moisture, blow drying the ear canal, or the use of an alcohol, or alcohol/acetic acid ear drop.

SYMPTOMS OF SWIMMER'S EAR

One can recognize swimmer's ear by the extreme discomfort it causes; even the movement of the jaw side-to-side can elicit intense pain in a full-blown case. It may also be noticed that the ear feels clogged, or full or has a "popping" sound, or that the hearing has become somewhat impaired.

Itching and, or pain are usually experienced. If pain is present, it usually is made worse by pulling on the ear lobe or putting pressure around the ear opening. At times, a malodorous discharge can come from the ear canal.

TREATMENT

To prevent further damage, resist any inclination to search the ear canal. Alcohol/acetic acid drops can aid a mild condition in that the drops produce three favorable conditions that would diminish the favorable environment for Swimmer's Ear: dehydration (the removal of water), disinfection, and the production of an acidic environment which inhibits bacterial growth. If the drops do not afford relief, a physician will have to prescribe an antibiotic/anti-inflammatory ear drop. Sometimes the prescription ear drop has a pain killer added. For serious infections, an oral antibiotic might also have to be taken.

For those who have had ear "tubes" inserted to equalize pressure between the outside and the middle ear, a constant opening is produced in the ear drum which precluded water sports unless the water can be physically barred from the canal as with silicon ear plugs.

CHAPTER 11

THE MAGNIFICENT BANANA

INTRODUCTION

In order to have a healthy lifestyle, consumption of at least five fruits and vegetables daily is something all athletes should strive for. And in my opinion, the best of all fruits especially for swimmers, is the magnificent banana. Any athlete worth his sweat and strain knows that there are several fine choices of this class of food that both satisfy taste and physical needs. But when one needs to really "fuel up," the choice should almost always be the banana. Research has shown that just two bananas can provide enough energy for a strenuous 90-minute workout, making the banana the number one choice among the world's top athletes. The banana constitutes almost a completely balanced diet in combination with milk. The two foods supplement each other in an ideal manner and provide nearly all the needed nutrients to the body. We know that most fruits are near ideal as food… Many are **fat-free** or nearly so, contain plenty of **water**, and have **natural sugars**. Some even have a few **natural organic** substances (hormones and proteins) that can positively affect various segments of the body's physiology. What, then, makes the banana such a standout among many beneficial choices and the most popular fruit in America?

PHYSICAL ASPECTS OF THE BANANA

First of all, the skin of the banana provides a natural covering to protect the fruit from exposure to potentially dangerous insecticides and other chemicals. (Even with washing, many fruits retain some contaminants that can present a potential problem down the road.) A medium-sized banana contains only about **110 calories (90 calories/100 grams** of fruit), yet provides at least *76% water in a pleasant-tasting, soft-consistent* package. There is no sodium (which could elevate blood pressure) and no cholesterol (that is indigenous to the animal world). Banana oil, as a flavoring, is quite palatable, is easily digested and rarely causes allergies. In fact, the banana is one of the foods of choice for the very young as it is used to help settle and regulate their sensitive digestive tracts. It can also be used to help control an acid stomach due to its natural antacid capacity. Up to four grams of fiber per banana can act to keep intestinal health a consistent condition. Many people suffer discomforting side effects taking in fiber supplements, consuming several bananas daily will most likely never be bothersome.

CHEMICAL ASPECTS OF THE BANANA

There are several important physiological substances that are found in every banana. The **carbohydrate** content is probably the largest single class of nutrient in the banana. As fruits mature and then age, their starch content converts to sugar content. A green banana, for instance, has about 7% sugars and 80% starch; the yellow banana has about 65% sugars and 25% starch. And the spotted and speckled banana is 90% sugars with only about 5% starch. The three quickly-absorbed natural sugars of the banana, *sucrose*, *fructose*, and *glucose*, allow for almost instant energy upon consumption. Since *glucose* is the prime sugar that the body needs to fuel the muscles and the only substance the brain can use as fuel for its functioning, it is a great choice for energy replacement. In addition, due to the sucrose and fructose content (which are transformed biochemically to *glucose*), the banana can also provide for an extended energy boost.

Bananas are famous for containing **potassium (470mg** each), an essential electrolyte that helps regulate blood chemistry and muscle activity. In fact, potassium (along with calcium and sodium) is extremely important in preventing the muscles from fatiguing and cramping during vigorous exercise. Potassium also presents something very important to sprint athletes: it helps to keep the acid content (pH) of the blood down. This has an important regulatory function when lactic acid builds up and causes the blood and muscle fibers to become too acidic. Too much acid (drop in pH) and the muscles shut down almost instantly. Anything that buffers this acid buildup will have the effect of allowing more vigorous muscular contraction for a longer period of time. The strong blood-pressure-lowering effect of potassium is such that the US Food and Drug Administration has now allowed the banana industry to make claims for the fruit's ability to reduce the risk of blood pressure and stroke. Research in "The New England Journal of Medicine" has shown that eating bananas as part of a regular diet can cut the risk of death by strokes by as much as 40%! And other research has shown over time that students can boost their "brain power" and stay more alert by taking in two to three potassium-packed bananas a day (before, during, and after schooling).

Bananas are also rich in **vitamin B6** (*pyridoxine*). This important vitamin is essential to the metabolic pathways of over 60 proteins, assists in red blood cell (RBC) production and helps regulate blood *glucose* levels. This together with its high *iron* content stimulates the production of *Hemoglobin* (Hb) which aids in the maintenance of a healthy blood picture to prevent *anemia* and carry oxygen to working muscles.

The banana gives you 17% of your daily value of **vitamin C** (*ascorbic acid*) though not heavy on this nutrient, it does contribute an antioxidant effect which neutralizes free radicals (harmful waste products or highly reactive elements that can damage many tissues with which they come in contact). Vitamin C is also very important to the making of collagen which is the base material of much of the body's connective tissue (ligaments, tendons, cartilage).

It was mentioned above that there are certain organic substances in the banana that can alter the body's physiology; in this case, brain physiology. Two substances: *tryptophan* and *nor-epinephrine* can act in consort to reduce anxiety and depression. The tryptophan is metabolized to *serotonin* which has a calming effect, and the nor-epinephrine acts as a psychic stimulant.

BANANA RECIPES

BREAKFAST:
Sliced bananas to cold cereal; banana pancakes or banana muffins; banana and yogurt shake; add bananas to bowl of mixed fruit with low fat yogurt.

LUNCH:
Add sliced bananas to fruit salad; eat a banana in addition to whatever you are eating; banana & peanut butter sandwich.

SNACK:
Banana by itself; make a "smoothie" with a banana and several other fruits and low fat yogurt or skim milk.

DESSERT:
Low fat banana milkshake; sliced bananas as a topping to fat-free frozen yogurt or low-fat ice cream.

CHAPTER 12

THE PHYSIOLOGIC CONSEQUENCES OF TOO MUCH STRESS

It is a common saying: *"stress kills."* More correctly, **unrelenting** stress can kill over time and when physiologic conditions allow. The body has mechanisms to handle stress. In fact small to moderate doses of physical stress actually does the body good when mixed with appropriate rest and recovery. But, as mentioned, when the stress mounts, doesn't stop, or becomes too much to handle, the amazing machine we call the human body breaks.

Our bodies have a built-in mechanism for protection from the effects of acute, immediate stress. This effect is called the *stress response.* It causes the body to produce and release hormones from the *adrenal gland* which act to allow the body to quickly adapt to its threatening environment Following this immediate *adrenaline rush* which functions to help us escape the present danger, massive amounts of *cortisol, the stress hormone,* is almost always released. The adrenal gland uses the base formative substance, cholesterol, to produce *adrenaline* and other stress hormones when tapped to do so under stressful and threatening situations. When the stress subsides, and the stress-related hormones are being broken down after use, cholesterol remains circulating throughout the body. We know the negative association cholesterol has when elevated in circulation over time, so excessive stress can cause this marker of troublesome physiology to produce pathology if not reduced in a timely fashion.

Nature provides a biological *circadian rhythm* for cortisol release dependent upon the "normal" cycle of human activity. It wanes to have the least amount normally available between midnight and about 4 AM. The body is supposed to be deep in the middle of restful and restoring sleep at this time so dealing with waking moments of stress is not built into this segment of our 24-hour day. This can help explain why going to bed with anxieties can interfere with a good night's restful sleep. Anything that is sufficiently troubling emotionally but has been put "on the back burner" of our consciousness during the day, can come to the fore and interrupt a normal sleep pattern in the wee hours of the morning when there is less cortisol to handle one (emotional) of several types of stress.

PHYSIOLOGICAL EFFECTS OF CORTISOL

Short-term bursts of cortisol are physiologically necessary to help the body recover from the damaging effects of short-term stress:

- Blood sugar levels are elevated, providing immediate energy supply.
- The immune system is bolstered in the short-term.
- Calcium is leached from bone and sent to muscle for contraction activity.
- The response to pain is reduced, helping to keep the focus on immediate survival.
- Short-Term memory is enhanced, enabling evasion of similar threats in the near future.

Short, intermittent bursts of cortisol helped protect our ancestors survive the wilds, and they still come to our aid today. But unlike what our ancestors had to endure, modern times present **chronic** physical and emotional stressful situations that are usually not able to be resolved quickly and thoroughly. Job loss, financial difficulties, troubling interpersonal relationships, academic pressures and various goal attainment interruptions are compounded with biological and public health difficulties such as obesity and environmental toxins. *If the stress lingers, elevated cortisol in the circulation lingers.* Having a physiologic situation where circulating cortisol remains high can threaten human health and longevity.

Chronic overexposure to cortisol can most certainly be devastating. Sustained blood sugar elevation can lead to excessive reflex insulin-stimulated release and beta-cell burnout of the pancreas. Substantial and prolonged loss of calcium from bone will lead to its honeycombing and weakening, a condition called *osteoporosis.* Constant stimulation of the immune system will lead to its breakdown, allowing the body to succumb to many illnesses. Hypertension requiring strong medication, loss of muscle mass, increased fat accumulation, and even diminished cognitive function are possible resultants from excessive cortisol exposure. A stark example would show a patient, having to endure chronic steroid therapy for various reasons of controlling inflammation, will most likely develop a round and puffy "moon face" due to fat and fluid accumulation. Also with extended steroid exposure, deposition of fat is also often times seen high on the upper back and has stirred the moniker of "buffalo hump." Stooped posture can result from bone loss in the spine as well as euphoria, depression and dementia from prolonged cortisol's effect on various segments of the brain.

ALLOWING THE GOOD, CONTROLLING THE BAD OF CORTISOL: THE USE OF *ADAPTOGENS*

So how can we preserve the *beneficial effects* of *short-term* cortisol elevations in response to acute, dangerous stress, while tamping down the *dangerous effects* of chronic, *long-tens* cortisol elevations? That is where plant-based compounds that improve resistance to stress come into physiologic play. They are called *adaptogens.* These organic compounds have undergone several preclinical (animal) and clinical (human) studies and have been seen to exert system-wide protective and restorative effects, increasing longevity and healthy life spans so far in experimental animal models. They have also been shown to favorably modulate the stress response, restore vital organ function, and boost immunity in humans. And they have shown activity to combat aging cognitive function, minimizing depression and anxiety. To no one's surprise, sports physiologists have now developed serious interest because of these *adaptogens* and their ability to enhance muscle contractive performance, increase its endurance and prevent resultant muscle-fiber damage while improving muscular blood circulation.

The concept of "adaptogens" goes back thousands of years in Chinese herbal medicine and was often sought to help the body withstand the slings and arrows of life. The term, *"adaptogen,"* was coined in 1947 by a Russian scientist who defined an "adaptogen" as *an agent that aides an organism in its effort to counteract and resist a variety of stressors.* In 2001, noted nutrition scientist Gregory S. Kelly, intrigued with this class of substances, updated and strengthened criteria for defining an adaptogen, requiring that any one of these substances must:

- Produce an increase in power of resistance against multiple stressors, including physical, chemical, biological agents, or emotional.
- Normalize physiology, helping the body maintain youthful function, regardless of the cause of stress.
- Normalize bodily functions beyond what is required to gain resistance to stress naturally.

Adaptogens exert a normalizing effect*:* They allow organisms to increase healthy functions that are impaired by stress, and to decrease unhealthy responses that can be triggered by stress without any risk of "overshooting" and creating an unbalanced response. Scientists use the term *"homeostasis"* to describe the body's ability to maintain physiological function within certain parameters, including temperature, respiratory rate, and blood chemistry within tightly controlled limits. In mainstream language, then, adaptogens simply enhance the body's ability to maintain *homeostasis* and fight age-inducing stress.

The main target of investigation has been the substance, *rhodiola,* which had been scarcely heard of in this country, but had been the target of increasing interest for quite a while in Russia. The reason for this was that Soviet scientists were looking for something to first give their cosmonauts to improve their endurance, concentration, and strength during extremely taxing space missions. As the cold war continued, the Soviets wanted to build on their lead over the Americans in the "space race" and began to intently study *rhodiola* and other adaptogenic herbs and how they could allow their space program people to endure (with quality) prolonged missions in the unfriendly environment of outer space. US astronauts were placed in the same dangerous environment but with much less demand for prolonged exposure. Our scientists were amazed as to the length of time the Russians could tolerate the out-of-this-world existence even when we chose the best of our best. They had *adaptogens;* we did not. Their military and elite athletic personnel were also enabled with these *adaptogens* specifically to handle situations where long-term stress was an issue.

Russian physiologists and medical researchers knew that high levels of cortisol initiate a dangerous cascade of stress and disease that would hamper the efforts of their best and brightest if allowed to suffer over time. They searched for, discovered, and took the pains to categorize *rhodiola's* adaptogenic powers such that they could lessen the mounting impairments often produced by chronic stress without interfering with the valuable short-term stress response. So far there are 16 scientifically established adaptogens, or plant extracts, endowed with the power to enhance system-wide function in the aging human. Present-day researchers are further validating *rhodiola's* ability to mitigate the negative impact of chronic cortisol elevations.

A large, phase III (human test subjects) placebo-controlled clinical trial was conducted in Sweden in 2009, studying participants aged 20-55 *years* with a diagnosis of stress-related fatigue and emotional burn-out. Those taking the actual *rhodiola* had significantly lower cortisol responses to chronic stress than did the placebo recipients, and, as a result, they had lower scores on scales of burnout and showed improved performances on cognitive testing.

A similar-protocol testing model was performed in China also in 2009. It revealed like results with stress-induced elevated cortisol but in otherwise healthy individuals. The target results here showed that subjects pre-medicated with *rhodiola* showed no increase in their cortisol levels, while levels rose sharply among placebo recipients when both groups were exposed to chronic stress in the form of endurance exercise. An added positive to this study showed that *rhodiola* also increased the efficiency with which subjects used oxygen, potentially reducing additional stress from oxygen radicals.

Advanced laboratory studies have demonstrated that *rhodiola* achieves its cortisol-lowering, stress-fighting effects through several different mechanisms. It directly interacts with the brain/adrenal gland axis to reduce cortisol production while enhancing stress-resistance proteins. It stimulates "stress-sensor" proteins to reduce the production and impact of cortisol, resulting in enhanced mental and physical performance and even longevity. And multiple studies have demonstrated the complete lack of side effects from *rhodiola* supplementation.

Modulating the Stress Response: Unlike any other compound, adaptogens condition your body to respond favorably to stress at the physiological level through a unique mechanism. Adaptogens deliver minute shocks of mild stress that condition your physiology to respond to more major stresses in a favorable way similar to the vaccine theory of inoculating the body with a small but harmless amount of a virus to help the body build the ability to fend off a major attack.

Experiments with *rhodiola* have repeatedly shown its ability to reduce fatigue and restore normal mental and physiological functioning, even in stressed humans categorized as having "burnout" as a presenting emotional state. Studies that took place in Russia in 2000 and 2003 of two highly-stressed types of individuals: doctors working over-night shifts and students studying for major exams, demonstrated improvement in fatigue level, neuro-motor performance, and perceptive and cognitive function, even when tested under ongoing stressful condition.

Another more recent study in 2010 of young to middle-aged women with significant impairment from living in psychologically stressful environments demonstrated improved scores on attention, speed, and accuracy during stressful cognitive tasks. And those positive effects were evident just two hours after a single dose of *rhodiola* combined with Siberian ginseng and *Schisandra chinensis.* And no serious side effects were reported in this or any other study of *rhodiola.*

A Powerful Weapon Against Anxiety*:* In addition to handling the above-mentioned symptoms of stress, *rhodiola* has shown promise in alleviating **stress-related symptoms** such as anxiety and a diminished appetite. A 2008 study (daily dosage of 340mg for 10 weeks, age range 34-55) shined a light on *rhodiola's* ability to circumvent the symptoms (difficulty concentrating, irritability, tense muscles, sleep disturbances, and trouble controlling worries) and severity of general anxiety disorder, a common condition characterized by frequent excessive worry that is out of proportion to external circumstances.

As researchers are wont to do, they investigated *rhodiola* in greater detail. They discovered that one of this adaptogen's key components, the phytochemical, *salidroside,* showed activity responsible for many of its anti-aging properties, as well as being an important factor in its ability to help combat anxiety. A 2007 animal study showed that *salidroside* produced notable sedative (calming) and hypnotic (sleep-inducing) effects in a dose-dependent fashion. A different 2007 study showed that administering pure *salidroside* to animals reversed stress-induced anorexia. When the study advanced to human test subjects, results were repeatedly seen to support *rhodiola's* ability to calm individuals subjected to mounting stress and to restore normal patterns of rest and eating. What seemed to be common folk-lore knowledge for hundreds of years in China and Russia seems to have been backed up with these recent studies.

Enhanced Longevity*:* Another amazing aspect to this adaptogen's activity is that it possess the power to *restore* malfunctioning biological systems, a key factor in reducing the detrimental effects of aging. In testing multiple organisms, *rhodiola* was found to enhance healthy responses to negative stressors in the environment by protecting human cells from premature aging when they were exposed to oxidative stress, acute and chronic heat shocks, and toxic chemical exposure. To ensure reproducible results, the investigators again worked with the isolated phytochemical, *salidroside.* The focus of one of these studies was the ability of *salidroside* to enhance aged skin cells' ability to reproduce in mice and, thus, produce, new healthy, vital skin. They also cataloged its ability to prevent various pathological conditions of aging by preventing the accumulation of inflammatory **A**dvanced **G**lycation **E**nd products **(AGEs).** This presents a rather remarkable fact in that, up till now, the only way to show reproducible prolongation of life in the animal model was to institute severe calorie restriction. The work with *salidroside* became the first studied activity to definitely prolong life outside of deliberate caloric restriction, and its mechanism of activity is independent of various diets.

Bolstering Heart Health: Heart disease has been the number one killer in America for many decades, and studies have shown that many cardiac events are absolutely stress-induced. Stress, whether physical, emotional, or chemical allows for the *adrenaline* reflex to occur. This powerful hormone, secreted by the adrenal glands above the kidneys, prepares the body for flight or fight and causes all sorts of internal physiological changes that are not conducive to well-being if allowed to linger unabated.

The link between the administration of *Rhodiola Rosea* extract and prevention of potentially dangerous abnormal heart rhythms (*arrhythmia*) has also been studied for years in Russia. Various animals were pretreated with this adaptogen for only a few days each in several studies, and they were found to be resistant to chemicals known to cause irregular heartbeats; they were also much less vulnerable to heart damage caused by experimentally-induced myocardial infarctions (frank heart attacks).

In follow-up studies where *rhodiola* was given to animal models having induced coronary artery disease with concomitant impaired oxygen delivery to cardiac muscle, the extract helped decrease the heart muscle's oxygen consumption needs while increasing oxygen supply to the functioning heart, helping to ensure that the cardiac muscle proper had enough oxygen required for optimal functioning.

With such positive investigative studies on animals, human trials are now being set up to clarify *rhodiola's* potential to protect man from the number one killer threatening his quality of life.

Vital Organ Function and Enhanced Immunity*: Rhodiola* has also shown specific activity to support natural antioxidant systems in the liver and to protect it from various toxins and the oxidative stresses it undergoes every day. Being the main organ of detoxification, anything that enhances the liver's main activity and protects it from day-to-day exposure to numerous toxins routed through it, will most certainly protect and enhance the quality of human life. As adaptogens, the *rhodiola* species also carefully modulate the immune system, increasing its response to real threats of infection or malignancy, while preventing excessive inflammation. It has been shown to lessen the amount of the inflammatory-induced marker, **C-R**eactive **Protein (CRP)** circulating in the blood. CRP can show either a generalized or cardio-specific inflammatory process. Obviously, if an elevated CRP can be reduced by *Rhodiola* so can an on-going inflammatory process. It was also tested to see if it had generalized enhanced immune influence, and it did. The adaptogen increased the positive formation of antibodies to a tetanus toxoid stimulus in rats, in a 2010 study.

Rhodiola also possess direct antiviral and antibacterial activities which were brought out in several lab studies over the past four years. These were performed mostly on animal subjects but studies with the flu had human subjects; all the responses were positive and reproducible. Of specific interest was the fact that *rhodiola* had the ability to block certain enzymes (e.g. *neuraminidase*) that flu viruses exhibit after exposure that enhances their ability to attach to and invade the cells of the upper respiratory tract. This is a major finding in infectious disease control since flu transmission is so rampant with modem international transportation and in congested populations.

Combating Brain Aging: The well-known neuro-degeneration in Alzheimer's and Parkinson's diseases occurs as a result of inflammation in the nervous system coupled with the accumulation of harmful, pro-oxidant (*beta-amyloid*) proteins that trigger even more inflammation and ultimately brain cell destruction. Constituents from *rhodiola* species such as *salidroside* display powerful antioxidant properties that prevent oxidative, pro-inflammatory effects, as well as the actual formation of these proteins and the subsequent inflammatory cascade. The results of several studies with several different test animal models have all shown that, under lab-induced oxidative reactions with hydrogen peroxide, fewer brain cells died from intense oxidative stress.

Several Chinese studies have shown that nerve cells in the memory centers of the brain resist age-related damage and produce more beneficial neurotransmitters after treatment with *rhodiola* in rats. Both short-term and long-term memory enhancements have been demonstrated with several *rhodiola* extracts on human models in Russia where mental performance and acuity (test-taking) under experimentally-induced adverse conditions (sleep deprivation) at sea level and at altitude have resisted deterioration. And, finally, *rhodiola has* helped aging humans fall asleep faster, stay asleep longer, and with improved quality of rest by increasing the amount of time in healthful REM (rapid eye movement) sleep. Greater blood oxygenation during sleep was also observed which is a key longevity factor.

PHYSICAL PERFORMANCE ENHANCEMENT

Whenever sports physiologists and physicians hear of anything that can enhance the functions of the human body, they think physicality enhancement. Increased performance under all sorts of adversity was studied for years by the Russians when their space program was in serious competition with the United States. Their military personnel and cosmonauts were given *rhodiola* extracts and observed for positive physiologic effects. They were not disappointed. This lead their researchers to test a third segment of human endeavor undergoing extreme demands of physical capacity: the building of world class athletes.

But with constant, repetitive, intense physical training comes a greater tendency to produce injury from oxidative stress, muscle cell damage, and generalized inflammation. If a substance with no deleterious side effects can induce resistance to all these dangers, it will generate great interest in laboratory study that is now going on.

When tested with elite-level rowers, rhodiola increased antioxidant blood levels and minimized oxidative stress-induced muscle damage for up to 24 hours after strenuous training. And the time to exhaustion in both an extended-yardage crew course and with extended yardage swimming was significantly increased due to marked increases in oxygen delivery to muscle tissue during the actual workouts.

Rhodiola species have been used for centuries by villagers living at marked altitude in the Himalayas to enhance their resistance to the effects of oxygen deprivation and to boost their endurance for strenuous tasks. This information has been distilled and clarified in various lab studies to show how the *rhodiola* adaptogens protect internal organs from low oxygen levels found at higher altitudes, and that can also occur if suffering a heart attack or stroke. These tissue-oxygen adaptations have also proven equally beneficial at more moderate altitudes all the way down to sea level. Physiologically, *rhodiola* helps exercisers work out longer, increasing their oxygen uptake and decreasing the markers for muscle damage post exercise. When long-term supplementation with *rhodiola* happens, energy storage capacity is boosted, and blood oxygen levels increase prior to exercise, further enhancing workout capacity and endurance.

A major 2011 study also revealed a significant helpful property of *rhodiola* by its prevention of a physiologic phenomenon known as **vascular remodeling** in lung tissue at high altitude. This deadly occurrence is defined by the thickening of pulmonary blood vessels that contribute to increased blood pressure in the lungs, known as **pulmonary hypertension.** The danger lies in the potential for a rapid production of congestive heart failure if not quickly corrected. There are also other causes of this dangerous condition: cardiovascular disease, obesity, and obstructive sleep apnea. *Rhodiola's* ability to prevent vascular remodeling represents the possibility of an important and much needed new approach to managing a major cause of death and disability in older adults.

Rapid Take-Home Points: Rhodiola is a cortisol-suppressing herb that is becoming an increasingly popular dietary intervention due to several lab tests proving positive effects protecting many organ functions of the human body. It is one of a handful of known **adaptogens... plant-based compounds known to support long, healthy lifespan in part by exerting system-wide protective and restorative effects.** Rhodiola has been shown to favorably modulate the stress response, restore vital organ function, and boost immunity. It is a low-cost nutrient that combats cognitive dysfunction, minimizing depression and anxiety, while enhancing muscle performance, endurance, and circulatory health.

Physiologic System Wide Benefits From Rhodiola At A Glance

Reduces Stress	**Lowers levels of cortisol; Restores normal physiological responses to stress; Fights stress-induced despair; Restores brain cells in areas damaged by stress-induced depression**
Protects the Heart	**Prevents stress- and ischemia-induced heart muscle damage; Increases heart muscle cell tolerance to reduced blood flow (ischemia); Prevents stress- and heart attack-induced arrhythmias; Reduces size of heart muscle infarction (tissue death); Promotes new cardiac blood vessel growth after heart attack**
Protects the Liver	**Prevents toxin- and oxidative stress-induced liver cell damage: Reduces serum markers of liver dysfunction; Restores depleted liver stores of natural antioxidants**

Prevents Cancer

Inhibits proliferation of human leukemia cells; Inhibits growth and induces death of human cancer cells (apoptosis); Reduces new blood vessel formation (angiogenesis) in tumors

Protects Against Radiation

Increases survival following otherwise lethal total-body irradiation; Reduces radiation-induced lipid oxidation (antioxidant effect); Scavenges radiation-induced free radicals; Prevents anemia from red blood cell membrane damage

Modulates the Immune System

Anti-inflammatory effects in settings of excessive inflammation; Stimulates appropriate immune responses; Boosts immune response to vaccines; Antiviral activity against hepatitis C, influenza, and Coxsackie virus (causes viral myocarditis); Antibacterial activity vs Staph aureus and tuberculosis; works to boost suppressed immune function following chemotherapy

CHAPTER 13

MITOCHONDRIA AND THE ESSENCE OF LIFE

This is my second paper on the energy-producers of the body. The fact of knowing exactly which elements at the cellular level are responsible for producing most of the body's energy and the new knowledge of how their metabolic actions are intimately related to preventing or at least lessening several diseases and dysfunctions as the body ages has absolutely captivated me. Only a few years back there were not very many articles devoted to *mitochondria*... their use, their development, when their dysfunction leads to disease. But bio-medical researchers have now come to the conclusion that as goes the *mitochondria*, so goes the quality of life. Almost 800 articles were published the last two years, and the topic has become the "stuff" of physiological investigations on several fronts. As our knowledge and understanding grow in studying the functionality of *mitochondria*, they are seen to be inexorably entwined with more and more pathology and the ravages of aging as their primary function diminishes or ceases, and the opposite shows true that physiologic problems either diminish or dissolve away as we generate more healthy vibrant *mitochondria*, and the body is able not only to move with more vigor but to thrive.

An overview of the interaction of *mitochondria* and the major organs and life systems will enlighten the reader as to the fact that fully-functional *mitochondria* is the key to longevity and the quality of life. Almost all energy (nearly 95%) in a cell is derived from the activity of intracellular *mitochondria*. Unlike most other cellular components, *mitochondria* are also able to divide and multiply *in-situ* (within the cell) such that as the numbers of vibrant *mitochondria* increase, the better the guarantee of healthy functioning throughout the body.

HEALTHY MITOCHONDRIA ESSENTIAL FOR PROPER BRAIN FUNCTION

While it has been shown that compounds like co-enzyme **Q10**, *L-carnitine*, and *alpha lipoic acid* support *mitochondrial* function and aid in their protection from their innate processes to produce the energy of life, early research centered only around keeping the *mitochondria* intact and functioning as they relate to cardiac activity. Overlooked was the large amount of energy required for brain cells to carry out their specialized functions and that of other vital organ systems. Dealing with just the central nervous system, researchers in 2010 at the University of California (at Davis) and a few other institutions have corroborated the role of abnormal *mitochondrial* dynamics with neuronal cell death and the onset of

Alzheimer's, Parkinson's disease, Huntington's chorea, and other neuro-degenerative disorders.

Those fortunate enough to make it into their eighth decade nevertheless have the Sword of Damocles hanging over them in that they face the danger of a 30% or more chance of suffering from Alzheimer's dementia. Specific pathologic mechanisms have been elucidated that reveal the role of *mitochondrial* dysfunction in the initiation and progression of this hideous disease such that most of the physiological investigators have concluded that *mitochondrial* protection and subsequent reduction of oxidative stress are important targets for prevention and long-term treatment of early stages of Alzheimer's disease.

The reader can see the compounded positive effects and the absolute pertinence and importance of ancillary research taking this a step further by demonstrating the activity of the first substance known to science *PyrroloQuiniline Quinone (PQQ)* to actually allow the body to create new *mitochondria*. *The* critical factor that we seek to keep the body moving with vigor as it chronologically ages is the *continuous generation of new vibrant fully-functional mitochondria* within our cells... *mitochondrial biogenesis*. We want the body to obviously age in years but not as much physiologically.

CARDIAC DIFFICULTIES WITH DYSFUNCTIONAL MITOCHONDRIA

Damage to the *mitochondria* of endothelial cells (composing the *inner* lining of the *coronary* arteries, in this case) is an underlying cause of atherosclerosis. Traditional risk factors for arterial disease such as smoking, obesity, high blood sugar, elevated cholesterol and *triglycerides* all bring with them various degrees of *inflammation* and subsequent *mitochondrial* injury. It is these localized inflammatory responses on the inner lining *(intima)* that allow for the fats circulating in the blood to become drawn to and forcefully-attached onto the insides of the arteries. Eventually, as the depositing of the fats become more entrenched over time, persistent coronary artery blockage ensues which can bring on a clot (thrombosis) for sudden and dramatic coronary circulatory blockage and damage or the gradual, but inexorably just as debilitating severe weakening of cardiac muscle that produces what is labeled *congestive heart failure*. Reduce the inflammation with a powerful antioxidant such as **PQQ** (5,000 times more biologically potent than vitamin C), and this process can be lessened or eliminated. Produce new vibrant *mitochondria* and we can alter the negative effects of dysfunctional and non-functional *mitochondria*.

A study published in 2010 looked at left ventricular heart muscle tissue in patients with end-stage heart failure vs. normal hearts. Compared to well-functioning hearts, *mitochondrial* DNA was DECREASED by 40% in failing hearts. This was accompanied by REDUCTIONS of up to 80% in *mitochondrial* DNA-encoded proteins of failing hearts. Thus if there is a paucity of *mitochondrial* DNA, there is no *mitochondrial* biogenesis in the failing heart. Nutrients like **co-enzyme Q10**, L-carnitine, and alpha lipoic acid have shown to improve clinical and symptomatic indicators of congestive heart failure. Add the ability of **PQQ** to promote actual *mitochondrial* biogenesis, and the possibility of even greater improvements in cardiac function are there to experience.

DYSFUNCTIONAL MITOCHONDRIA CONTRIBUTING TO HUMAN CANCERS

With the human element, in some cases, many years can pass from carcinogenic exposure to clinical occurrence. The "something-plus-something" coupling is usually the cause and effect. The first "something" is the exposure to the chemical or physical substance that can disrupt DNA functionality; the "plus-something" is the body's resultant physiologic reaction to it. Cancer is fundamentally connected to *mitochondrial* dysfunction. A dramatic decline in *mitochondrial* energy production with progressing dysfunction from damaging exposure or the inevitable processes of aging is associated with the allowance of increased free radicals which cause cellular mutations throughout the body including those of *mitochondria*. These mutations can grossly interfere with and inhibit the immune system and the normal cell-removal process known as *apoptosis.*

A critical factor in protecting against cancer is the ability to eliminate *damaged* cells through *apoptosis*. Much research is now focused on the huge energy-dependent processes required to eradicate faulty or abnormally-growing cells. Physiologically, dysfunctional *mitochondria* deny cells the ability to go through normal apoptotic removal processes, thus sowing the seeds for cancer initiation and inevitable progression. In addition, *mitochondria* are the source for several apoptotic proteins that activate desired cell death in the quest to eliminate damaged tissue.

Mitochondrial dysfunction that occurs as a result of normal aging has a major influence on the body's ability to produce cancer cells. A major study completed in 2010 showed that the more *mitochondrial* dysfunction, the greater the prediction of progression of prostate cancer in those undergoing surgery for it. While the *reversal* of *mitochondrial* senescence in non-tumor cells using **PQQ** as the sole strong cellular antioxidant produced cells more resilient to tumor initiation, cancer cells that have already evolved are better controlled by *tumor suppressor genes* activated by *vibrant mitochondrial* cell-signaling.

MITOCHONDRIA INSUFFICIENCY PROMOTES TYPE 2 DIABETES

One of the three chief maladies of the **metabolic syndrome,** *insulin resistance*, is, sooner or later, the foundation for developing frank diabetes. A host of dangerous sequelae ensue over time that can negatively impact several organs and systems as elevated circulating blood sugar continues to ramble out-of-control. There is usually found a genetic component that steers the physiology toward an inability to *glucose* tolerance along with physical inactivity.

When studied, several young, lean sedentary children with insulin resistance whose parents had developed type 2 diabetes were discovered to have, on average, 38% LESS *mitochondrial* density in their muscles than counterparts from normal parents. These metabolically-challenged children also showed increased amounts of fat content in the musculature, which also contributes to insulin resistance. This supports the concept that *hereditary mitochondrial* dysfunction contributes to the development of inflammation, insulin resistance, and subsequent type 2 diabetes.

The encouraging aspect to this study is that those genetically predisposed to type 2 diabetes may be able to avert this calamity through either rigorous physical exercise and, or supplementation with **PQQ**, both of which have been shown to promote *mitochondrial* biogenesis. There are even a few types of anti-diabetic drugs, metformin and the thiazolidinedione's, which work to produce *mitochondrial* biogenesis as a desired side effect through other pathways of pharmacology and physiology.

THE NEED FOR FUNCTIONAL MITOCHONDRIA TO REJUVENATE STEM CELLS AND CELLULAR DNA

The human body possess an innate remarkable ability to renew and repair many tissue and organ systems allowing most of us to enter into maturity and old age. Ideally, this activity is vigorous and comprehensive throughout most of life but it often wanes after entry into maturity. As aging progresses, and life's experiences cross our paths, exposure to toxins, inflammation, moderate to strong oxidants, and physical and emotional trauma all challenge the physiologic ability to continue to thrive. Nature has provided for this life-preservation by way of *somatic stem cells.*

Research completed in 2010 has shown that *intact, vigorous mitochondria* are essential for maintenance of strong functioning stem cells. In response to *mitochondrial* impairment and insufficiency, there always develops increasing amounts of free radicals accompanied by stem cell compromise. Further research has shown that stem cell populations do not necessarily decline with advancing age, but instead, lose their *restorative* potential. This *functional* stem cell decline is usually followed by organ malfunction and increased incidence of disease. *Mitochondrial* dysfunction therefore underlies a progressive, degenerative cycle that robs aging humans of the **renewal** benefits of their own stem cells.

It is a short leap of logic that the researchers looking into the importance of *mitochondria* to the quality of life have proposed that absolute integration of processes to produce large amounts of functional vigorous *mitochondria* into the very core of the "axis of aging" will yield successful therapeutic strategies designed to rejuvenate tissues of the aged. As long as we have enough strong working *mitochondria* we should have vigorous physiology for most of our existence.

WHEN MITOCHONDRIA DETERIORATE

There are various downward spirals in physiology. When there is muscular pain there are spasms; spasms make more pain that make more spasms. We see the same negative spiraling at the cellular level that can portend dangerous outcomes. Glycated (proteins cross-linked with sugar molecules) or otherwise damaged proteins can bind to functional *mitochondria* and render them dysfunctional. The resultant accumulation of dysfunctional *mitochondria* results in a vicious negative cycle whereby increased oxidative and glycation reactions disable more *mitochondria*, eventually leading to a cell's demise.

Research in 2010 highlighted the fact that the accumulation of **inactive** *mitochondria* in tissue drives the lethal cascade first to cellular damage then to cellular death as mostly seen in the elderly; it also showed the counterbalanced effect of the protection provided to the cells by L-carnitine, carnosine, alpha lipoic acid, resveratrol, and PQQ. The fortunate young with virtually no *mitochondrial* damage experience a vigorous existence.

MITOCHONDRIA AND THE HUMAN HEALTH SPAN

The aging of the American society is upon us with an accelerated impact on healthcare expenditures. Present-day conventional medical practitioners are taught to focus mostly on what they can see immediately in front of them. They treat the apparent signs and symptoms of disease but fail to correct the major underlying cause at the cellular level... *mitochondrial dysfunction.* The number of articles published since 1980 centering around this topic has exponentially exploded into the scientific literature as knowledge builds upon knowledge in our understanding of this cellular organelle and how it can sustain a healthy life span.

The consumption of the above-mentioned supplements has been shown repeatedly in peer-reviewed scientific analyses to either maintain *mitochondrial* integrity or increase their number by the process of *mitochondrial biogenesis.* With the discovery of the unique properties of **PQQ** and its ability to promote *mitochondrial* formation, a missing link to the puzzle of degenerative aging has been uncovered.

Pyrroloquinoline quinone [PQQ]

156

CHAPTER 14

THE IMPORTANCE OF PQQ... THE FIRST NEW VITAMIN IN 35 YEARS

Energy is required to keep all living things just that way... living. Simply being alive continuously takes thousands of complex processes preceding, succeeding, and augmenting each other such that enzymes, hormones, muscles, organ tissue, and bodily fluids are able to produce movement, force, heat, repair, and end-of-reaction by-products. In the grand scheme of division of labor, Nature has assigned the task for energy-formation in the remarkably complex body to ubiquitous small segments of each cell... the *mitochondria.*

Unfortunately for those wanting to experience a long, active, productive life, it has been determined that *mitochondrial damage, dysfunction, and deterioration link to many illnesses that can manifest themselves with the aging process.* As we age, overall energy dissipates, and the zest for life can fade with the morning mist. The up-side approach from recent physiologic analyses shows that *the more healthy, functional mitochondria we can manufacture and preserve in our cells, the greater our abilities to endure and partake vigorously of what life lays before us.* The simple muscle-tissue analysis of an aged man in his eighth decade can produce up to 95% damaged and dysfunctional *mitochondria* while that from a five-year-old presents with almost no damage to these energy-producing elements. How many of us have wondered where the "little ones" get all their energy compared to how we need to pace and recover.

As a coach and competitive masters swimmer, I personally consume and have offered to many of my athletes, substances (l-carnitine, alpha-lipoic acid, and co-enzyme Q10) to protect from oxidative destruction what *mitochondria* we produce from consistent, vigorous training. Up until now, the two main avenues for *mitochondrial* production have been gross caloric deprivation (the body trying to keep alive while sensing greatly reduced caloric intake and to compensate, upping the production of cellular *mitochondria*) and, much more conducive to the athletic world, pushing past the comfort zone with appropriate enzyme, hormone, and tissue adaptation, aided and abetted by correct hydration and "re-fueling" (eating) along with rest and recovery. Even with all the care and fore-thought needed for good physiologic adaptation, much of the *mitochondrial* production is destroyed by its own ongoing oxidative processes while producing energy. It can be a long and difficult process "climbing the mountain" over many months into years to produce noticeable increases in adaptation of strength, power, and condition. But add the potential for the first time ever of being physiologically able to induce the body to produce *new mitochondria* even in aging cells, and the possibilities become mouth-watering.

Though most of the recent hands-on lab research involving PQQ with pertinent physiology and biochemistry has used preclinical models (rats), so many of the experiments have evolved with success that the jump to the human model has started in earnest within the past few years and is taking place with increasing frequency now and will continue in the immediate offing.

MITOCHONDRIAL GENERAL FUNCTION AND ACTIVITY THROUGHOUT THE BODY

Mitochondria are the only cell components, other than the nucleus, to possess their own DNA. This provides for their ability to continually replicate allowing for strongly increasing their numbers. Depending upon tissue function, ambient oxidative states, and appropriate nutrient, and other physiologic factors, *mitochondrial* content in various organs and tissues can range from a few to a few thousand. Physiology dictates that the more *mitochondria* produced, the better to help withstand stresses, provide for more power and enhance endurance, and to possibly extend viability... life.

The problem aging presents to all of us is that our *mitochondria* degrade and become less capable of producing energy. This type of deterioration occurs more rapidly than with other cellular components. To distill this down to its essence: for most of us, *it is the loss of* **FUNCTIONAL** *mitochondria that can ultimately spell our personal demise.*

PQQ (PYRROLOQUINOLINE QUINONE)

The body cannot synthesize PQQ, thus, it is considered an essential nutrient. It has now been classified as *the first new vitamin (placed within the B-complex grouping) in 55 years.* It is found in many plant species, bacteria, the animal kingdom, and can be present in human milk. It functions as an extraordinarily potent anti-oxidant and has shown to be excellent in defense against *mitochondrial* decay. PQQ's structure is sufficiently sturdy to enable it to withstand exposure to oxidation up to 5,000 times greater than vitamin C. Early findings have elucidated PQQ's central role in growth and overall development across multiple forms of life. Studies have already revealed that when deprived of dietary PQQ, animals exhibit stunted growth, compromised immunity, impaired reproductive capability, and most emphatically, fewer *mitochondria* in their tissue. When PQQ was introduced back into the diet, these deficiencies were reversed, restoring systemic function while simultaneously INCREASING *mitochondrial* number and energy efficiency.

When combined with the anti-oxidant, Co Q10, physiologic research has shown that just 20 mg per day of PQQ can significantly preserve and enhance memory, attention, and cognition in aging humans. But an exciting revelation on PQQ emerged in early 2010 when researchers found it not only protected *mitochondria* from oxidative damage, it actually stimulated growth of NEW *mitochondria*. New *mitochondria* = new cells possibly anywhere in the body.

158

PQQ'S ACTIVITY AT THE CELLULAR LEVEL

Mitochondrial bio-genesis can be defined as the growth and division of preexisting *mitochondria* to produce more. Actual physical numbers of *mitochondria* not only increase but also their size and mass.

This bio-genesis requires the coordinated synthesis and import of up to 1,500 proteins. The process occurs through the combined effects of "alphabet-soup-labeled" genes activated by PQQ via the following three mechanisms:

- PQQ increases expression of *peroxisome proliferator-activated receptor gamma co-activator 1-alpha* (PGC-1a). This is a master regulator gene that mobilizes your cells' response to various external triggers. It directly activates genes that boost *mitochondrial* and cellular respiration, growth, and reproduction. This capacity to modulate cellular metabolism at the genetic level favorably influences blood pressure, cholesterol, and *triglyceride* breakdown and can delay the onset of obesity.
- PQQ activates a signaling protein known as *c-AMP-response element-binding protein*(CREB). This gene plays a pivotal role in embryonic development and growth. It also beneficially interacts with histones... compounds shown to protect and repair cellular DNA. CREB also stimulates the growth of new *mitochondria*.
- PQQ regulates a recently discovered gene called DJ-1. As with both PGC-1a and CREB, DJ-1 is intrinsically involved in cell function and survival and has demonstrated its ability to prevent cell death by combating the intense stresses placed upon antioxidants. This is of particular importance to brain health and function. DJ-1 damage and mutation have been conclusively linked to the onset of Parkinson's disease and other neurological disorders.

PQQ'S ABILITY TO PROTECT AGAINST MITOCHONDRIA-GENERATED FREE RADICALS

It is a physiologic irony that, as the primary energy engines of our cells, the *mitochondria* rank among the structures MOST vulnerable to destruction from what they produce: oxidative damage. You would think Nature would have provided more protection for her own tissues as we evolved over the millennia. But with these physiologic processes, there is substantial deficiency in protective activity. The chief oxidative apparatus is quite susceptible to severe damage from its intrinsic functionality.

As the cell's power generators, *mitochondria* are the sites of enormous and constant oxidative activity that spews out gross amounts of toxic free radicals. To make matters worse (relative to nuclear DNA in all cells that have a nucleus) *mitochondrial* DNA possesses few defenses against free radical damage. The DNA in the nucleus proper is protected by several "guardian" proteins that blunt the impact of free radicals. No such repair systems exist to protect *mitochondrial* DNA.

We see nuclear DNA enjoying superior structural defenses by being housed within a protective double-membrane that separates it from the rest of the cell. This protective barrier is complemented by a dense matrix of filamentous proteins called the *nuclear lamina*... a kind of hard shell casing to further buffer nuclear DNA from external impacts.

By comparison, *mitochondrial* DNA is left almost entirely exposed. It attaches DIRECTLY to the inner membrane where the *mitochondria's* electrochemical furnace rages continuously, generating an enormous volume of toxic reactive oxygen species. This is why supplementation with substances like Co-Enzyme Q10, Lipoic Acid, L-Carnitine, and now PQQ is so important. The extraordinary antioxidant capacity of PQQ represents a powerful new intervention that should effectively reinforce the mitochondria's meager defenses.

PQQ'S ABILITY FOR NEURO-PROTECTION: WORKING AGAINST BRAIN AGING

PQQ has been shown to optimize function of the entire central nervous system in rodent models. It reversed cognitive impairment caused by chronic oxidative stress when lab rats were tested, improving their memory performances. PQQ can also greatly diminish dangerous toxic oxidative elements that can arise from physical damage to the Central Nervous System (CNS).

These toxic elements, ***Reactive Nitrogen Species*** (RNS) and ***Reactive Oxygen Species*** (ROS) impose severe stresses on damaged neurons. They arise spontaneously following stroke and spinal cord injury and have been shown to account for a substantial proportion of subsequent long-term neurological damage. PQQ directly suppresses RNS in experimentally-induced strokes. It also provides additional protection by blocking gene expression of inducible *nitric oxide synthase*, a major source of RNS, following spinal cord injury.

PQQ also demonstrates activity to protect brain cells against damage following *ischemia-reperfusion injury*... the inflammation and subsequent oxidative damage that result from the sudden return of blood and nutrients to tissues deprived of them by blood-flow blockage. Given immediately before induced stroke in animal models, PQQ significantly reduces the size of the damaged brain area. *This physiologically implies that if a person were to suffer a temporary loss of cerebral blood flow due to cardiac arrest, stroke, or trauma, having PQQ circulating in their body would afford considerable protection against permanent brain damage when restoration of the blood supply is allowed to occur.*

PQQ can also protect against a phenomenon called *excitotoxicity*... a response to long-term overstimulation of neurons that is associated with many neuro-degenerative diseases (e.g. ALS) and seizures and it can protect against other neuro-toxins like mercury.

A growing body of evidence points to PQQ as a potent intervention against Alzheimer's and Parkinson's diseases for other reasons. Both diseases are triggered by accumulation of abnormal proteins that initiate a cascade of oxidative events resulting in brain cell death. PQQ prevents the development of *alpha-synuclein*, the protein responsible for Parkinson's. It also protects nerve cells from the oxidizing ravages of the Alzheimer's-causing *amyloid-beta protein.* A recent study revealed that PQQ could prevent formation of *amyloid-beta* molecular structures by the mechanisms of gene-modification listed above.

PQQ has recently demonstrated its activity to protect memory and cognition in aging animals AND HUMANS. It stimulates production and release of nerve growth factor in cells that support neurons in the brain. In humans, supplementation with a daily 20 mg dose of PQQ resulted in improvements on tests of higher cognitive function in middle-aged and elderly people. These effects were significantly amplified when these subjects additionally took a daily dose of 300 mg Co Q10.

PQQ'S ABILITY FOR CARDIO-PROTECTION: KEEPING THE HEART FUNCTIONAL AND STRONG

As seen with the vascular blockages in the central nervous system from some strokes, increased damage to cardiac tissue is also inflicted by a resurgence of blood flow after it is temporarily blocked (ischemia). This *ischemia re-perfusion*, though at first blush might seem the exact condition we want to occur as quickly as possible, actually brings with it a storm of cellular trouble. Dedicated intake of PQQ reduces this damage potential. And it works whether PQQ is given before or after the ischemic event itself.

To further investigate this cardio-protective potential in humans, researchers compared PQQ with metoprolol, the standard protocol medication given post-heart attack. PQQ administered alone proved more effective in many patients by allowing the ventricles to pump more efficiently than with metoprolol alone or when given with it, thus demonstrating PQQ's presumable overall superiority to metoprolol in protecting cardiac *mitochondria* from ischemia-reperfusion oxidative damage.

PQQ'S ABILITY TO ENHANCE VIGOROUS ACTIVITY: MORE ENERGY = MORE MOVEMENT

It is my hope that the reader has grasped the important take-home points of this chapter, and by so doing, can easily extrapolate the concept to the human condition that *if we consume a product that produces more functional mitochondria throughout the body, we have the increased intrinsic capacity to focus on training harder, the physical capacity to recover more easily and thoroughly, and the ability to command quality muscular movement.*

The heart will be adequately prepared and protected to handle its charge as the prime driving pump to force as much oxygen-rich blood as necessary to wherever it is needed. The brain will have increased capacity to focus, conceptualize, and remember all the demands extended vigorous movement requires. And, of course, living the very essence of having as much *mitochondria* as possible will allow us to rise above our DNA and produce amazing physicality... legally, safely, and reproducibly upon demand.

Pyrroloquinoline quinone [PQQ]

CHAPTER 15

MORE ON WHAT TO EAT WHEN AND WHEN TO FUEL-UP AND RE-FUEL

Though proper eating is vital for those wishing to push their bodies to perform well in their chosen sport(s), correct supplementation is a very important add-on. Some foodstuffs are absorbed more quickly and thoroughly than others (whey protein); some are needed to re-fuel "hungry" body parts throughout the day (dairy, egg and soy proteins). Others are added to aid the psychology of consumption (dark chocolate)… it is absolutely true: many athletes emotionally need certain foods and tastes to soothe their psyches after pushing so hard in training. *Circadian rhythm* also dictates certain needs in athletes used to training at certain times. Grape juice should be consumed before and during vigorous exercise to help prevent platelets from sticking that allows the blood to circulate more quickly to the muscles that need to be fueled.

If you train mornings before 10:00 AM	If you train lunchtime between noon and 2 PM	If you train from work between 5 and 8 PM
Pre-workout fueling 30-60 minutes before training	**Breakfast** flavored oatmeal with mixed fruit; liquid yogurt; energy drink of mixed proteins	**Breakfast** mixed grain cereal w/berry fruit + skim milk, whole grain toast + jam peanut butter; coffee/ tea to taste
Most intake should be in liquid form 12 oz Accelerade liquid or powder mix of same into liquid; 1 banana or 2 slices watermelon, or small bowl oat-meal with skim milk and banana and 12 oz whey protein/Egg Beater/ soy milk mixture; bring 32 oz of energy drink or grape juice/ Powerade mix if workout is longer than 60 min.; consume throughout	**Mid-morning/pre-workout snack** about 1 hour before training; 12oz Accelerade liquid or powder into liquid; or a tall glass fat-free chocolate milk; glass of grape juice	**Mid-morning snack** 12 oz mixed protein + yogurt energy drink
Western Omelet; **Breakfast within 1 hour of workout** 3-egg equiv of Egg-Beaters omelet + mushrooms and onions if tolerated + Canadian bacon; 12 oz fresh juice; coffee or tea to taste; 12 oz Endurox	**Lunch** following workout within 1 hour; tall glass of juice; 12 oz Endurox; Chocolate milk; fruit-flavored sherbet; 12 oz	**Lunch** soup; chicken breast sandwich w/tomatoes; roll & butter; juice; coffee or green tea
	Mid-afternoon snack couple handfuls of mixed nuts with dark chocolate M&M's	**Mid-afternoon snack** tall glass of apple juice; 3-4 squares dark choc; banana
Mid-morning snack Flavored liquid or solid yogurt; choice of fresh fruit preferably in the berry family; at least 12 oz of Fusion juice;	**Dinner** hearty bowl of soup; sliced lean roast beef open sandwich; potato + mixed greens and/or carrots; mixed salad with plenty of tomatoes flavored with olive oil-based salad dressing; fat-free ice cream or sherbet	**Pre-workout snack** 12 oz Accelerade or equiv amnt of skim chocolate milk; glass grape juice
Lunch Caesar salad with tomatoes, onions, grilled chicken, turkey or omega-3-rich fish (tilapia, salmon); or tuna salad sandwich on whole wheat; or sardines and anchovies over a salad; 24 oz of liquid from juice, skim milk And/or green tea		**Dinner** within 1 hour of training session: grilled salmon or tilapia or sirloin steak, sweet potato + mix veg; 12 oz Endurox drink
Mid-afternoon snack Nut-supported with either peanut butter on crackers; or a few hands-full of almonds/cashews/raison mix; can take 2 to 3 squares of dark chocolate, 12-16 oz coffee, tea, and/or juice		
Dinner Grilled fish, chicken or fresh turkey, or 12 oz lean red meat; creamed spinach or green beans and corn; choice of tomatoes, onions, peppers, or a mix of same with olive oil dressing; sherbet or non-fat ice cream		

CHAPTER 16

STEROID ABUSE IN ATHLETES... A VERY BAD CHOICE

An athlete, by description, is one who chooses and is able to be trained in acts of strength and agility. An athlete is also one who usually shows proficiency in a sports environment and often in more than one physical activity. And, finally, a truly competitive athlete is one who seeks various ways to help carry his physical potential as far as it will take him to meet success in his chosen effort. It is this last correlative that has become worrisome in the last two decades or so. Seeking ways to increase physical potential is a very serious business. With good guidance and correct and sufficient research, most choices for supplemental energy consumption are safe, effective, and appropriate, but there are a few that are as bad as they are seducing.

I would like to capture the thoughts from the title of an old "spaghetti-Western" (made in Italy) from the 60's starring Clint Eastwood: The Good, the Bad, and the Ugly, to describe the effects of a class of very potent biologic chemicals and their actions on many of the basic processes of the human condition. These chemicals are **steroids**, and they deeply effect the most basic processes of the body's internal environment. Mother Nature has provided for this both in appropriate amounts and times throughout the circadian cycle (daily rhythm).There are different types of steroids produced and secreted by the body to help keep its functioning on an even keel in dealing with life's stresses: to control inflammation, to regulate the mineral content of our internal fluid environment, and to influence sexual characteristics and tissue building and repair. But when we fool with nature's ways, we often pay the price for our folly.

Some things in life, when first implemented, present early as perfect or nearly so. They can even astound their discoverers. Often the hard science has to play catch-up with the discovery to paint a clearer picture as to cause and effect. Steroids are powerful hormones and produce very profound effects. Effects that, at times, can alter the very nature of the body's physiologic processes and appearance and produce astounding, even frightening results. This usually ties into the realm of the medical and, or pharmaceutical world and has offered up the concept that if a little does so much good naturally, why not play adventuresome physiologist and pep up the dose of certain steroids to produce biologic "super-men and women."

My extensive backgrounds as pharmacist, biochemist, and physiologist have prepared and grounded me over the years to help keep my biological wits. Very potent chemicals, when ingested, must be treated with the respect they command. In good conscience and practice, the three main tenets of *ergogenic* (a substance taken to help the body perform work) consumption must be respected and followed: (1) does the substance WORK AS DESIRED; (2) is it LEGAL TO USE under the auspices of the various sports governing bodies, and (3), most importantly, is it SAFE FOR THE ATHLETE to take, especially over time? Of the several classes of steroids found naturally in the body, only one will be discussed at length because of its inherent ability for abuse to build muscle tissue along with desired ancillary characteristics found beneficial to those athletes participating in vigorous training, competitions requiring power, and body-building. This class of steroid is labeled, depending upon slight molecular differences, either *androgenic* or *anabolic.* I will also discuss the other seducing bio-chemical that has reared its ugly head in sports in recent years: **natural growth hormone** and explain a major physiologic difference between the two.

ANDROGENIC AND ANABOLIC STEROIDS

When extracted and isolated from its natural state in the body and tested for its specific activity, the prime male characteristic hormone, *testosterone,* shows its signature overt effects for masculine maturity: deepening of voice, all-over increase in body hair, thickening of skin and bones, and maturation of genital organs. This is the **androgenic response.** The relatively rapid effect of thickening the body with lean skeletal muscle tissue comes about from what is biochemically called a **positive nitrogen balance.** This, in turn, produces the tissue-building response called *anabolism.* Because the building blocks of protein (amino acids), and protein itself have the element *nitrogen* attached, the more protein brought to the body, the more nitrogen comes along for the ride. A positive nitrogen balance therefore is synonymous with tissue-building. On balance, the body can also experience protein breakdown in its daily functioning when enduring vigorous exercise on a regular basis. If insufficient protein replenishment ensues tissue-breakdown (*catabolism*) results. This condition is also seen with wasting diseases like AIDS, the metastases of cancer, the atrophy of multiple systems in the poorly-nourished elderly, and with frank starvation. If allowed to proceed without appropriate daily protein replenishment, this **negative nitrogen balance** would produce severe tissue wasting to the point of death. Combating wasting disease is the "good" of *anabolic* steroid ingestion.

But science and human curiosity being what they are, organic chemists began manipulating the basic testosterone molecule to magnify and specify its biochemical actions. Just a few slights-of-hand and we had products that exhibited as much as 1000 times the muscle-building (*anabolic*) potential of the original natural parent hormone yet with less androgenic (*masculinizing*) effects. How quickly and how emphatically a positive nitrogen balance could be developed became more a matter of the chemists' skills in the lab with an agenda to produce chemical "super-beings" than a philosophical reckoning as to where all this would lead. Lean-body tissue-building (mostly muscle) amazed researchers and seduced them into thinking that many dysfunctions of the human process could be corrected quickly and dramatically and with little or no untoward effects. Those engrossed in athletics felt first-hand the steroid's ability to accelerate power output, enhance the ability to recover more quickly from strenuous training, and produce both an extended emotional state of euphoria and an exaggerated aggressiveness to beat the competition. But life was found to be not so kind nor so simple. Add to this a mix of ignorant, gullible youth and highly competitive adults with self-serving agendas, and we move through the "bad" with the Eastern-European Block drug-doping scandals of their female swimmers of the 1970's into the Chinese duplication of abuse of the 1980's and early 1990's to arrive at the present-day environment surrounding professional and highly desirous amateur athletes and others who choose to gamble on their long-term health to deal with pressures to excel beyond their potential by consuming potent androgenic steroidal medications.

THE DOSING AND EXTENT OF ILLEGAL STEROID ABUSE

It has only taken about two decades for steroid abuse to grow into the national scandal it is today. The problem is such that the federal government had one of its agencies, the National Institute on Drug Abuse, develop a website that deals in great depth trying to dispense impartial, hard-nosed facts on the dangers of this practice.

The full extent of abuse is understandably unknown. Few want to admit illegal usage in competition, and none wants to suffer the consequences of illicit possession. But experts in epidemiology estimate upwards of three million current or former abusers in the U.S. alone. With high-schoolers alone, next to creatine (the most highly-abused supplement) *anabolic* steroids place a strong second and are strongly associated with various sports. It is also known that much more than the admitted 15% of high school boys have taken "roids," but as mentioned, dealing with probable reprisals for this troublesome behavior has kept the experts guessing.

The majority of abuse comes from participants in football (almost 30%), track and field events (21%), wrestling (15%), weight training and power lifting (10%-15%).

Abusers have developed numerous dosage schemes to minimize adverse effects, avoid detection, enhance efficacy, and prevent the development of tolerance. **Stacking** refers to the practice of taking more than one steroid concurrently hoping that 1 + 1 will equal 3. In **cyc**ling abusers set a standard period of time for their cycle, such as anywhere from six to 16 weeks. They can sometimes take high doses for one cycle, moderate down for a cycle, then stop for a cycle. Repeating of this periodic usage over time presumably allows the body to acclimate to the hormone's benefit but not succumb to its dangers. In the method called **pyramiding** (also known as "stacking the pyramid"), abusers use a cycle to try and escalate the doses and, or the number of steroids used to reach a self-set peak at mid-cycle. Then, the abuser tapers the dosage and, or the steroids until the end of the cycle. This can get quite complicated and usually requires help and the wrong kind of "guidance." When the abuser stops using the steroids altogether during the cycle, it is called a "drug holiday."

As mentioned above, the swimming world was deeply tarnished for several years as records have shown once the former Communist Block countries had their secret files on such things brought to light. Thousands of elite female athletes from all areas of sport were dosed repeatedly with *anabolic* steroids, many not knowing what they were given. The most obvious recipients of *anabolics* were the female field-event participants. They presented as anything but female, many with vastly more bulk than contour. The hulking Russian, Tamara Press, world record holder and Olympic gold medalist in the shot putt, seemed Bunyonesque compared to her competition who, in their own right, were the best representatives of their respective countries.

The 1976 Montreal Olympics proved to be the most blatant example of illegal drug abuse during high-level world competition. Several of the USA female swim team complained repeatedly that the East Germans and other Communist-run teams had women that seemed more like men. Deep voices, inordinate musculature, square jaws, "Adams Apples" and other androgenic physical features predicated extremely powerful performances throughout the competition. While the USA men had their best swimming Olympics in history, the USA women, also with a very talented team, were only able to win one gold medal in all of the swimming competition… the last event: the 4 x 100 free relay. And they (the USA girls) were not treated kindly by the U.S. press. The team and their coach, Jack Nelson, were unfairly blamed for "embarrassingly" leaving the USA without gold medals. This negativity hung over this team for years.

Once the cheating coaches, managers, and administrators of the Eastern Block teams were forced to resign in disgrace, all thought this insult to sportsmanship would never be of concern again. Not so. It took several years for the same type of subterfuge to rear its ugly head again. The cheaters simply went where they were welcome: Communist China. And they brought what they knew about pharmacologic cheating with them.

All of a sudden, seemingly out of nowhere, the Chinese girls were breaking world records without the appropriate build-up to fast times in international competitions. Bells, whistles, horns went off signaling the same problem that came from Eastern Europe years before. Expected denials and angry countercharges ensued all to again tarnish a noble sport and deprive deserving athletes of their just rewards. Enough negative publicity was generated that once again the steroid problem and its perpetrators thinned out and seemingly just blew out to sea. But man's brilliant though devious nature once again allowed a new chemically-enhanced approach to inspired performance. The use and abuse of the most powerful endogenous substance Nature provides, **growth hormone**, was explored and expounded. Since the young healthy growing body naturally relies so dearly on this physiologic wonder, why not intentionally utilize it in a planned training regimen in mature athletes that would allow recovery from vigorous training so much more quickly and provide inordinate amounts of energy and power to train at a higher level that athletic superiority would be almost a given. Well, that is just what happened.

GROWTH HORMONE

Growth hormone has now been used (and abused) in most sports requiring endurance and power since it affects muscle growth in a special way. In swimming, all efforts (and energy costs) are at least four times the requirement than for running. And the property of water is such that as the swimmer moves more quickly through it, the water holds him back by increasing its resistance by the **square of the effort** to move. If the swimmer doubles his speed, for example, he is expending at least four times as much energy to move through the water, which holds him back by a factor of four: 2 squared = 4. To illustrate by times: Michael Johnson set the world's record in the 200 meter dash at 19.32; Alexander Popov has the swimming record for 50 meters at 21.64. Johnson has the fastest 400 meter run at 43.18 while Pieter Van Den Hoogenband covered 100 meters freestyle in 47.84.

When swim racing 100 meters or more, even the best slow down towards the end of their events because of how the water treats them. The idea is to train to slow down less than the competition, and this utilizes the sciences of physiology, biochemistry, and biomechanics plus talent and determination. If we add growth hormone to the correct training protocol, you can imagine the results.

Physiologic flags go up when we see power swimmers actually accelerate towards the end of their races. You see, with growth hormone, we actually have more muscle fiber cells being formed... A greater "army" of muscle tissue from which to recruit power. With steroids what, muscle fibers we have are simply made bigger. This also provides more power but the endurance factor is not as pronounced as with growth hormone since there are less cells to help along the way. Again, the size or bulk of muscle groups will enlarge with both hormone classes, but for obviously different reasons; one because of greater density of substance (steroids), the other because of greater numbers of cells (growth hormone). The muscle group that has more muscle fibers from which to recruit will not tire as readily and the athlete will be able to finish his event not only with more power but with enhanced endurance over those not so "anointed." Thus, if given the choice, growth hormone has the greater effect on performance.

Up till now it has been very difficult to test for growth hormone abuse. Being a naturally-found substance, amounts could be regulated up and down as major competitions approached, and any questionable amounts found would bring about the usual individual variation response. Sports administrators had to be absolutely sure of bad intentions if positive results were found. Litigation, or the threat of same, was almost a reflex response from the accused athlete to almost every drug-testing scenario.

But now there is a means to observe "footprints" or "markers" in the blood and urine. If growth hormone is found naturally produced by the body (*endogenously*), it shows as remnants with scalloped edges or irregularities under examination. If abuse has taken place and outside sources consumed (*exogenously*), the edges of the remnants are perfectly smooth with no irregularities. Of course, the hormone could have been utilized illegally for several months during intense training and stopped well in advance of competition. But that is why the governing bodies have instituted un-announced body-fluid testing to which all competing athletes must agree.

The human condition being what it is; it is almost a sure bet that drugs that will mask growth hormone's presence, or some other protocol that will be geared to enhance the possibility of cheating will be sought and tried.

ADVERSE EFFECTS

Adverse effects could be and usually are profound since the abusers could be taking from 100 to 1000 times the amount of hormone or steroid normally found in the body. This is the "ugly" of this whole topic. Some produce mainly cosmetic effects though rather intense; others can cause permanent disfigurement and organ dysfunction, and some lead all the way to death even in healthy young, vigorous athletes.

A. **Cardiovascular effects:** blood pressure has been seen to spike uncontrollably; lipoproteins (cholesterol and all its "cousins") become totally unfriendly to the internal environment with the "good" cholesterol, *High-Density Lipoproteins* (HDL's) being lowered as much as 70%, and the "bad" cholesterol, the Low-Density Lipoproteins (LDL's) being raise as much as 100%; the actual structure of the heart can become negatively altered with the enlargement of the left ventricle and resultant poor diastolic function (the lower number of the blood pressure reading being too high); this results in not allowing the heart to rest in between beats because of the constant back-pressure being created; this abnormality can persist for years after usage is stopped and is what probably killed the former NFL great, John Matusack, 12 years after his playing days were over while he enjoyed a budding acting career; acute myocardial infarctions (major heart attacks) are not uncommon even after short-term usage due to an exaggerated response of the left ventricle to a hypertrophic stimulus such as vigorous exercise; steroids can also increase the risk of acute vascular thrombosis (blood clot) in peripheral, coronary, and cerebral vasculature. The athlete's degree of atherosclerosis (clogging of the artery) is directly related to elevated plasma *homocysteine* which is induced by steroids.

B. **Hepatic (liver) effects:** some *anabolic* steroid structures (methyl testosterone, fluoxymesterone) have greater adverse effects on liver tissue than others; at first there is a reversible deterioration of the active liver tissue, then it becomes non-reversible; what can arise is increased liver tissue to cause painful swelling, inflammatory reactions of this tissue (*jaundice*), blood-filled cysts, benign tumors, and cancerous growths;

C. **Reproductive effects:** since reproductive tissue had its origin from birth using testosterone as a starting point, both reversible and irreversible changes in function can arise; since this system is heavily influenced by feed-back mechanisms, if supra-therapeutic doses of testosterone or its relatives are given, the body senses that it no longer needs to produce these vital sex-related hormones (testosterone, luteinizing hormone, follicle-stimulating hormone); the sex organs are deemed not necessary and lose their capacity to function properly; **hypogonadism begins to develop within 24 hours post-administration** which produces these far-ranging negative responses: reduced sperm count, poorly-shaped and ill-functioning sperm, testicular atrophy (wasting away) and infertility; recovery may take as long as a year or may never happen.

D. **Behavioral/psychiatric effects:** often causes inappropriate aggressive behavior patterns called "roid rage;" severe changes in mood such as depression, paranoia, hypomania, schizophrenia, steroid dependence, psychotic symptoms, the risk of homicide and homicide; often seen is a condition called **reversed anoxia syndrome** where the victim senses his body is not as well developed as it actually is; this can lead to an inappropriate and all-consuming perception that more work must be done to build muscle, called the **Adonis syndrome.**

E. **Miscellaneous adverse effects:** with supratherapeutic doses of anabolic steroids are administered, the excess is converted to estrogens; male abusers may discover that their breasts have begun to grow resulting in a painful condition called **gynecomastia.** Surgery may be needed to reduce breast tissue if this does not resolve once abuse ends; females experience male-pattern baldness, permanent lowering of the voice, shrinking of the breasts, enlargement of sex organs, menstrual irregularities, and increased body hair; tumors can arise almost anywhere; the famous NFL all-pro defensive lineman, Lyle Alzado, knew he was dying from a steroid-induced brain tumor and made several public health commercials warning of this; any growth, whether benign or cancerous can be induced to spread much more quickly when growth hormone is abused; an benignly-enlarged prostate gland can become quite troublesome in response to excess growth hormone.

PENALTIES FOR STEROID POSSESSION AND TRAFFICKING

It seems the famous have been able to dodge bullets when it comes to the long arm of the law. Some are stripped of their title, and promise of wealth and stardom as the most recent Tour-de-France winner found out so unceremoniously. Some endure controversy and persevere: an elite American female sprint swimmer of the early 1990's tested positive for testosterone 1000 times greater than she claimed her birth control pills caused. She was initially banned for life by United States Swimming, but somehow found her way back to elite competition within two years.

But some actually bask in the heat of notoriety. Jose Conseco's recent book about steroid abuse running rampant in Major League Baseball brought the expected controversy especially when he named as co-chronic abusers some of the greatest home-run hitters of all time. Everyone's icons. Those who have been prosecuted for selling and distributing to these professionals and have named names and situations are doing time and paying fines, but, again, the famous, are free to roam about. And to their shame, they have never owned up to the obvious. Mark Maguire entered the league in his early 20's at 6'5", 180 pounds, and retired at 6'5", 240 pounds, not looking at all soft and fat. Bobby Bonds similarly "thickened up" to aid his ability to power the ball over the years to be presently positioned second only to the fabulous Henry Aaron who relied on natural gifts, hard work, and longevity. And there are plenty more now undergoing scrutiny.

For anabolic steroids, individual states may have harsher penalties than allowed by the Anabolic Steroid Control Acts of 1990 and 2004. However, both acts specify that the first offense of possession of anabolic steroids obtained illegally carries a maximum penalty of one year in prison and a minimal $1,000 fine. If trafficking is found to be the game, the maximal penalties for a first offense are five years in prison and a $250,000 fine; these both double for a second offense.

This seems harsh enough; you would think the negative notoriety would cause the potential offenders to pause and think of the legal consequences not to mention the great risk to bodily health. But the perception of all this does not seem to be as negative as we would hope because the allure of greatness still calls so many of the young and talented (and, oh, so foolish) to try anything that just might give them that edge up on everyone else.

SECTION III:

INJURY PREVENTION AND THE TREATMENT OF SOME... BEST TO AVOID THE "HIT"

This section will enlighten the reader as to knowing when enough is enough. What happens when we exceed this threshold and how to regenerate and rejuvenate, including appropriate diagnosis and treatment, therapeutic massage, correct pharmaceutical applications... bringing in the various members of the community health team. Outlining the various pitfalls of mechanical improprieties in the weight room, the pool, on land, and on the bike will serve to put the reader on guard as to what he or she will face and how to prevent same.

CHAPTER 1

HELPING THE BODY HEAL

OVERVIEW

The body can handle many types of stresses. Nature has provided for this or else none of us would age into maturity, let alone grow out of adolescence. A highly trained athlete can usually handle the physical stresses demanded by his sport to a greater extent than the so-called "weekend warrior." *The body can train to train, but can it train to greatly improve or excel? That takes in-depth knowledge of human physiology mixed with good coaching, accommodating genetics, and a little luck.* But there is one circumstance that has nothing to do with athletic prowess or good coaching or even high-minded determination which could make or break a competitor... especially if circumstances present poor timing with regards to a major athletic event. And that circumstance deals with *physical trauma,* whether sustained from an accident, overuse injury or the need to recuperate from reparative surgery.

THE BODY'S RESPONSE TO PHYSICAL TRAUMA

The body's response to sustaining wounds is to first isolate, and then adapt the affected tissue to try and lessen the extent of damage. Then, *regeneration* begins which takes time and energy, nutrients and hydration, rest and recovery. *The most critical nutrients involved with wound healing include protein, enzyme co-factors. Glucosamine, Omega-3, zinc, vitamin A, vitamin C. vitamin E. and iron.* The fact that these substances can all be purchased (OTC) affords the athlete and, or coach the opportunity to help the healing process quickly.

When the body is injured, its normal operating functions can become compromised. Depending upon the severity and, or the extent of physical trauma, **the body's need for high-quality protein is substantially increased. The immune system is extremely dependent upon quality protein** to have manufactured all its important elements for keeping infection and inflammation from getting out of control. To emphasize, several studies have shown that about 25% of hospitalized patients and as many as half of general surgery patients exhibit protein malnutrition. This can significantly lengthen the time of healing by allowing inflammation to linger and infection to fester. Also, the building of new blood vessels *(revascularization)* and the actual remodeling of tissue can both be delayed and impaired. Anyone undergoing major surgery can attest to the body's need for help in recovery by experiencing a dramatic, sustained increase in overall weakness. Much of this can be alleviated by the simple intake of quality protein starting about a week before elective surgery and the assurance of adequate fluid intake before and after surgery.

174

(A rather amazing story of recovery, exhibited by Jeff Farrell, America's premier freestyle sprinter in 1960, is made all the more remarkable in light of what was stated above. He only had seven days after abdominal surgery for appendicitis before Olympic Trials that year. His high level of physical fitness and his obviously strong determination to make the team have become the stuff of legend.)

PROTEIN SUPPLEMENTATION

Prime sources of protein include fish, lean meats, eggs or a quality vegetable protein, such as soy. Soy is also available in powdered form that can be mixed in drinks or in yogurt. Supplements of several individual amino acids can provide an additional protein benefit. Increased intake of *sulfur-containing amino acids such as cysteine and methionine (as found in eggs. for example)* shorten the inflammatory stage and decrease the amount of protein destroyed during inflammation.

Two other very important amino acids that have an intimate relationship with the healing process are *arginine* and *I-glutamine***.** *Arginine* functions as an antioxidant to kill bacteria and increase T-cell-mediated activity, which, in turn, also enhances immune function. Supplementation with *arginine* has been shown to significantly increase the amount of collagen deposited into a wound site during the healing process.

Requirements for *I-glutamine* increase dramatically during critical illness or trauma. It is considered "conditionally essential" in that as physical stress increases, so does the body's need for *glutamine;* depending upon how vigorous the stress or intense the trauma, the body's ability to produce *glutamine* in skeletal muscle can fall short of need. Endogenous (from within) sources are soon depleted with generalized sepsis (infection), extensive burns, major injury, surgery, intense exercise, and over-training in athletes. Exogenous sources (outside the body... from diet or as a supplement) are needed to help in the healing process and /or recovery. *Glutamine* is the most abundant amino acid in skeletal muscle protein, and as such, its uptake during stress exceeds that of any other amino acid. Because it is an effective *nitrogen donor* (all amino acids must have the element nitrogen as part of the molecular structure) and a precursor for protein synthesis, *glutamine* is also extremely important in helping to rebuild wounded tissues.

MINERAL SUPPLEMENTATION

The mineral *zinc* is another powerful ally in supporting immune system function and speeding healing. *Zinc* levels decline dramatically during stress from the same causes listed above. *Zinc* concentrates in wounds during the period of collagen synthesis and helps to strengthen new tissue. The simple application of *zinc* topically (in either spray or ointment form) can reduce the size of the wound and shorten healing time even in patients who are not *zinc* deficient. But those who are *zinc* deficient can suffer a compromised immune system which can delay closure of wounds and ulcers, and cause newly-produced collagen (connective tissue) to have a weaker tensile strength.

Iron is the other essential mineral nutrient for new cellular growth and wound healing. The enzyme *ribonucleotide reductase*, which requires iron as co-factor, is essential for DNA synthesis. Since cells cannot divide without prior DNA synthesis, iron deficiency can impair the proliferation of all cells involved in wound debridement (removing dead or dying cells and other contaminants) *and healing. Iron-deficiency anemia is relatively common in menstruating women, and anemic patients of any age will exhibit delayed wound healing.* Some salts of iron are absorbed better than others, and some are more irritating to the gut than others. As a rule, it is also best to have vitamin C taken along with the iron supplement to insure the proper oxidation state of the mineral for best absorption. Consultation with a pharmacist should bring about the best selections.

There are some minerals that are needed only in small concentrations to have a positive effect on many metabolic *processes...* micronutrients. *Copper* and *manganese* are examples and act as co-factors for enzymes involved in collagen synthesis. If, for some reason, a deficiency existed for either of these two minerals, the overall healing process would be compromised.

VITAMIN SUPPLEMENTATION

Vitamins, especially J, C and E, play a significant role in wound healing. Administering Vitamin A for seven days after surgery increases *lymphocyte* (infection-fighting) activity, collagen synthesis, and enhances the bursting strength of scar tissue. Large doses of A (100,0001U/kg/day) can reverse post-surgical suppression of the immune system and speed up healing but should only be taken at this level for no more than one week. During the recovery period from severe injury or infection, A in dosages ranging from 10,000 IU to 25,000 IU daily can be safely used for a few weeks' duration. The reason for caution here is that Vitamin A is fat-soluble and is readily stored in the body. Toxic levels can be reached much sooner than with water-soluble vitamins that are excreted daily through the kidneys.

The water-soluble Vitamin, C, meanwhile, increases the strength of new collagen formation and the rate of healing, and it enhances the immune system and helps fight infections. Severe trauma such as burns, fractures or major surgery cause a substantial decrease in plasma Vitamin C levels. The stresses associated with injuries and wound healing dramatically increase the body's overall need for C Amounts as high as 1000 mg/day can safely be ingested for a few weeks. The caution here, even though the vitamin is able to be excreted daily, concerns the kidneys. Since about SO% of Vitamin C degrades to a molecule called *vacillate,* there is always the potential for kidney stones in the form of *Calcium Oxalate*, the most insoluble substance known in physiology. Adequate hydration with non-calcium and **non-oxalate**-containing liquids (water is best) will usually dilute the urine enough to help prevent this type of stone formation. A few studies have shown that as much as a 42% reduction in blood Vitamin C levels can develop by the third day following major surgery if extra C is not ingested.

Vitamin E supplementation also enhances immune function and increases resistance to infection. But special benefit comes from its ability to help prevent excessive free-radical destruction that seems to surround wounded tissue, thus reducing secondary damage and improving the healing process. Topical Vitamin E has been touted as preventing or at least lessening scar formation if applied directly to a wound. But scar formation is probably more a function of genetics than vitamin effect since some patients produce more scar tissue than others. It has also been shown that Vitamin E can possibly inhibit collagen formation suggesting that there may be somewhat of a cosmetic effect with Vitamin Vs. but if the strength of a wound closure is important, topical E should probably be avoided.

ANCILLARY SUBSTANCES SUPPLEMENTATION

Two substances have been hyped into the common pool of knowledge regarding their ability to help heal damaged tissue. Glucosamine is a natural compound produced within the body that acts as a natural precursor of important large molecules needed to keep connective tissue functioning healthy and to help heal any damage that can occur. The substances that *glucosamine* produces are *glycoproteins*, *glycolipids*, and *glycosaminoglycans* or *mucopolysaccharides*... complex words that describe the content and substance of the various tissues that make up ligaments, cartilage, *synovial fluid*, mucous membranes, and blood vessels. In cases of serious and, or extensive trauma, whether from an accident or training overuse, the body's store of *glucosamine* may not be sufficient to meet the demands of tissue needing to synthesize these macromolecules for wound healing.

The essential fatty acid compound, Omega-3, is a powerful antioxidant. Found naturally in several species of "fatty" fish, it not only is beneficial to keeping a healthy blood lipid profile, but it is also an intimate component of cell-wall architecture; a deficiency of *Omega-3* compromises the transport of important substances across cell membranes, which can contribute to poor wound healing.

Water, the simplest of all the substances mentioned here, is so vital that it is *second only to oxygen* in keeping the body functioning the way nature intended; it should NEVER be overlooked, taken for granted, or assumed to be adequate. Waiting for the **thirst alert** is wrong. People suffering trauma can help speed their own recovery without much effort by forcing fluids. As adequate hydration is crucial to wound healing, patients should be encouraged to **drink two to three quarts of quality water daily during the healing process.** Nutrient delivery, tissue repair, detoxification, and pain are all directly influenced by hydration, and injury and wound healing greatly increase the body's need for water. Adequate hydration positively influences circulation that enhances nutrient delivery and waste removal during the time of healing.

Whether it be vitamins, proteins, minerals, natural body substances or simple water, there are numerous options available (in addition to appropriate medication) to assist the trauma patient in healing. It has been stated by those in the medical field: THE BODY NEVER FORGETS. We realize the possible long-term effects of various trauma but hope for the best. Time may heal, but it can always use some help.

CHAPTER 2

CONTROLLING THE CAUSE OF ALL DISEASE: INFLAMMATION

Much has been written over the years, especially with the change from prescription to over-the-counter of various non-steroidal anti-inflammatory drugs (NSAIDS for short), about inflammation and how to keep it in check. Let me first state that, in general, *inflammation* is not a good thing... Better not to have it happening at all if possible, but on occasion it is a necessary process that the body endures to help it return to *homeostasis* (original biologic condition of adequacy) after some bad physiological things happen.

Many of the body's healing processes have *inflammation* as a component of the cascade of events to bring a condition to resolution, and this is as it should be. We can find our way into trouble, though, if the *inflammation* is not resolved, or if it becomes acute to where the body needs to marshal much of its inner natural energies to get on top of the situation. If *inflammation* is not resolved in a timely fashion and becomes chronic, then other physiologic processes appear; none of which is good for athletic performance, and general quality of life.

To that end, it is wise to seek proper medical intervention be it medication, physical rehabilitation, a healing diet, a more healthful lifestyle, or even simple rest. This chapter hopefully will make the athlete aware, no matter the age, of the "three C's" of human biology: the **causes**, the **consequences**, and the **cures.**

DESCRIPTION OF INFLAMMATION

Using basic concepts, inflammation is a gathering of cellular elements (white blood cells, *histamine* and other chemical factors) that the body releases into circulation to the affected area involved either with **trauma**, **infection**, **overuse**, or **toxic exposure**. In an **acute** situation, the elements released cause a whole cascade of events to occur which nature provides to, at first, try and isolate the trouble to as small an area as possible, and then to immobilize the area to hopefully prevent further spread. An often-seen consequence of this is "The Three Musketeers" of *inflammation*... from the Latin: *calor (heat), dolor (pain), and rubror (redness). Swelling (tumor)* is a common addition to the above trio... all done with Nature's best intent to heal what is wrong. But this intent is often not compatible with the athletic goal of *"swifter, higher, stronger."*

If the *inflammation* is allowed to become **chronic,** a situation can emerge where the body sort of allows a "Mexican standoff" to occur. Here the main elements of the above cascade of *inflammation* subside but not totally disappear. The bad news here, even though

178

the body may feel somewhat better, is that since total resolution has NOT occurred, tissue damage is allowed to continue, and a festering, if you will, begins to invade the affected site. What is even more disturbing is the possibility of altered tissue integrity… The loss of functioning capacity and even progression to a state of damaged DNA that can lead to pre-malignant or malignant states.

CAUSES AND CONSEQUENCES OF INFLAMMATION

Causative elements can come from any or all of the following: **infective micro-organisms, sudden and intense trauma, unhealthy lifestyle or diet, chronic overuse, or toxic exposure.** About microorganisms, Mother Nature has provided proper compartmentalization for resident bacteria in the body. If bacteria like *E. coli,* which usually are harmless in their intended place of origin (the lower gut), find their way into an area not intended for their residence (upper gut) through either contaminated food or water where swimming is allowed, those exposed can develop severe gastrointestinal *inflammation… gastritis.* We can also have the situation where several types of bacteria, which normally reside ON the skin, can produce serious *inflammatory* reactions if allowed to penetrate into deeper tissue areas due to trauma. Some to the extent that the skin can actually be eaten away, and a dangerous generalized septicemia (systemic bacterial blood poisoning) could develop that can kill.

A somewhat "high-profile" bacteria have come to the public's awareness of late: **Helicobacter Pylori,** better known *as H. pylori.* This is not a normal resident of the stomach, but when found there, it has shown a correlation of almost 100% in those with gastric ulcers. People can have *H. pylori* and not have an ulcer, but those with ulcers from otherwise unexplained causes will almost always test positive for this stomach invader. What is even more distressing is the fact that the chronic *inflammatory* condition the bacteria produces in the gut tissue could lead to a strong association between *H. pylori's* presence and stomach cancer. Infection with *H. pylori* is increasing in numbers throughout the population to where we see the older one gets, the more likely he/she will test positive. Signs or symptoms to watch for are **sudden chronic stomach upset, acid reflux** (which can cause its own *inflammatory* response in the esophagus, or food channel), **intolerance for foods that never gave problems before,** and surprisingly, **a constant low reading of HDL's** even with devout aerobic training. It seems the *inflammation* the bacteria causes interferes with the body's ability to metabolize fats properly. In fact, a few studies have shown that getting rid of *H. pylori* in the gut allows for an almost 25% rise in HDL's (the good cholesterol). A logical action if an athlete constantly comes up short on HDL's would be to request a blood test for *H. Pylori* even if no symptoms out of the ordinary appear.

Science is not sure how infection is spread with *H. pylori,* but we see several avenues emanating from the gastrointestinal area: dentists are quite susceptible due to constant proximity to their patients' mouths. The bacteria can be found in poorly treated pools and can spread to those who unfortunately swim through a contaminated area. Food handlers can also be focal areas of spread.

Intense trauma that effects bony structures can most definitely produce *inflammatory* reactions. Bone is a constantly changing structure, gaining and losing calcium, but it is a relatively-slow healing organ. Unlike most soft tissue trauma (other than vital organs), bone pain can last for months with severe trauma, and *inflammation* can find a "home" in relatively quick time. Any involvement with bone leaves the potential for prolonged and serious consequences. In fact, it is almost a given that the body will produce an arthritic condition which causes calcium to be deposited at the site of injury. Even sub- acute constant trauma will eventually produce an osteoarthritic condition that makes the victim pay the price with reduced mobility and range-of-motion. To say nothing of the constant discomfort. And age is not a specific factor of the condition. High school athletes, for example, may think they've healed from a physically traumatic experience (it's good to be young). The immediate, intense discomfort has dissipated, but eventually they pay the price. The **"the body never forgets"** its mistreatment, and they are left with a body "older than its years."

There is one soft tissue involvement, however, that can have very severe consequences, and it does not usually come from trauma, per say. When the coronary arteries become *inflamed*, the body's response is to send, by way of the circulation, the elements listed above, plus it increases the chances for calcium to be deposited *in-situ (at the site)*. The calcium actually produces an irregular surface on the inside lining (intima) of the arteries which then allow for elevated circulating cholesterol and other fats to cling, harden, and finally occlude. Thus, it should be the goal of those seeking a healthy lifestyle to try and keep the coronary arteries from becoming *inflamed,* so this potentially deadly cascade of events is prevented or at least diminished.

There is now an easy to obtain blood marker (test) that can be used with some degree of medical certainty to spot *inflammation* in the body. In fact, it can show itself with most types of systemic *inflammation,* but if there are no other *inflammatory* processes going on, and this marker is elevated, then prudent medical analysis would call attention to the possibility of coronary artery *inflammation.* This blood marker is called C-**R**eactive **P**rotein **(**CRP**)**. Though it was first discovered in 1930, *CRP* has only recently been confirmed in an important association for potential coronary artery risk.

Many physicians are now using the CRP enzyme to establish heart-attack potential. Almost half the heart-attack and stroke victims each year in the United States have essentially normal cholesterol levels. Even a moderately elevated serum cholesterol may not be considered as potentially dangerous as in the past if the CRP is below a certain threshold. **Low risk: CRP less than 1 milligram per liter (mg/L); moderate risk: CRP 1 to 3 mg/L; high risk: CRP above 3mg/L.**

Unfortunately, in our modern multi-task society many seem to be deprived of the quality of life needed to lead a healthy lifestyle. The main deprivation from this way-of-life is **adequate rest**, especially **quality sleep**. There have been a few studies of late that have shown the *C-Reactive Protein* to rise to potentially heart-damaging levels in a sleep-deprived state. Someone who subsists on 4 to 5 hours of sleep when 7 to 8 are needed over an extended period of time can develop an elevated CRP. This probably results from increased *cortisol* (the anti-stress hormone) being spilled into the circulation. Add to this dietary practices that allow for excess cholesterol and *triglycerides* to enter the circulation, and you create the potential for **Coronary Heart Disease (CHD).**

Just about every athlete who trains intensely to get to a higher level becomes at risk for **overuse injury**. Each sport has its vulnerable body parts. With swimmers it's mostly the **articular joints of the shoulders, knees, and neck (**in that order) that present targets of discomfort and **inflammation. Swimmer's shoulder** is the most common injury for aquatic athletes, and it involves the most important areas of the body for moving through water. Performing thousands of repetitive motions day-in and day-out will tax most anatomical areas to their breaking point. Once the *shoulders* become *over-stressed,* the elements of *inflammation* emerge… All wreaking havoc in a small enclosed space that was never really designed to perform these intense overhead actions repeatedly. The shoulder girdle is not even a well-developed stable ball-and-socket joint. The elements that compose the inner workings of the shoulder have little space in which to navigate comfortably through the optimum **R**ange-**O**f-**M**otion (ROM) needed for correct form and fast swimming. If development of improper technique ensues whether from fatigue, ignorance of proper mechanics, or poor coaching, and it is not corrected (and kept from returning), the athlete is at risk for developing a full-blown *inflammatory* condition. Constant rubbing and continued irritation, but lacking appropriate rest and recovery… All contribute to the development of the items listed above to produce what could wind up as an aquatic-terminating condition.

The *knees* in breaststrokers are the most vulnerable, with the *shoulders* a secondary concern. The knees for obvious reasons: the requirements of the breaststroke kick, if done optimally, place much pressurized torque on the medial (inside) aspect of the knees. Ideal form requires "high heels"…where the ankles must reach all the way back, and the heels approach the butt with each kick to move as much water as possible. Any *inflammation* that develops in the knee could lead to the condition of *crepitus…* Where "sounds" are heard upon movement; eventually the "sounds" are joined by pain, weakness, and reduced range-of-motion… All due to arthritic (calcium) deposits. This can happen at any age but is usually seen after several years competing in breaststroke.

The shoulders in breaststrokers (flyers, too) can develop problems due to repetitive open turns at the walls. If done correctly, one arm sustains more compression against the shoulder girdle than the other… Usually the top arm on an open turn. If one turns from right to left, for example, after the touch, it is usually the right arm (the last to leave the wall) that deals with compressing the humerus (upper arm bone) into the inner workings of the shoulder structures (mostly the *supraspinatus…* one of the *rotator cuff* muscles).

Toxic exposure as a cause of **inflammation** should not be any more common to aquatic athletes than to athletes in other sports, but it is. Any athlete can experience toxins released with certain contaminating bacteria in food, and everyone must be vigilant to prevent this potentially debilitating condition. But the aquatic athlete, by nature of his sport, is exposed to either chemically-treated pools and, or non-treated open water. Inflammatory reactions to the skin and mucous membranes (eyes and respiratory tract) often occur in poorly maintained aquatic venues; mostly with too **little** active chlorine and too much chlorine-breakdown metabolites. The body biochemically can handle an acidic environment (pH 1.0-6.8) better than it can handle a basic one (pH 7.5-14). When one smells chlorine, and the nose and eyes become irritated, it is usually from a highly **basic** condition. Asthma in swimmers has become more prevalent. Whether it be cause-and-effect from training in a contaminated environment or the athlete bringing the condition to the sport, *inflammation* of the respiratory tract is the resultant.

TREATING INFLAMMATION

Some treatments are obvious and straight-forward: anti-infectives for infections; anti-inflammatory medication for simple *inflammation;* removal from toxic exposure or treatment of same with medication; simple lessening of movement or complete rest with overuse symptoms.

For the most part, we would be fortunate indeed if the above procedures work. To varying degrees they do, but in-depth true resolution of the **inflammation syndrome** at times requires some medical sophistication and biological logic. Sometimes exotic multiple antibiotics and ancillary medications are needed with complex dosing regimens to eliminate resistant strains of infecting organisms. We see this with the above-mentioned gut-invader, *H. pylori.* Leaving this bacteria to fester in the gut is just asking for trouble. It is not a normal gastrointestinal resident; eliminate it!

Since we are after-the-fact in treating trauma, isolating the damaged tissue and treating it vigorously is the most logical approach. Down time for an athlete is usually all negative. As mentioned in the opening paragraph, there are now several potent over-the-counter (OTC) non-steroidal anti-inflammatory drugs (NSAIDS) that can bring about inflammatory resolution in a receptive patient. There are also new prescription medications that claim to reduce side effects while performing their seemingly miraculous work. None are without long term risks.

But there are several research studies going on presently where the anti-inflammatory substances come from natural sources. **Phytochemicals** (chemicals from a plant source) have presented an exciting avenue of research with their anti-oxidant and anti-inflammatory activity. Plants such as milk thistle, turmeric, garlic, onion, and gingko biloba have all shown to possess substances that lessen *inflammation* when ingested. A rather well-known natural substance now used by several Olympic teams is the enzyme *bromelain.* Bromelain aids in muscular recovery after intense training, and it also aids digestion. Most tropical fruits possess this with *pineapples* having the most. The enzyme is now available in capsule form with concentrations much higher than can be ingested consuming reasonable amounts of the natural source.

Another natural anti-inflammatory that is showing great promise is the **omega-class of fats.** Two forms of the free-fatty acid are seen: **omega-6** and **omega-3.** The former comes from plant sources like corn, safflower, and sunflower oils. The latter is derived from certain fatty fish: salmon, tuna, sardines, rainbow trout and sea bass, and plants sources: flaxseed oil, walnuts, and canola oil. Research has shown that it is the **ratio of omega-6's to omega-3's** that has the effect of either producing *inflammation* or reducing it. Too much omega-6 and inflammation is allowed to occur. With a dietary ratio of omega-6 to omega-3 in a 2:1 up to a 4:1 intake, the *inflammatory* response can be lessened. The same research is also combining these natural anti-inflammatory substances with NSAIDS to see if lower doses with less side effects can produce the same benefits over an extended period of time.

Those swimmers constantly exposed to irritating chemicals in their pool environment can developed definite breathing difficulties. Chronic exposure can lead to chronic *inflammation* of the respiratory tract. Anti-inflammatory inhalers and, or oral medication, bronchiole dilators, and other related medications can only treat the symptoms. Once asthma has taken hold, it usually becomes a permanent condition with variances in severity day-to-day. Some days... Pretty good; some days even medication seem not to help much. Much better not to develop the condition in the first place. Therefore, it is incumbent upon all places that have **C**ertified **P**ool **O**perators (CPO's) responsible for healthy pool conditions that the aquatic environment is kept in a swimmer-friendly condition at all times.

Some things in life can and should be prevented. Most *inflammatory* reactions and conditions fall into this category. When *inflammation* does occur due to circumstances beyond our control, it is best treated heroically and with all good intent to resolve it; letting *inflammation* linger, or taking a cavalier attitude about its systemic resolution could place the sufferer in a precarious position to say the least.

CHAPTER 3

ATHLETES NEEDING TO TREAT SORE MUSCLES AND TENDONS; TENNIS ELBOW AND THE "SUITCASE SYNDROME"

One would think that Mother Nature, having lots of time and practice to work her magic, should have provided for a trouble-free mechanism allowing the body to move through life. Unfortunately no. As a chemist, I had to learn the periodic table of all the elements, but I am still learning about one: the human element. The body is the most miraculous consequence of living evolution. Having evolved millions of years ago with no choice but to handle severe ambient threats every day, our ancestors adapted and were able to progress to where most of us today put our musculature and related structures to the test voluntarily either to earn a living or to "enjoy" leisure time.

Muscle and tendon soreness sooner or later will affect virtually everyone, regardless if the patient is a serious athlete or engages in exercise on an intermittent, recreational basis. The wide-spread appearance of muscle discomfort is due partly to the various activities that produce it and partly to the muscles not being adequately conditioned to handle stressful loads repeatedly placed upon them. Those who think they are in "shape" usually suffer consequences of pushing through bouts of increasing intensity on a too-much-too-soon basis. They can feel the effects of this as quickly as two hours later or as long as the next day or two. Those of the "weekend-warrior" ilk often develop delayed discomfort (DOMS) a few to several hours later. It is also never a surprise to see tendons become inflamed and sore either right along with muscle tissue or noticeably before. Tendonitis is a common though certainly undesired musculoskeletal complication of overuse, improper use through faulty technique, or an imbalance of use from having some muscle groupings pulling harder against others.

WHAT EXERCISE DOES TO DAMAGE MUSCLE

Vigorous bodily movement that can produce muscle soreness and pain causes structural damage to the contracting muscle fibers and their surrounding membranes; this allows for increases in muscle enzyme leakage into the blood that act as easy markers for detecting tissue damage directly related to trauma. Inflammation usually follows quickly and surrounds the traumatized area as the body tries to protect the injury from becoming more intense by making movement painful and difficult.

Some exercises and movements are more damaging to intact muscle tissue than others. Activities that cause a forceful lengthening of the fibers (eccentric movement) will usually produce more concerted damage than those only requiring contraction since that is what muscle tissue was fabricated to do: contract forcefully. When an athlete engages in activities that produce extraordinary lengthening of muscle tissue like running or hiking downhill, descending stairs, lowering weights back to a starting position and proceeding through the recovery cycle in each of the swim racing strokes, micro-tears occur. This allows for a cascade of events starting off with bleeding *in situ* (at the site) which then adds leaked fluid volume to the already crowded area of swelled (with blood from the circulation) fiber tissue. Increased swelling produces increased pressure against nerves in the immediate area which then signal the brain to discomfort, then to pain, then to weakness and reduced range-of-motion. And an injured muscle fatigues more readily than an intact fully-functioning muscle. Activities that only require fiber contraction do not usually cause this type of damage and produce much less muscle soreness since, as stated above, muscle tissue is designed to contract. A popular example of this type of activity is cycling.

Abnormally-lengthened fiber undergoes increased tension against resistance compared to the same fiber in an un-stretched or contracted state. The elongated fiber must endure an increased load-to-fiber cross-sectional ratio (not enough tissue) acting against a resistance and is much more susceptible to damage (picture a tight-rope walker bending the rope and swaying precariously as he tries to move) whereas a contracted muscle has an increased fiber-to-load ratio and can more easily handle the load with much more tissue to move a resistance (picture the same person walking more stably on a heavy steel beam with no give or swaying).

WHAT EXERCISE DOES TO DAMAGE TENDONOUS TISSUE

Tendons can become irritated and inflamed leading to fraying of the fibrous material if they are caused to rub against hardened surfaces in a crowded joint capsule as in the shoulder of a swimmer or baseball pitcher. An inflamed tendon then swells taking up more room than Nature intended in areas not designed to accommodate lots of tissue. Tendons, all of which attach muscle to bone, can also become overly-stressed and even tear from its insertion into the muscle if too great a resistive load is placed on the muscle fibers which would then need to be prevented from pulling it out of its normal range of motion. And finally, tendons can be damaged simply by applying repeated pressure against them as in someone constantly leaning on their knees causing the main connective tissue running over the knee cap, the patella tendon, to become inflamed. This condition, generically called "housemaid's knees" from the constant pressure of excessive force against the knees proper can develop in high-jumpers, participants in basketball and volleyball, weight lifters who excessively and incorrectly stress their knees with deep-knee bends and leg-lifts at the wrong angle of attack, and anyone else having to endure the force of body weight transmitted through the knees against gravity and immoveable ground.

Tendonous tears, as with muscle tears, come in various degrees of severity. It is usually an easier road to healing if a muscle sustains a minor to moderate tear than a tendon. Muscle has more tissue to help it sustain a resistive load and with appropriate rest and physical rehabilitation can have the damaged tissue re-join together, though scar tissue and calcium deposits can ensue, while a tear in a stringy tendon, even one somewhat enhanced due to the adaptive processes to training, could much more easily produce a complete or near-complete separation requiring surgical repair.

CHARACTERISTICS OF MUSCLE AND TENDON SORENESS

Generally speaking, after a single intense bout of vigorous activity where too much exercise in a short period of time has been endured, muscle soreness could occur at the highest level about 24 to 48 hours after the fact, reaching a peak within 48 to 72 hours, and noticeably disappearing five to seven days after the activity. Inflammation also increases to reach its peak in a few days after the bout that usually delays healing. But as the body becomes exposed to repeated physical effort, recovery happens sooner and full and even increasing strength return more quickly as adaptation becomes manifest. In short: the body is getting in "shape" and is becoming used to the rigor of intense physical activity.

Another cause for muscle and tendon soreness occurs when muscle groups are repeatedly used under force in a certain way day after day with no or very little change in routine. This is known as *repetitive use injury* or *cumulative trauma disorder.* This has been the method utilized by the military in "boot camp" for many decades. The young men and women are pushed through grueling body movements every day during the hellish eight to nine weeks officially listed as basic training. Prescribed increases in physical demand are presented and expected to be handled which, thankfully, is usually the case, but we are dealing here with the situation of intense exposure to physicality at the expense of everything else. In addition the prize of human existence: sweet youth approaching physical maturity, is the commanding reality. With scholastic and collegiate athletes a balance must be sought between the choice of intense physical participation and academic and social demands. And attention should be placed upon appropriate recovery so the incidence of having injured athletes becomes less of a factor rather than more of a concern.

There are several syndromes (signs + symptoms) actually designated to body parts and activities where muscle and tendon become adversely affected due to excessive usage: tennis elbow (outside aspect of the elbow joint), golfer's and breaststroker's elbow (inside aspect of elbow joint), jumper's knees, breaststroker's knees, bowler's thumb, and swimmer's shoulder just to name a few. These usually occur around and in the actual articular systems (joints) proper which bear great force against which the athlete must propel himself. Beginning tendonitis associated with muscle over-usage usually presents itself as localized pain after a few minutes into a training session. Early on in the injury process, discomfort often eases a few hours after training. As the condition worsens, pain, weakness, and loss of range-of-motion in the affected area become more constant to the point of continuous discomfort throughout the day. This also can present with a strong negative psychological component to where the athlete sees training as a source of misery and has to deal with mounting avoidance. I as a concerned coach do not want to see my athletes endure the intense physical abuse the actor Bruce Willis portrays as the character John McClane in the

"Die Hard" series of movies so prevention becomes paramount with additional concern for enhanced aided recovery and treatment.

TREATMENT OF DAMAGED MUSCLE AND TENDONS

Though an ounce of prevention is worth much more than a pound of cure, nowhere more so than in athletics, it is usually after the athlete begins to notice pain, suffer weakness, and endure limited mobility and maneuverability that he and, or his coach realize that additional steps are needed to get things turned around. If constant technical guidance is neither possible nor provided throughout all training sessions, and it usually isn't, the next best thing to try and prevent the need for rehabilitation is to make the musculature as strong as possible along with all the supportive connective tissue. In addition, rest and recovery (even with specific workouts geared to provide this) are always appropriate to allow the body to catch up with the adaptation process. If the need for medicinal and, or physiotherapy intervention becomes a given, then the following suggestions should be heeded. We are now guided by the anagram PRICE where the letters stand for the five activities that should begin as soon as possible after perceived injury: "protection, rest, ice, compression, and elevation (above the heart)."

Obtainable from the local well-supplied pharmacy... the EXTERNALS: cold-application packs, heat-application products, supportive bandaging products; the INTERNALS: (NSAIDS), analgesics, and supplements.

EXTERNALS

As a practicing pharmacist for 30 years I have never found rubs of any kind that provided substantial reproducible pain relief and none has helped in the repair process. I do not believe external irritants benefit athletes in any way except to provide a superficial short-acting warming sensation where applied. Familiar proprietary names include *BenGay, Myoflex, Aspercreme, Sportscreme, Mobisyl, Zostrix*, and *Blue Stuff*. The active ingredients include *menthol, eucalyptol, camphor, methyl salicylate, trolamine, capsicum*, and *capsaicin*. They all carry the potential to do more harm than good. They can irritate the surface of the skin more than provide relief to the underlying muscle and can produce contact dermatitis at the place of application, and fumes and fragrances can be a source of respiratory irritation especially in youngsters and those with asthma. A sore muscle needs relief to get to the damaged site. Medications applied externally do NOT penetrate deep enough to reach muscular tissue; it is like scratching an itch... Superficial only, and not getting deep enough to the affected site will neither provide tangible relief nor cure. It is a total waste of time, effort and money and will only delay what truly needs to be done.

What does work is *cryotherapy* (application of cold) utilized immediately after trauma to reduce swelling and lessen tissue damage at the immediate site. Cold therapy should not be utilized after the first few hours after injury is perceived, and it is not the treatment of choice for non-acute muscle problems, such as muscle soreness and the repetitive-use syndrome.

Here we need heat application that dilates blood vessels and increases blood flow to the affected area to provide true warmth and soothing and to allow certain enzymes and cellular types carried in the blood to be sent to the injured site to help in the clearing away of damage tissue.

Sandy Kolfax, the great left-handed fast baller for the Los Angeles Dodgers of the 1960's was famous for having photo ops of ice packs strapped to his elbow immediately following his appearance on the mound. This probably provided some relief to the tendons in his elbow region by delaying the formation of the inflammatory response and lessening swelling to some degree, but in the long run, heat would have been better on a repetitive basis to enhance the blood supply. Unfortunately, many athletes were often given injectable steroids at the site of injury to control inflammation and render the area insensitive to the distress it was undergoing. Though this might have extended playing time in the short term, it most likely hastened the end of careers by allowing tissue damage to ensue in an unhealed area while it was forced to endure severe physical stress.

The application of heat can be brought about in several ways, some more efficacious than others. Moist heat penetrates tissue better than dry heat, so a moist heating pad is more helpful than a standard one but caution must be taken to prevent skin burns. An extended hot shower provides good relief if only for a relatively brief period. What has proved to be the best source of heat application is the recently-developed therapeutic heat wrap such as ThermaCare. This product with its discs of iron salts becoming oxidized when the package is open provides a safe 104 degrees of sustainable heat which should not burn the skin over the extended eight-hour wearing time. This product can also be worn during work and many recreational activities, affording the patient an uninterrupted session of therapy. After the eight-hour wearing, most patients usually experience pain relief for a full 24 hours. Some elderly patients, those with circulatory problems, and with sensitive skin might need a thin layer of clothing over which the heat wrap is placed to prevent discomfort from skin irritation.

INTERNALS

When injured, the damaged tissue emits pain which causes most muscular tissue to go into spasm, which then brings about more pain, all falling into a discomforting and escalating cycle that needs to be broken. Administering analgesics is not just to provide physical and emotional relief; as mentioned. If we can obtund the pain sufficiently, we can go a long way to preventing unwanted muscle spasms and further damage. The most common relatively safe product is *acetaminophen* (e.g. *Tylenol*). Four grams (4,000 mg) is the maximum safe daily dose for an extended period with half that or less if this drug is consumed in proximity with alcohol to prevent liver toxicity. Aside from this and no allergy to the active ingredient, *acetaminophen* should be the first product taken for pain relief on the road to recovery.

Along with *acetaminophen*, the NSAIDS can be taken to enhance analgesia with no contradictions. The two medicines act in different sites, in the brain and the body and actually provide a positive synergistic effect. The NSAIDS have an added benefit of providing an anti-inflammatory effect which helps to keep swelling and internal damage somewhat under control. These enhanced pain and inflammation antagonists bring a few cautions with them. Since they interfere with blood circulation and tissue repair throughout the body they must be taken with food to protect the stomach lining which constantly needs new tissue laid down to handle constant exposure to digestive enzymes and acid, and they also carry a caution on limiting the number of days taken because they can diminish blood circulation to the kidneys over time. It has now been realized that the number one cause of kidney failure in the United States came from overuse of NSAID medication right from their discovery even before they went over-the-counter. A safe suggestion is to administer for five consecutive days, if needed, with a two-day "drug holiday." If continuous treatment is needed, then this cycle usually can be safely repeated up to two more times in otherwise healthy patients with no intestinal ulcerations or decompensated kidney function. The drug holiday is to allow the body to rid itself of the drug and prevent potential serious adverse reactions. As stated above, since NSAIDS as a class interfere with circulation throughout the body, it can have a delaying effect in the absolute healing process; it presents as sort of a two-edged sword: reducing inflammation, which is what we want, but, with continuous use, delaying total healing at the injured site. This, again, emphasizes the need to be cautious with administration over several days.

There is another class of products that has as its primary use, the lessening of symptoms of allergy and colds but extrapolating its effect on the body has shown that it can produce a positive outcome on healing trauma. *Antihistamines* act, as the name implies, to reduce the release of *histamine* that is usually secreted in areas of inflammation whether in the nasal passages or at any site of trauma. The sooner it is taken, the better. *Histamine* causes blood leakage into the affected area with concomitant swelling. An *antihistamine* that can reduce swelling can aid in the body's ability to recover. The stronger *the antihistamine*, the better it can perform but this brings along the side effect of drowsiness, so much so that some products in this class are used to aid in sleep production. An example of this is the long time popular product *Benadryl* (*diphenhydramine*). Since it can easily cross the blood/brain barrier, it can cause drowsiness. The milder products that don't pass into the brain may not make the patient sleepy, but they really don't have much of an effect in reducing trauma.

There are also a few supplements that can enhance the repair process. The body makes its own joint-bathing substance, *glucosamine*, a complex sugar molecule, that presents as a thick gelatinous "ooze" coating the space between joint bones. It is responsible for providing nutrients and moisture to keep the joint areas functioning smoothly. In a healthy joint, it is associated with an enzyme (chondroitin) that helps in its production. When damage occurs or due to aging, adding an exogenous supply helps provide for good functionality.

The one healing supplement that truly works to help the body heal is found naturally in tropical fruit, mostly pineapples. It is the enzyme *bromelain*. Initially found to aid in digestion especially in "nervous stomachs," subsequent research proved that the enzyme helped the body clear itself of dead and damaged tissue almost anywhere, thus accelerating the healing process. It has proved its worth in athletes training hard, aiding them to recover from injury and the "planned" trauma of intense workouts when consumed regularly.

MORE ABOUT WHEN TENDONS GET DAMAGED

OVERVIEW

Tendons; afforded enough importance to have special mention in Greek mythology. The warrior, Achilles, was dipped in the river Styx by his mother, Thetis, to render his body invulnerable to future harm. Every inch was coated except where he was held by his ankle covering the tendon area named for him. This relatively small area would prove his fatal weakness. Are tendons, then, important enough to be concerned about their health when we ask the body to withstand rigorous training and competitions? Yes. And what if they do sustain definite injury, is it something to take seriously? Yes. Should we push past they're telling us something is amiss with increasing pain and weakness when they are brought into play? No.

This topic falls within my "keeping-the-athlete-healthy" research and is something everyone associated with athletics needs to understand and respect. Too many people, even the health and coaching professionals whose areas of expertise include how the body reacts to vigorous training, have utilized the wrong term more often than not in describing the painful and weakening condition when damage occurs to the all-important tendons attached to vital muscles for movement in chosen sports. To immediately clarify: **tendons attach muscle to bone; ligaments attach bone to bone.**

Due to their important function regarding the body's ability to move with force by attaching to less dense muscle as opposed to heavier, thicker bone, tendons have more elasticity than ligaments; they need it due to the inherent contraction (*concentric*) and extension (*eccentric*) of muscle movement. And they are not built as thick and strong as ligaments which usually allows them to suffer more injury due to irritative or incorrect **repetitive** activity as opposed to acute traumatic injury for ligaments. **To keep tendons in a healthy state and prevent the cascade of overuse into injury are vital responsibilities of both the athlete and the director of training.** Keep in mind the fact that just about every disease condition in the human body is caused by some type of initial inflammation. If it is not treated appropriately and thoroughly with a quick resolve, the initial diseased inflammatory response can progress to several possibilities, all leading to inevitable entrenched tissue damage over time. This almost always leaves its repeated "calling card" of tissue destruction which lessens the ability to optimally generate force.

The first word that usually comes to mind as a simple and rapid "diagnosis" either from the suffering athlete or the care-giver examining same is "*tendinitis*" especially when pain increases with specific repetitive movement, and an increasing sense of weakness emerges. The suffix "*-itis*" medically implies that an inflammatory condition has developed. This may be the correct initial call, but more often than not, the condition that *continually* presents

190

itself morphs away from true inflammation, per say, The major cause of *lingering* tendon pain has been found to be a failed healing response with tendon tissue degeneration. The inflammatory response should not be considered a stagnant or slow-moving condition. It is a serious warning which the body is broadcasting that the quality of the affected tissue has been compromised and diminished to varying degrees and cannot hold up its task of adequately handling sufficient force for continuous vigorous exercise. The major cause of **lingering tendon pain has been found to be a failed healing response with tendon tissue degeneration.** Ideally, as mentioned above, the patient's condition must not be treated casually, but rather thoroughly and vigorously to prevent what medical specialists now label this connective tissue damage as *tendinopathy and tendinosis.*

Chronic tendon injuries are most often a result of *repetitive* exposure to excess mechanical load or incorrect movement. Eventually, the damaged tendon tissue becomes weakened and unable to adequately respond to this load. While almost any tendon can become overburdened, the most common and important ones in sports are:

- "Swimmer's shoulder" where the possible involvements are tendons of the four *rotator cuff* muscles and the bicepts brachii;
- "Tennis elbow" involving tendons located at the outside (distal) aspect of this joint and "breaststroke" or "suitcase" elbow settling at the inside (medial) aspect.. .all allowing movement as common wrist extensors;
- Forearm where the tendons allow for flexing and extension;
- Wrist and fingers supported by the abductor (away from) pollicis longus tendon and long finger flexors;
- "Jumper's knee and "breaststroke knee" involving the patella (kneecap) and quadriceps (largest single muscle mass in the body) tendons;
- Lower leg extension and flexion affected by the Achilles tendon;
- Foot and ankle movement involving the Tibialis posterior.

Both intrinsic (from within) and extrinsic (from outside the body) factors contribute to the development of tendinopathy. Intrinsic factors predisposing an athlete to these tendon issues include an inherent "crowding" of the joint space where the internal elements of a joint are constantly forced to rub against one another with demanded range-of-motion; increased age with concomitant loss of flexibility; and male gender. As inevitable aging ensues, tendons become stiffer and less capable of handling high loads, and tendon injuries can occur with only moderate exertion. Estrogen may play a protective role, as females have a lower incidence of tendinopathy, and post-menopausal females taking hormone replacement therapy experience less tendon damage than those who do not.

Extrinsic factors that can hurt tendons include the training error of allowing incorrect repetitive movements through various joints, inappropriate use of equipment (e.g. swim paddles that place constant excessive forces throughout the shoulder, improper footwear for distance running), and the simple but, oh, so very important premise of not allowing the athlete adequate rest and recovery throughout the training cycle.

PATHOLOGY AND PRESENTATION

There are many ways to describe the pathology of an injured tendon. The most recent model utilized by orthopedic specialists suggests that there is a continuum of tendon pathology progressing through three stages: from the asymptomatic tendon to the tender-to-the-touch tendon to the degeneration-of-tissue tendon.

The first stage of injury and overuse is called the **reactive phase** which is a short-term adaptation of an acutely overloaded tendon. No inflammation is seen yet but a thickening of the tendon develops. No overt symptoms are presented yet, even with misuse, but the smart play would entail appropriate rest and recovery from intense and prolonged use. A correct stretching protocol would also be indicated here. Remember, even with no symptoms, damage can be working to undermine the tissue integrity of the tendons.

The second stage of injury comes into play if the overload on the reactive tendons is not reduced sufficiently, the tendon(s) may progress to a state of disrepair. **Tendon disrepair,** or failed healing, is characterized by an increase in a disorganized breakdown of the functioning tissue matrix. Pain becomes constantly noticeable with movement and palpation. Weakness increases even with the will to try and hold movement to a quality level.

As the tendon disorder progresses, what develops is the third or **degenerative stage.** Here, the functioning tissue matrix becomes more disordered with areas of cell death and loss of quality tissue. Tendons in this last stage of the continuum are past the point of spontaneous healing and are much more likely to rupture with continued demand for force. It is virtually impossible to continue on with vigorous training and competition if the condition has been left to get to this state.

Since tendinopathy is often a clinical diagnosis, proper treatment requires a thorough history of training routines, movements, and intentional increases in exercise demands. In the weight room, as examples, with swimmers the motion of a bench press with serious weight resistance can have the shoulder elements press against each other causing the rotator-cuff tendons to rub against bone and cartilage producing damaging impingement. The land-based athlete who wants to develop his legs and build strong quadriceps for speed and power must be careful to use an easy angle of lifting when doing leg extensions so as not to put excessive pressure on and damage the patellal (knee cap) tendon. When running over distance and non-level paths, having to deal with gravity and the hardness of the roadway, over three times gross body weight can be brought down with each stride onto each articular joint (knees, hips, ankles). This can cause the Ilio-Tibial Band (ITB), Achilles, and all the other tendons attached to the driving musculature to become overstressed, inflamed, and begin degeneration. If there is question as to absolute diagnosis and extent of damage, the use of sophisticated diagnostic procedures (ultrasound, MRI imaging) may be beneficial in confirming the existence and extent of tendinopathy, identifying any macroscopic tears and determining the extent of involvement of surrounding structures. Obviously, once an affirmative diagnosis has been made, treatment should be quickly instituted and any modifiable extrinsic factors should be corrected. Unless absolutely pointing to the need for surgery, utilizing more conservative management should be the first path to rehabilitation.

APPROPRIATE CONSERVATIVE MANAGEMENT

Staying out of the OR should be the hands-down first approach. Although conservative treatment regimens may be unsuccessful in a sizable portion of patients (up to 45%), it is accepted medical protocol to have them attempt diligent physical therapy for up to six months along with other conservative approaches prior to surgical intervention. Of course, if we are dealing with professional or aggressive elite athletes, getting them back into competition status becomes the most pressing issue. Having them wait several months to see if health and functionality can be restored in these cases is usually not the approach that will be tolerated. Both non-pharmacological and pharmacological protocols will be listed and discussed below.

NON-PHARMACOLOGICAL PROTOCOLS

Rest: It is NOT recommended to force absolute rest and immobilization in chronic tendinopathy. Some tendon loading is necessary for collagen repair and tendon remodeling. RELATIVE REST, which allows for maintenance of activities with reduced intensity and mechanical load, is the preferred approach. Activity that elicits pain from the tendon and the original activity that caused the injury should be absolutely avoided during the acute phase of recovery.

Cryotherapy: Application of ice or sustained cold to an acute injury is a common practice. The cold provides an analgesic effect with the additional benefit of reduced metabolic rate and blood flow in the tendon, leading to decreased influx of cells that are caused to circulate and bring about an inflammatory response and acute swelling. Though the benefits of applied cold to a chronic condition is less pronounced, it has been common practice over the years where we see many times a hard-throwing baseball pitcher (e.g. L.A. Dodger's Sandy Kolfax) or football quarterback (Oakland's Kenny Stabler) undergoing an elaborate ice-packing wrap after the game which seemed to have taken down the swelling and lessened the perceived inflammation for a quicker healing response.

Exercise and Stretches: When discussing movement with regard to muscle and attendant components during rehab of injured tendons, it is important to first differentiate between the two most common exercise regimens: ECCENTRIC and CONCENTRIC. The former utilizes active *lengthening* of the muscle/tendon unit. Alternatively, the latter involves application of a load to *shorten* the muscle/tendon unit. During vigorous exercise it is the eccentric (lengthening) movement of the muscle under stress that causes problems like **D**elayed **O**nset **O**f **M**uscle **S**oreness (DOMS) due to micro tears with attendant bleeding and swelling pressing against nerves. But to better help heal damaged tendon tissue, lengthening eccentric exercises under mild force appear to positively alter the structural and mechanical properties of the tendon proper. Increased collagen cross-linking and tendon remodeling through regeneration of healthy tissue is superior to tendon scarring which is the more common outcome with concentric exercises.

Several trials with eccentric exercise and modalities have shown definite positive results. Several tissue types, when damaged, tends to shrink and close in as the healing process ensues. This is Nature's protective mechanism to try and prevent excessive use in the subsequent stages of healing after-the-fact. But with elements of the body that work to produce range of motion, this is counter-productive... absolutely not what we want.

The idea of instituting a pre-stretching protocol to increase the actual length of the damaged tendon is good. Stretched tissue will lessen the strain on the tendon proper during subsequent elongation movement; this will allow for better adaptation toward desired tissue healing. Then progressively increasing the load with contractive force applied against the tendon will result in increased integrity of tissue and, thus, strength. Finally, causing the tendon to contract with increasing speed leads to the development of greater force... everything we need to try and get back to where we were pre-injury.

The exact protocol to elicit the best results is still being perfected but positive outcomes will only occur when patients become highly motivated and adhere to the rigorous regimen which entails, for a good-working protocol, twice-daily repetitions of exercises, seven days per week for as long as 12 weeks. Also, the fact that definite discomfort into pain will most likely develop with this type of physical rehabilitation is not an absolute contraindication. Unless totally debilitating, the patient should emotionally incorporate the discomfort as simply part of the healing process. But as with instituting any extended protocol, consulting with and getting medical approval from any and all of the pertinent medical team is strongly suggested. Some patients bring other medical issues to the table and might need modification so as not to do the patient more harm than good. Most cases also require pharmacological (medication) treatment to lessen the discomfort and enhance the healing procedures.

PHARMACOLOGICAL PROTOCOLS

For the past several decades, the most common choice of medication to treat what was thought to be simple inflammation was from the class of medications called *NSAIDS*. These are *prostaglandin*-inhibitors which innately reduce inflammation by lessening the effects of *prostaglandins*, powerful substances that are brought into play in the inflammatory process. Unfortunately, *prostaglandins* are also needed to ensure adequate perfusion of blood into organs and the regeneration of various tissues to continuously heal and repair stressed areas of the body. The first of this class of drugs, the prototype, was simple aspirin (*acetylsalicylic acid*, ASA) discovered in Germany by Frederick Bayer in 1899. For decades, scientists had no definitive idea how this "miracle" drug worked at the cellular level. But once elucidated, several derivatives were quickly manufactured by the big pharmaceutical houses. As their classification implies, they provide mild to moderate anti-inflammatory activity and were used for such thinking that in most cases inflammation was the root cause. Maybe early on in the diseased state but, as outlined above, not chronically. When the inflammatory response is no longer the presentation, these medications can actually do the patient more harm than good.

As eluded to above, because of its inhibiting effect on *prostaglandins*, it has been shown at the cellular level that NSAIIDS can actually delay the healing process, make the target tissue weaker over time and negatively affect several other organ tissues. Though this class of drugs can provide mild to moderate analgesia, controlling most pain associated with this type of injury, historic medical investigation has shown that since their wide-spread use for all types of aches and pains dating from the 1970's, NSAIDS have become the number one cause of kidney failure, a major cause of gastrointestinal irritation into frank ulcer formation, and potentially serious cardiac distress in the American populace. If the patient finds the analgesia produced by this class of medication adequate and can tolerate the proper dosages without having to endure the potential untoward effects, the emotional burden of not having to endure constant pain is worth the short-term exposure. A recommended dosage protocol is an adequate daily dosage according to labeled directions per drug for up to five days with a two-day "drug holiday" to clear the body and allow all organs to function properly with adequate blood supply and tissue regeneration. If progress in pain relief and ability to move with gaining strength and range-of-motion is present but not at a totally-healed level, a repeat of the dosage protocol can most times be tried. A more serious class of medication entails the use of very powerful anti-inflammatories called *corticosteroids.*

CORTICOSTERIODS

True steroid anti-inflammatory medications are usually reached for when the attending physician feels more "heroic" treatment is needed to quickly reduce what is thought to be the inflammatory process, even though this is usually not the major pathological feature. These drugs are injected *in situ* (right into the sight of pain and weakness whether it be soft tissue or an actual joint). Most evidence supporting the use of steroids is anecdotal, and the limited clinical evidence suggests that local corticosteroid injections have varying effects at different tendon locations. For *rotator cuff* tendinopathy or tennis elbow, short-term pain relief and range-of-motion benefits have been reported but no long-term benefit has been repeatedly and consistently shown. As for Achilles tendinosis, there has been no clear benefit proven, and numerous reports of tendon failure (rupture) have been sustained when the patient reverted too quickly back to intense training. Below is a small listing of available corticosteroid preparations for joint and soft tissue injection.

Generic Name	concentration	Dose	Duration of Action
Hydrocortisone acetate	*25mg/ml*	*5-50 mg*	*36 hours*
Methylprednisone acetate	*40 mg/ml*	*4-80 mg*	*weeks to months*
Prednisolone acetate	*25mg/ml*	*5-25mg*	*weeks to months*
Dexamethasone phosphate	*4mg/ml*	*0.4-6mg*	*weeks to months*
Triamcinolone acetonide	*10 mg/ml*	*2.5-15mg*	
	40mg/ml	*5 -40mg*	*weeks to months*
Triamcinolone hexacetonide	*20mg/ml*	*2-30 mg*	*weeks to months*

SURGICAL INTERVENTION

For tendon lesions most experts recommend soluble, shorter-acting *hydrocortisone* preparations to decrease the long-term negative effects on protein synthesis and connective tissue metabolism. These types of medications usually produce intense localized pain upon administration and are usually combined with local anesthetics which, unfortunately, more often than not don't seem to provide the desired obtundent effect.

GLYCERYL TRINITRATE (NITROGLYCERIN)

"Nitro" is mainly associated with treating cardiac conditions by relaxing vascular musculature to open up circulation to a damaged heart to reduce chest pain (angina) in either quick-dissolving tablets taken sublingually (under the tongue) or by ointment application right on the skin over the heart. But in this medical situation, studies have shown that **N**itric **O**xide (NO) is produced when nitroglycerin is metabolized, and NO enhances tendon healing by causing more collagen synthesis to occur from specific tissue (*fibroblasts*); more collagen = stronger, quicker-healing tendons.

Several studies and analyses have shown repeated positive effects in reducing pain associated with performing activities of daily living in people taking this medication with chronic tendinopathies. When used in conjunction with the elongation exercises mentioned above, positive pain relief has been long lasting and seen in a majority of cases. The most improved tendinopathy was with the Achilles. Patches of glyceral trinitrate are applied directly to the tendon area in doses of 1.25 mg to 5 mg per day. Patches are changed daily, and as seen whenever this drug is administered, varying degrees of headache are always a trade-off.

SCLEROSING INJECTIONS

The chronic condition of tendinopathy is associated with areas of increased vascularity. An excessive amount of vascular infiltration to the affected sight is seen to occur at the damaged areas of the tendon which, despite what might be thought, does NOT aid in tendon repair. On the contrary, it has been the major cause of pain at the sight. Injections of sclerosing chemicals act to strip away excess vascularity or to produce a thrombus (clot) in the formed vessels to prevent them from allowing excessive blood to go to the affected tendon tissue. The most pronounced successes have been with the Achilles and patellar (knee cap) tendons. Very few side effects have been noted with this treatment protocol, and patient-return to a modified training regimen have been as soon as one to three days.

Patients suffering persistent symptoms after about six months of conservative therapy are considered candidates for surgical correction. Though procedures are dependent upon the surgeon's training and experience, there are two main approaches to the problem. The most invasive and intense has the total removal of the affected tissue with replacement of healthy tendon tissue from other areas of the body. Recovery with rehab takes dedication and patience. This is better known as the Tommy John procedure for the professional baseball pitcher who was the initial highly successful recipient. The other protocol is less severe and requires less recovery time and effort and revolves around "scraping" away as much affected tissue as is possible while still maintaining sufficient tendon for regrowth and a return to appropriate activity.

TAKE HOME POINTS

Tendinopathy, or tendinosis, results from **chronic** tendon injuries. Not being able to tolerate **repeated exposure to mechanical stress** is a sure path to this condition. The initial tissue involvement can present as an inflammatory response which sometimes forms even before symptoms arise. If the training and, or competition regimens continually over-stress the ability of the tendons to handle demanded vigorous movement, chronicity of condition moves the tissue into a state of tendinosis or tendinopathy which is more difficult to treat. Initial treatment can, and often does, include the NSAID class of drugs but only for a week or two since the benefit-to-risk ratio heads in the wrong direction, and most of the time inflammation moves into another plateau of tissue disease that presents differently. With many of the NSAID class of drugs available over-the-counter allowing the patient to self-medicate, if they don't take advantage of appropriate medical consult, either from a physician or pharmacist or knowledgeable trainer, they could unwittingly risk over-exposure to serious medications.

It is now considered a better path to healing to include an *eccentric (lengthening)* exercise program, initial cryotherapy (cold applications) then applied heat if it feels better, and, of course, adequate and appropriate rest. Other conservative pharmacological treatments include topical glycerol trinitrate and sclerosing agents which have shown promise in several studies.

CHAPTER 4

ATHLETE'S KNEES (DIFFERENTIAL DIAGNOSIS FROM VARIOUS SYMPTOMATIC MOVEMENTS)

The second area of the body that is most vulnerable to overuse injuries is the knee. Repetitive strain injuries happen when the body cannot take the constant repetitive movements that cause inflammation, damage, and impairment to proper functioning of any muscle group or joint. Swimmer's shoulder is the most notorious; what we might call "breaststroker's knee" falls into this category of injuries, right behind the shoulder in frequency.

It is widely assumed that swimming is the almost perfect non-impact athletic endeavor in an anatomy- friendly gravity-free environment. And this is exactly the problem. The body has a tremendous ability to adapt to its surroundings, though in some cases it may take as long as 2 or 3 years. The more the body swims, the more it gets used to gravity-free conditions—not having to deal with the pounding and stresses gravity can produce on the body day after day.

Cross-training on land can thus set the swimmer up for a fall by placing too much pressure on the rather delicate joints of the ankles, knees, and hips. All too often, swim coaches have their athletes do various vigorous activities on land (running steep banks of steps, long runs up and down hills, continuous-walking deep-knee bends, and the like); these coaches are so convinced this cross-training will produce a positive holistic effect that movement on land becomes a mandatory part of their swimmers' daily training. This routine may work for some, even more than some, but in the long run (no pun intended) this practice is putting the swimmer in harm's way. The only exception to my premise is the obvious training of triathletes, which, by the nature of their chosen events, must bridge the gaps among watery (gravity-free), mechanical (bicycle), and gravity (land-based) environments.

Unfortunately, epidemiological studies indicate an increased incidence of osteoarthritis—the wearing a way of bone, cartilage, and other joint elements— in all age groups, particularly the damage that is now being seen in many of the articular (joint) areas of the body. Remember this rule of trauma and overuse: *The body never forgets.* Trauma, no matter how seemingly trivial, can leave its "footprint" on the body, and the older the athlete, the less able he will be to remove these markers of damage and fully repair the physical insults.

With each step taken on land, the moving body puts pressure about equal to three times its total weight on the knees and hips. Add weights to knee- bend exercises or movements and the pressure can mount to 13 times body weight. The soft cartilage actually needs some of this pressure to squeeze it and push out the fluid that bathes the surrounding area. As a sponge is squeezed, once the pressure is released, the surrounding nourishing liquid is absorbed back into the cartilage tissue, bringing in nourishing substances that allow it to thrive and function properly. That is all well and good, as Nature has adapted humans to functioning on land, but within limits of intensity and endurance. If land-based exercise is not overdone and if no trauma is sustained, the knee can function as designed for many years.

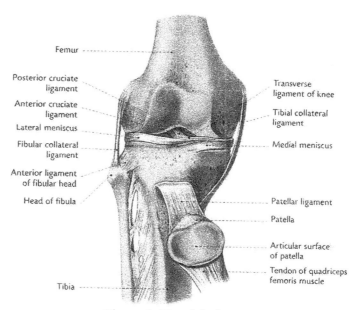

Figure 1. The right knee

Water, on the other hand, is not supposed to place the joints in this type of peril. But the knees still endure a slow, continuous barrage of mechanical insult with increasing intensity as swim training is increased over time. Intermittent discomfort can lead to continuous pain and then damage, often becoming permanent. Some athletes are blessed with cartilage and connective tissue substance and design that adapts appropriately to the mechanical stresses place upon them, but most are susceptible to varying extents. Add the stresses of land-based movements, and many a promising career can be placed in jeopardy or at the very least pain and discomfort endured as daily burdens—not something to look forward to before coming to the pool. Chronic pain usually leads to permanent injury and dysfunction. Pain should be respected for what it does: alarm the sufferer. Have the pain treated to prevent its recurrence, and dysfunction may be prevented.

Of all the racing strokes, it is breaststroke that forces the knees to endure the greatest tension. The stroke requires the legs to snap crisply together through a motion that is truly not joint-friendly. The greatest stress is placed on the medial (inner) aspect of the knees as they whip toward each other to produce forward propulsion. In addition, the torque (twisting) effect upon the knee joint at each wall for each open turn can place the knee in a position that stretches and twists the ligaments, tendons, and *menisci* within the knee capsule to cause inflammation, swelling, and osteoarthritis. The *menisci* are *fibrocartilaginous*, crescent-shaped discs at the inner (medial aspect) and outer (lateral aspect) areas of the knee joint that act to separate the cartilage ends of each bone and cushion their movement (see Fig. 1).

How to Distinguish Meniscal from Patellar Syndromes

What you notice	Meniscal	Patellar (kneecap)
Symptom site	Localized on side of knee	Pain in front of knee; pain right under kneecap
History of locking	Sometimes locks with pain	Grating, ratcheting, no locking
Weight-bearing activity	Pain during activity	Pain after activity, sometimes for hours
With "cutting" sports	Pain with rotation	Less pain, diffuse if any
When squatting	Pain going down in a squat	Pain coming up from a squat
When kneeling	Rarely painful	Pain with direct pressure on knee
When jumping or pushing off walls	May be painful	Definite pain, difficulty pushing off hard surfaces
Doing stairs or hills	Painful going up	Painful going down
When sitting	No pain	Pain in front of knee
Strengthening the supporting quads	Helpful but usually won't cure	Often the solution, with leg lifts
Swimming breaststroke	Pain as the legs come together as kick finishes	Pain as legs bend and heels come up to buttocks
Swimming other strokes	No real pain with dolphin and/or free or back kicks	Pain in the knee as it bends with kick
Pushing off wall in turns	Twisting off wall causes pain on sides of knee	Pain at knee with any turn leaving the walls

Pain with any type of movement is a sure sign of trouble. Normal movement of the knee (mostly up and down or with some slight side twisting) should be smooth, pain-free, and silent. I mention "silent" because a clicking or grinding noise emanating from the knee joint as it moves through its range of motion—called crepitus—is sometimes benign, sometimes a harbinger of trouble, especially if accompanied by pain. Sometimes you can actually feel the grinding more than hear it by placing your hand over the knee (or any joint for that matter) as it is moved. Normally, as Nature has intended, the movement of the patella (kneecap) in its groove as the leg is extended and contracted includes the two most slippery surfaces in the human body.

CAUSES OF KNEE PAIN

Deciphering knee pain, knowing which symptoms involve which internal structures, is extremely important for both coach and swimmer. The chart opposite might help in deciphering where and what the damage may be, but the sooner trouble can be properly diagnosed by the appropriate professional (usually a sports medicine or orthopedic practitioner), the sooner the proper treatment can be implemented and healing can occur or at least further damage from training can be halted.

Extensor-chain pain is by far the most common source of knee distress. Leg extension is the movement of the bent leg toward a straight position; the extensor chain is the series of muscles, tendons, cartilage, and bone that connect the thigh to the lower leg and hinge at the knee. The large quadriceps muscle attaches around the front two-thirds of the knee for natural protection, while the hamstrings attach in back of the knee. The kneecap (patella) is attached by means of its own tendon to both long bones of the leg (femur and tibia). If there is any defect (pain or diminished function) in the ability to extend the leg at the knee, the ability to explode off the starting block or spring off the walls in a streamline fashion will be hampered, as will the ability to kick with force in most positions, especially breaststroke.

As a "poor man's" guide to differential diagnosis, I will describe the most prominent types of pain, their causes, and the associated symptoms with movement. This is by no means intended to be used by coach, parent, or athlete in place of qualified professional care. This is simply a good quick outline that raises awareness and places caution at the center of the training regimen. As mentioned above, a swimmer with pain, injury, or difficulty in this area should be taken to a skilled practitioner who is experienced in treating injuries of this sort.

The *meniscus* gets involved when a twisting stress is placed upon the knee joint. This can happen acutely on land with a misstep or a quick cutting motion or a forceful sideways movement against the knee. It can also arise from chronic and repetitive stress on the knees (as is seen with veteran swimmers), producing slow degeneration and tearing. *Meniscal pain* is localized to the side of the knee with the tear. It allows the tear to produce a flap of tissue that can get caught and compressed between the long bones of the leg. This can give the knee the sensation of a painful "locking." This type of discomfort is usually sharp and happens with twisting and cutting movements of the knee.

A *meniscus* tear causes pain with a full squat, hurts when climbing up stairs, and can produce swelling at the knee. Twisting tests for a *meniscus* tear will produce a painful, palpable "clunk." Exercising and strengthening the joint-protecting quadriceps will help in recovery, along with appropriate rest from the offending movements, only if the tear is very small and the internal damage is minimal. But if the tear is moderate to severe, surgery will probably be needed to repair the damage.

Patellar pain, on the other hand, stems from damage to another internal structure of the knee joint. The kneecap is a wedge-shaped structure that normally slides up and down in its groove during extensor chain movements. When the kneecap tracks poorly in this groove, painful overuse problems usually result. Normal motion of the patella in the groove does not cause degeneration or pain. Pain with lessened mobility is often characteristic of patella inflammation. This inflammation is usually related to chronic stress at the site from on-land exercise or movement: leaning directly on the knees, running downhill, deep-knee bends, or squats with or without added weights. Kneeling puts direct pressure on a sore or inflamed patella and will produce definite localized pain. Jumping and landing against rigid things (ground, cement, wood flooring, etc.) will also produce knee pain.

A condition peculiar to women is the *bowstring effect of the kneecap.* This comes about when women's wider hips force the kneecap to track outward from its natural groove. Sometimes quadriceps atrophy is the culprit, allowing the knee joint to move out of line of the groove Nature intended. Pain or discomfort starts diffusely directly behind the kneecap. There is no locking of the knee joint *per se,* but a "ratcheting" sensation is felt with movement. Pain is often noticed after physical movement even if the athlete is at rest. An easy diagnostic test for patella pain involves dropping down to a full squat: there should be no pain dropping down, but rising up again will definitely be uncomfortable. The pain is felt right under the kneecap.

What helps in rehabilitation of kneecap inflammation is to strengthen the supporting musculature around the knee joint to keep the bending of the knee in proper alignment. Anti-inflammatory medication and ice after trauma, and then heat the next day or two when trauma has subsided some, can work to get the inflammatory condition under control.

TECHNIQUE AND WELL-TIMED REST

I would have to say, and I think most who know the sport would agree, that the single most important element in injury prevention in swimming is correct technique. It helps to have been taught the right way early on; *neuromuscularly*, this is a big advantage. Good technique is something that should stay with you forever. Sports people call it "muscle memory"; scientists call it "neurological adaptation." Put any name to it you want, but it is the coach and athlete who must understand that this requires constant reminding and training, because the human element brings in mistakes and faults over time unless we take great care to prevent them. Call it laziness, call it carelessness, call it lack of focus: it all comes down to taking the time to do it right and not settling for just moving through water. One need not be a born swimmer: I have seen highly motivated, talented athletes who have come to swimming relatively late make it their business to learn quickly and correctly how to perform the most efficient movements through water, which seems to emphasize how much a positive attitude means.

I would be remiss if I didn't include the one thing that requires no exertion of the athlete: *complete rest.* Correctly timed rest periods allow the body to heal itself and recover sufficiently to adapt to the stresses it has been put through, and ultimately to achieve a higher level of condition all around. With proper recovery nutrition, this is what allows the athlete to rise to higher and higher levels of condition and performance.

SWIMMER'S SHOULDER

Injuries or weakness in other body parts can be nemeses for the various strokes in competitive swimming, but the shoulders are by far the most important areas at risk for injury among aquatic athletes who train vigorously on a regular basis.

The cause or causes of swimmer's shoulder can be either endogenous (from within the body) or exogenous (arising from a source outside the body). The possibilities range from lack of flexibility, strength, and endurance in the supporting musculature of the shoulder to an unfortunate genetic body type in the shoulder girdle proper, which allows for impingement of tendons—all endogenous. Faulty technique or overuse in a particular repetitive athletic movement, on the other hand, would be considered exogenous.

Swimming in general promotes flexibility, but those who compete as triathletes, for example, and overemphasize running and biking tend to concentrate on stretching and strengthening only their lower extremities. As a result, most runners and bikers have relatively weak upper bodies that also lack flexibility. This double whammy can easily contribute to shoulder problems and hinder the development of good technique in the water.

Training for Shoulder Safety To train all the competitive swim racing strokes most efficiently, one needs to incorporate more than just the shoulder muscles into training. The body's core muscles must be trained as a group: abdominals, external and internal *obliques*, and lower, middle, and upper back muscles, which include the latissimus dorsi, trapezius, and rhomboids (see Fig. 2-a and b). Muscles trained as a group enable the body to roll side-to-side in a level position through the water for long-axis strokes (freestyle and backstroke) and to make the smooth and rhythmic undulation (dolphin-like) from the hips for short-axis strokes (breaststroke and butterfly). In this way, the pressure is taken off the shoulders, and the large muscle groups can help move the body through the water more efficiently. Once this side-to-side rolling motion or up-and-down hip motion is mastered, the swimmer can get more distance-per-stroke and slip through the water at an energy savings that is astounding.

In addition, it is most prudent to develop the smaller but very important supportive muscles in the back of the shoulder, the *rotator cuff*. The four muscles that make up the *rotator cuff* are, from bottom to top of the shoulder girdle, the *subscapularis*, the teres minor, the *infraspinatus*, and the *supraspinatus* (see Fig. 2a and b). It is this last muscle's tendon that takes the brunt of "hits" when the head of the humerus (upper arm) is forced upward into the shoulder girdle against a bony prominence called the acromion processes. (The acromion is the bone you feel when you pat yourself on the shoulder.)

A good example of this occurs when a swimmer "bounces" off the wall in open turns. Both shoulders would be expected to take the "hit" when the arms are jammed against the wall, as they should be for a quick, crisp turn in breaststroke, butterfly, or individual medley transition, and then the power arm (the arm that goes over the water) gets a second "hit" because it is used to push the body off the wall with more force as the body changes direction. If someone is turning from right to left, as is usual with right-handed swimmers, the right shoulder is the one at risk. This second "hit" seems to produce the greater compression damage over time, as it gets repeated over hundreds into thousands of times during a training season.

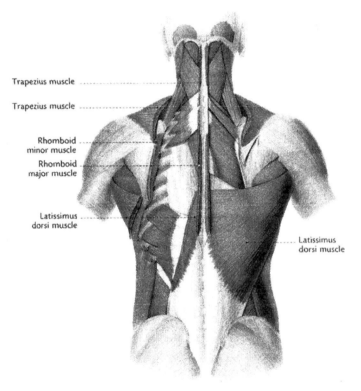

Figure 2a

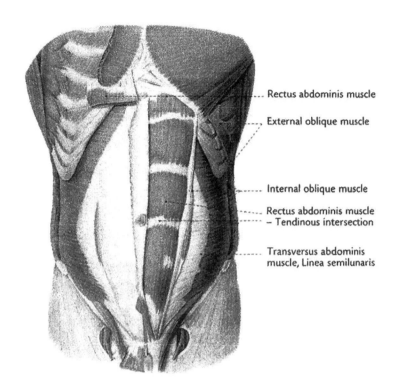

Rectus abdominis muscle

External oblique muscle

Internal oblique muscle

Rectus abdominis muscle
– Tendinous intersection

Transversus abdominis
muscle, Linea semilunaris

Figure 2b

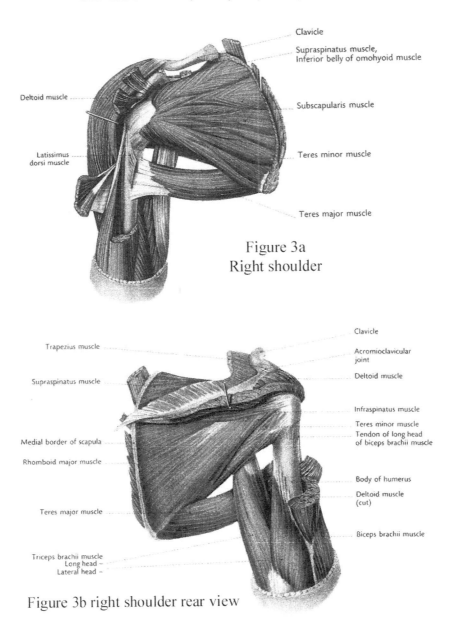

Clavicle

Supraspinatus muscle,
Inferior belly of omohyoid muscle

Deltoid muscle

Subscapularis muscle

Teres minor muscle

Latissimus
dorsi muscle

Teres major muscle

Figure 3a
Right shoulder

Trapezius muscle

Clavicle

Acromioclavicular
joint

Supraspinatus muscle

Deltoid muscle

Infraspinatus muscle
Teres minor muscle
Tendon of long head
of biceps brachii muscle

Medial border of scapula

Rhomboid major muscle

Body of humerus

Deltoid muscle
(cut)

Teres major muscle

Biceps brachii muscle

Triceps brachii muscle
Long head –
Lateral head –

Figure 3b right shoulder rear view

This compression from excessive movement of bone against muscle and tendon can be decreased by strengthening the musculature within and around the shoulder girdle. Impingement of this muscle and its associated tendon can also occur with repeated overhead movements in freestyle, butterfly, and in backstroke if there is naturally (genetically) not enough room for all the structures to move freely without rubbing against each other, or with overuse and the inflammation and swelling that follow.

Specific shoulder strengthening exercises with latex tubing and light weights done on a regular basis (three times weekly works well) should prove effective for preventative strengthening of both the shoulder girdle proper and the *rotator cuff* underneath, as well as for rehabilitation of an already inflamed condition. Flexibility exercises should be introduced as well. This has a twofold benefit: (1) to break up any adhesions that may develop as the body's response to inflammation and injury and (2) to increase the range of motion. It is so much easier to move through water with an increased **R**ange-**O**f-**M**otion (ROM) from the shoulders that increased distance-per-stroke is almost a given. Also, the potential for muscle tears is greatly reduced if we stretch the muscles gently but thoroughly, holding each stretch for about 30 seconds before vigorous exercise. It is much easier to stretch muscle fibers, which are designed for elongation, than the corresponding connective tissue (tendons) which are not. Anti-inflammatory medication should be considered to help reduce any swelling already in place and to prevent it from increasing.

CHAPTER 5

LACTIC ACID AS FOE

You swim fast, your muscles go anaerobic (without oxygen), and lactic acid forms. You continue to swim with intensity, and lactic acid builds up; your muscles burn, and you involuntarily slow down. This is because as the acid content rises above a certain threshold, the muscle fibers simply cannot perform the functions of contraction to produce force… they shut down. Pretty straightforward, right? Not anymore. Recent studies have shot down the notion that lactic acid accumulation is determined only by the supply and demand for oxygen, as George Brooks, PhD., and colleagues at the University of California, Berkeley, develop new ideas about lactate. You need to train fast not only to improve your anaerobic capacity, but to get rid of lactate faster, and even use some of it for energy. Several investigators and researchers have written that lactic acid in not an adversarial component to muscular activity; they have stated that they consider it an energy source that needs to be appreciated. My contention is that as it is being actively produced *in situ* (at the site of muscular activity) during anaerobic (without enough oxygen) activity it is an adversary because it is causing a building of an unfriendly internal environment at the cellular level. Once the pH starts dropping (acid environment) due to the buildup of lactic acid, the energy enzymes begin suffering and laboring to produce what we want from the musculature: power drops dramatically and quickly. Down the road biochemically and physiologically lactic acid may be considered a "friend" to the muscles, but as it is being made, it is a declared adversary.

HOW LACTIC ACID IS PRODUCED

Carbohydrates are broken down in your body first to simple sugars, usually *glucose* which is most easily handled by the body's energy systems. Then *glucose* (a six-carbon chain molecule) is further metabolized, mostly to pyruvate (a three-carbon chain molecule) if there is an adequate supply of oxygen. In your muscle cells during aerobic activity, pyruvate is either oxidized to produce energy in the *mitochondria* (the cells' powerhouses) or reduced to lactic acid through the action of an enzyme called **L**actate **D**e**H**ydrogenase (LDH). Again, production of pyruvate is favored with a preponderance of oxygen. Lactic acid is favored more and more as the oxygen supply becomes less and less. Brooks and others have shown that the key to lactic acid formation is not only the presence or absence of oxygen; you can also produce lactic acid simply because the rate of *glucose* to pyruvate conversion is greater than the rate of pyruvate use by *mitochondria*. Add in an environment where there is insufficient oxygen (sprint muscular activity), and lactic acid would start to accumulate.

LACTIC ACID ACCUMULATION

The concentration of lactate, as lactic acid is called in the blood, represents a balance between lactic acid production by your muscles, diffusion of same into your blood, and finally its consumption by your muscles, heart, liver, and kidneys. You produce and consume lactic acid even at rest, but as long as production equals consumption (called clearance), lactate in the blood does not increase. As you progress from rest to easy activity, then to more intense movement, the rates of lactic acid production and clearance in the muscles both increase… the better the condition of the athlete, the longer the balance of production and clearance can exist. Although the absolute blood concentration of lactic acid (lactate) does not increase at this point, the rate of turnover (production and removal) may multiply several fold.

When you exercise at increasing intensities, you reach a point at which muscle and blood lactate levels begin to climb. As you pick up pace and begin to sprint, the rate of lactate production continues to increase, but the rate of clearance cannot keep up.

Lactic acid is still being produced and cleared, but the two processes are no longer in balance. As clearance further falls behind production, blood lactate increases; the point at which this begins to occur is called the **lactate threshold.** There are several hypotheses proposed to explain this change in balance during high intensity muscular movement.

LACTIC ACID DIFFUSION AND CLEARANCE

Your body has several pathways that can clear lactic acid from the muscles, but the percentage of acid that follows each path varies, depending upon whether you are resting, exercising, or recovering from activity. Some lactic acid is oxidized to produce energy in your working muscles, while the rest eventually diffuses out of the muscles and into the blood. If lactic acid is produced and consumed to the same extent in the same muscle, it never reaches the blood stream, and cannot contribute to any rise in blood lactate. With quick-action high-intensity muscular movement, however, there is the inevitable delay between the lactic acid concentration immediately being formed in the muscle fibers and the concentration that cascades into the blood as lactate during intense exercise for at least several seconds.

Within the muscle proper, lactic acid may be oxidized either within the same muscle fibers that produced it (if they have a blood supply) or may migrate between the type of fast twitch fibers with a blood supply (high intensity activity) and the blood-laden slow twitch fibers (used for endurance). Be aware that the absolute quickest-reacting muscle fibers (all out sprints) have no blood supply at all, and any lactic acid that develops here **must be diffused out to other areas for oxidizing.** (This is the main reason that after a swim race, the **exact muscle fibers** that were utilized for propulsion must be used in a **similar** but **less**

intense recovery swim to help move the lactic acid more efficiently out to where it can be handled by the body's oxidizing systems.

THE FATE OF LACTIC ACID

As explained above, the body's reaction to lactic acid is not one of complacency; it works very hard to eliminate this by product of muscular activity. Eventually, if the muscular activity is pushed high enough and long enough, the concentration of lactic acid will rise sufficiently to cause a migration of the excess into the blood.. This can be ascertained by **blood lactate readings.**

After diffusing into the blood stream, lactate is either converted to *glucose* in the liver, or is oxidized in the skeletal muscles or heart. If there is no immediate need for *glucose*, the liver makes glycogen (a complex carbohydrate made up of long chains of *glucose* molecules) as a storage form of energy to, again, re-produce *glucose* for muscle and brain to use upon demand. (*Glucose* is the primary source of energy that the brain utilizes).

Liver glycogen formed this way can be looked upon as being re-cycled lactic acid from muscle contractions, and is called the **lactate shuttle.**

This overview shows the role of lactic acid during exercise as not being as simple as once thought. Blood lactate concentration doesn't only reflect lactic acid formation, but also the relative rates of lactic acid production, diffusion into blood, and clearance. The **anaerobic threshold** is still important because it signals the limit of aerobic endurance performance. But this doesn't necessarily represent a rapid increase in lactic acid production itself, but rather may be the result of exercise intensity at which lactic acid clearance can no longer keep up with lactic acid formation. In other words, you train at high intensity partly to improve your lactate clearance, and partly to teach the muscles to tolerate more lactate before they shut down.

YOUTH: A STATE OF MIND

Youth is not a time of life; it is a state of mind, a product of the imagination, a vigor of the emotions, a predominance of courage over timidity... a craving for adventure.

Nobody grows old by living a number of years. you grow old when you desert your ideals.

Years may wrinkle your skin, but to give up enthusiasm wrinkles your soul.

Worry, self-doubt, fear and anxiety... these are the culprits that bow the head and break the spirit.

Whether 18 or 80, there exists in the heart of every person who loves life the thrill of a new challenge, the insatiable appetite for what is coming next. you are as young as your faith or as old as your doubts.

So long as your heart receives from your mind messages that reflect beauty, courage, joy, and excitement, you are young. when your thinking becomes clouded with pessimism and prevents you from taking risks, then you are old... and may god have mercy on your soul.

CHAPTER 6

SKIN DAMAGE FROM THE SUN... "THERE IS NO SUCH THING AS A HEALTHY TAN"

Nearly everyone has experienced the pain of sunburn at some point. The insidious effect of being out in the sun on a nice warm day preoccupied with whatever activity is at hand can bring about great skin discomfort in a matter of what used to be measured in hours but now in minutes. Science tells us that the protective ozone layer is dissipating, and what once would give the average medium-skinned toned person a definite reddening in, say, two to four hours (depending upon locale, altitude, time of day and calendar date), can bring about the same damage and discomfort in less than half an hour. Though exact rates of sunburn are difficult to determine from the populace, a 2007 study of 10,000 teenagers showed that 83% admitted to at least one burn experience the previous summer, with as many as 36% reporting three or more. Though public awareness of the need to protect the skin and eyes from damaging Ultra-Violet (UV) radiation has increased, the large number of varying products for sale and the procedures needed to actually protect the body have done more to confuse and confound than to definitely and distinctly help. The main thing to remember here is that from the moment the sun rises until it sets, its rays can do damage, though to varying degrees. And that the longer and, or more often the skin is exposed to the sun, the more the damage can mount. Once again that old saying in medicine comes into play here: "the body never forgets; many things are cumulative."

Those who have carried on their lives on the Earth's surface for several decades can bring to mind some of the amazing nonsense that used to be practiced in the sun. Lifeguards, beach boys, stone masons, cabana boys, or whoever spent their working hours in the sun's hot rays thought they had to endure the ritual of getting past that first bad burn. The ensuing peeling and itchy skin that produced a tight and constricting feeling on muscle movement was the price they had to pay for that so-called healthy bronzed look. Some even went further in "ritual preparation" by anointing every square inch of exposed skin with "the lifeguards' magic potion:" a bottle of baby oil that had several drops of iodine tincture shaken through it. Incorrectly thinking this concoction would cause the sought-after bronze, it actually fried the skin like a potato chip, causing the damage we now see in the form of premature and excessive skin aging, alarming increases in precancerous and cancerous lesions of various kinds, and the formation of cataracts (when adequate eye protection was not worn). What was once considered an old-person's syndrome, are now being seen in increasing amounts in youngsters in their late teens and early 20's.

ULTRAVIOLET (UV) RADIATION... FROM WHICH WE NEED PROTECTION

UV is a type of invisible (to the human eye) light emitted by the sun and artificial tanning machines. The Earth's surface and its inhabitants are exposed to the entire spectrum of UV radiation, which consists of wavelengths of 290 nanometers (nm) to 400 nm. Visible light is composed of:

a. violet/blue (400 nm)
b. blue/green/yellow (500 nm)
c. yellow/orange (600 nm)
d. red (700nm)

For the purpose of this discussion, UV radiation will be divided into two segments: UVA (wavelengths between 320 nm and 400 nm) & UVB (wavelengths between 280 nm and 320 nm). **UVB radiation generally penetrates epidermal cells causing DNA and protein damage, and is largely responsible for sunburn. UVA is absorbed by skin cells in the same way as UVB but it penetrates deeper into the dermal layers.** It has been shown that UVA radiation exposure results in a wide variety of dermatologic consequences, such as DNA and tissue damage, while also contributing to early accelerated skin aging.

SUNBURN PROTECTION FACTOR (SPF)

Simply put, SPF is the numeric measurement of how effective a sunscreen is at preventing sunburn. It is calculated by dividing the amount of UV rays required to produce minimal erythema (reddening) on skin to which a sunscreen product has been applied by the amount of UV rays required to produce the same reddening on unprotected skin. Historically, SPF values listed on products have ranged from 2 to greater than 100. But this has led to an assumption that products with higher SPFs offer significantly better sun protection (i.e. SPF 30 being twice as effective as SPF 15). In fact, for example, SPF 15 blocks about 93% UVB radiation whereas SPF 30 blocks only a bit more at 97%. Another confounding situation is that historically SPF was only involved with UVB rays where many times a product didn't concern itself at all with UVA.

FDA SUNSCREEN REGULATIONS

To enhance consumer knowledge and understanding of how sunscreens actually function, and to standardize manufacturing requirements with the growing number of products, ingredient-listing, and marketing claims, the FDA proposed new labeling guidelines for sunscreen manufacturers back in July 2011 that were supposed to take effect in July 2012. But manufacturers have presented a problem in that they will not be able to comply by this deadline with the new labeling restrictions. So in order to have product available for consumer use without disruption, the FDA has moved the line in the sand to mid-December, 2012. These regulations specify which tests and results are necessary for sun protection claims and will be discussed below. Key aspects are listed for quick reference in table 1.

TABLE 1
Summary of New Sunscreen Guidelines

Cardiovascular

Label Terminology	FDA Regulation
Broad Spectrum	*The only statement permitted to indicate dual UVA & UVB protection.*
	The product must protect against at least 90% of UV rays 290-400 nm.
Water Resistant	*Product must be reapplied after 40 minutes of swimming or sweating And immediately after towel drying.*
Very Water resistant	*Product must be reapplied after 80 minutes of swimming or sweating And immediately after towel drying.*
Maximum SPF	*SPF 50+ is the maximum SPF claim allowed for any product.*
Water/Sweat proof	*These claims may not be used.*
Immediate Use	*This claim may not be used.*
Prolonged Protection	*It may not be claimed that protection lasts greater than 2 hours.*

Broad-Spectrum Status: The term *broad-spectrum* has been included on sunscreen product labeling in the past, however, there was no universal definition of what this claim represented. A specific broad-spectrum test is now mandated by the FDA to assess protection against **both** UVB & UVA wavelengths.

In order to now carry this claim, a product must pass a standard test measuring coverage against at least 90% of the absorbable UV spectrum from 290 nm to 400 nm. *Broad-spectrum* is the only term that may be used to indicate **dual** UVB & UVA protection. The new guidelines are intended to prevent false labeling claims.

Sun protection products that are not broad spectrum or are broad spectrum but with an SPF of 2 to 14 must state: *"These products have not been shown to protect against skin cancer and early skin aging. They have been shown only to help prevent sunburn."* Products that are broad spectrum and have an SPF of 15 or greater may state: *"If used as directed with other sun protection measures, this product reduces the risk of skin cancer and early skin aging, as well as helps prevent sunburn."*

Water Resistance: The guidelines also clarify labeling requirements for *water-resistance* claims. A sunscreen product must undergo immersion testing to qualify for specific statements regarding water-resistance. To be labeled as such, a product must retain the labeled SPF during two 20-minute immersion tests with 15 minutes of drying time between immersions. A product that retains the stated SPF during four 20-minute immersion with 15 minutes of drying time between immersions may be labeled *very water-resistant.* The labels of water-resistant products must include directions to reapply sunscreen after 40 minutes of swimming or sweating; those for *very-water-resistant* must have the 80-minute time limit listed. Both must have the advisory to reapply immediately after towel drying. **No product may claim to be water-proof or sweat-proof.**

SPF Claims: Addressing the confusion about SPF numbers and what actual protection they provide, among the FDA's new regulations is the stipulation that the maximum labeled SPF is to be 50. The FDA has stated that there is a lack of evidence that products with SPF exceeding 50 provide additional clinical benefit compared with SPF-50 products.

Additional Factors: The new regulations also emphasize the importance of administering sunscreen products 20 to 30 minutes before initial sun exposure. If people apply sunscreen and then immediately go swimming, for the most part they leave an oil slick as they move through water. The sunscreen will be washed away before it has had sufficient time to be absorbed into the layers of the skin for adequate protection. Other cautions include reapplying sunscreen at least every 2 hours, with more frequent reapplications (every hour) following swimming, sweating or towel drying. Products also may not state that they are for *"immediate use"* or provide protection for longer than 2 hours unless the manufacturer submits data to support these claims and receives FDA approval.

FDA-APPROVED INGREDIENTS

With all the sunscreen options on the shelves today, there has grown a wide assortment of active ingredients on product labels. It is important to distinguish which active ingredients various products contain and how they act. Some products offer only UVA or UVB coverage and some claim extended activity. As a rule, chemical (organic) absorbing elements work by converting UV radiation into energy before it can cause harm. Physical (inorganic) blockers work by actually reflecting and scattering UV radiation over an extensive range of wavelengths. Currently 17 active ingredients are approved by the FDA.

TABLE 2

FDA-Approved Sunscreen Ingredients

UVA FILTERS	UVB FILTERS	PHYSICAL BLOCKERS
Avobenzone	*Cinoxate*	*Titanium Dioxide*
Dioxybenzone	*Ensulizole*	*Zinc Oxide*
Ecamsule	*Homosalate*	
Meradimate	*Octinoxate*	
Oxybenzone	*Octisalate*	
Sulisobenzone	*Octocrylene*	
	Para-amino Benzoic Acid (PABA)	
	Padimate O	
	Trolamine Salicylate	

CONTROVERSIES ASSOCIATED WITH SUNSCREENS

Even though the American Academy of Dermatology (AAD) recommends that everyone use broad-spectrum SPF 30 products in addition to other sun-protective strategies, the long-term benefits of sunscreens have not been clearly established. There are also concerns about adequate and appropriate repetitive use and misconceptions about current claims. The following controversies should be discussed with an appropriate health care provider such as a knowledgeable pharmacist or a dermatologist so that the patient may come away properly advised and educated.

Skin Cancer: The two most common types of skin cancer are *melanoma* and *non-melanoma*. The latter skin cancers, characterized as *basal cell carcinoma* and *squamous cell* *carcinoma*, are the most common type of cancer in the United States with more than 2 million patients diagnosed in 2010 alone. The number of new non-melanoma cases exceeds the number of all other cancer diagnoses combined, and the incidence rate continues to rise rapidly. Non-melanoma skin cancers are rarely metastatic and generally have a good prognosis, but the *squamous cell* has the inherent potential to be more invasive than the *basal cell*. They can cause substantial local destruction and disfigurement if allowed to remain at the site for an extended period which is the prime reason to have them destroyed by deep freezing the site, burning the affected tissue with electro-spark cauterization, or extrication by surgery. There are many identified risk factors, but sun exposure remains the most recognized. A few studies have demonstrated that daily adequate applications of an appropriate sunscreen have shown promise in preventing the development of squamous cell carcinoma, yet other studies have yielded conflicting results.

Melanoma, the more dangerous classification of a skin cancer, has a higher mortality rate with an estimated 68,000 new cases diagnosed in 2010 and about 8,700 deaths in the USA. Melanoma ranks second to leukemia in terms of lost years of potential life per death, since the average age at diagnosis is only 59 years. Incidence rates of melanoma have continued to rapidly increase and is alarmingly demonstrated by these facts: the lifetime risk of developing melanoma in 1930 was 1/1,500 patients, compared with the lifetime risk of 1/55 in 2005.This dramatic increase may be attributable to the increasing dangers of a more "powerful" sun, now able to release much more UV radiation landing on the Earth as the dissipating upper ozone level loses its ability to filter out and dissipate UV rays. An analysis of many studies using sunscreen for its protection against melanoma have produced disquieting conflicting results.

The danger with a melanoma, which can arise almost any place on the body, is that unlike most invasive situations which produce some markers of inflammation that the immune system can recognize, this type of cancer can remain at the invading site and not arouse the body to its presence until metastases (aggressive spreading throughout the body) have done their dangerous deed. And this cancer, though known for its potential for spreading deadly cancer cells rather quickly, can act unpredictably. A lesion can remain *in situ* (at the site) for many months with no metastatic activity, yet some can spread so quickly as to cause death within weeks.

Overall, randomized trials evaluating the beneficial effects of sunscreen application in reducing cancer rates inherently contain many confounding variables, including unknown sunscreen SPF, insufficient information about appropriate sunscreen quantity, and time in the sun without reapplication. Although evidence supporting the use of sunscreen to prevent skin cancer is relatively weak, experts agree that public education should focus on appropriate sun protection to reduce the burgeoning rates of skin cancer.

Vitamin D Absorption: The need for Vitamin D is essential. For the body to synthesize it naturally, exposure to UVB is necessary, and up to 90% of one's required functional amount is formed with UVB radiation to the skin. The AAD has revised its stance on the effect of sunscreens and the inhibition of Vitamin D formation. This interference with the vitamin's formation by skin irradiation of UVB can be obviated by increased consumption of appropriate D supplementation. People dwelling in the sun belt latitudes around the Earth have the advantage and option of choosing a safe intermittent UVB exposure almost year round. An appropriate dose of rays for the average person would be about 10 to 20 minutes of decent skin exposure at least three to four times weekly.

Sensitivity & Toxicity: Both sensitivity and toxicity from regular sunscreen use are uncommon and subjective and usually manifest as localized burning and stinging. True contact dermatitis is rare with sunscreen ingredients but there are two which can occasionally bring this about: **P**ara-**A**mino **B**enzoic **A**cid **(PABA)** and *oxybenzone.* Organic filters such as *avobenzone, sulisobenzone, octinoxate,* and *padimate O* are better tolerated. Specific individuals at greater risk for this type of dermatitis include those with physiological photophobias or those from medication and those with generalized biologic hyperactive skin responses to the environment such as eczema. If a dermatitis does arise, there are many products with various ingredients such that a suitable substitute can most likely be found.

SPF and Sun Exposure: As mentioned a few times in this discussion, it is wrong to think that simply applying sunscreen, particularly the ones with a higher-SPF labeling freely allows one to stay in the sun longer with no increased risk for sun damage. Estimating the safe allowable time in the sun by using the SPF alone is asking for trouble, if not immediately, then surely down the road in time. If it is known that it would take about 10 minutes to bring about a reddening of skin, and application of a sunscreen with a SPF of 15 is the choice, the math says sun-protection is automatically (10 x 15) = 150 minutes (2.5 hours). But these figures are for the testing lab under controlled repeatable conditions. In the functioning world, we now know better. These important variables come into play: is exposure during the day at the height of the sun's power; what are the weather conditions at the time; is it during mid-summer at a latitude where the sun is at its strongest; at what altitude does the application take place (the sun's rays are more intense at altitude); what quantity of sunscreen was applied on the exposed skin? The bottom line here... patients could be doing themselves more harm than good if they remain exposed for prolonged periods without reapplying sunscreen at least every 2 hours.

Application Thickness: Many consumers believe that simply applying just enough sunscreen to cover exposed skin is sufficient to protect against sun damage. A standard application thickness of 2 grams per square centimeter of skin is the amount tested for in the lab for quantifying SPF. If less is used, the actual SPF can be drastically diminished. Under-utilizing an SPF 30 sunscreen could mean reduced protection as if provided by a SPF 15 product with much less safe time in the sun. Studies have documented that real-life application practices produce only about 0.5 gram per square centimeter of skin. To fully cover exposed arms, legs, neck, ears, and face, two tablespoonful's (1 oz.) is needed and an equal amount more for the chest and back.

APPROPRIATE PREVENTIVE MEASURES WITH SUN EXPOSURE

The goal of appropriate sunscreen use is to keep people safe in the sun while preventing damaging conditions from arising. Sun protection measures are listed in table 3 for ready reference. Monthly self-examination of common sun-exposed skin areas may help identify early signs of damage, particularly of the most dangerous type: *melanoma*. Patients should be educated about the "ABCDEs" of skin cancer:

(**A**)symmetry, (**B**)order irregularity, (**C**)olor variation, (**D**)iameter greater than 6 mm, (**E**)volution of lesions) so they can examine their body each month for any new or changing moles or growths. Furthermore, a patient with a family history of *melanoma*, any previous skin cancers, or a large number of moles should be referred to a dermatologist for a complete skin exam at least twice a year.

TABLE 3

Sun-Protection Strategies

Avoid or limit sun exposure, especially during midday (10 AM -2 PM), or use the "shadow rule": The sun's UV rays are strongest when your shadow is shorter than you are.

Always try to seek shade.

Wear sun-protective clothing including a large-brimmed hat to cover as much of the head and neck as possible and UV-coated (or polycarbonate) lenses that are also polarized.

Apply SPF 15+ sunscreen 20-30 minutes prior to sun exposure.

Exercise caution around water, snow, and sand, which reflect damaging rays even more strongly than the originating radiation presenting the condition for doubling down on the problem.

Reapply sunscreen every 2 hours while being exposed to the sun; sooner if swimming or sweating.

Conclusion: Having had the public endure so many products with so many unsubstantiated claims for so long, the FDA has finally drawn the line in the sand as to what sunscreens are efficacious, how to utilize these products, and to truly know what to expect from them in dealing with potentially very serious conditions of sun-exposed skin that have escalated alarmingly in recent years.

CHAPTER 7

THE IMPORTANCE OF THE WARM-UP AND COOL-DOWN IN RELATION TO VIGOROUS EXERCISE

Unless you are an experienced athlete or someone exposed to same, there is a better than even chance your warm up/cool down ritual might be lacking in content and extent. Logic would dictate that SOMETHING be done to prepare for vigorous exercise. But, what, exactly? And how much? And when? And, of course, why? The WHY is very important, for I have found that teaching and EDUCATING directly correlates with understanding the reasons for. Once understood, the athlete will most always respect the importance in the training regimen that this protocol renders and institute it as equally important as the training sets themselves.

If you do not partake of these preparatory and recovery activities, you are at greater risk for injury, and you will simply not perform up to your potential. The body must be prepared, conditioned if you will, to summon its energies and mobility for intense physical activity if you want a quality effort, and it is most wise medically to afford the body adequate time and ability to approach recovery even during a training session or between repeated competitive efforts.

Of major consideration is the allowance of the musculature's full range of motion for the different body movements per event. To stretch the muscles when "cold" is to ask for trouble. Muscles have but one action: to contract with force. If they are asked to perform this activity with no opportunity of easy sport-specific preparatory activity and the concomitant increase in blood flow *in situ* (at the site), their range of motion and the force produced will usually be diminished. We want long powerful movements to allow the covering of distance per stroke, step, throw or leap to be as much as our trained bodies can muster. Also, muscle fibers, when properly trained over time to become powerful, usually develop more force than the connective tissue (tendons) to which they are bound. Not allowing them adequate warming and not having them sufficiently elongate to their full range of motion can produce an environment for muscle and tendon tears when immediate demand is sought. But the body actually tries to prevent its muscle fibers from stretching. It develops an inhibitory stretch reflex which tries to keep the fibers of muscle in their steady state of length thinking if the fibers are stretched, imminent damage will ensue. To effectively stretch muscle, one has to hold a static (non-movement) stretch for as long as 30 seconds to break this inhibitory reflex. Best if the muscles have been somewhat pre-warmed with easy movement. After about 20 seconds the athlete can feel the resistance to the stretch ease up, and a comforting sense of elongation and relaxation of the muscle begins. Sometimes, with really tight muscle groups or in a cold environment, multiple 30-second stretching bouts work best to bring about the desired elongation. Of course, there is a two-edged sword in place here: if the muscles are stretched just before use, they can become weakened by as much as 30%. And because of this, many coaches and athletic trainers are now having their athletes forgo stretching altogether as long as the easy and sometimes prolonged movements in a prescribed warm up make the athlete feel ready to compete. It has been demonstrated that if the athlete's muscles are kept warm, a stretch session can have its desired effect for up to two hours. Thus, stretching along with a prescribed warm up about 45 to 60 minutes before vigorous activity should not contribute to weakening the musculature, yet allow for optimum movement.

The second, and medically more important reason to warm up and cool down encompasses the cardiovascular system. The heart and blood vessels must be conditioned appropriately with progressive increases in the demands placed upon them to fulfill the needs of increasing physical activity. Heart rate and blood pressure need to be increased to have the physical being ready to go when the athlete needs to perform. There are no absolute set distances to be covered during a warm up but physiologic consensus has shown that the older the athlete, the more the need for the warm up and the longer it needs to be. The greater the muscular development, the greater the need for the warm up. The more intense the upcoming athletic effort, the greater the need for a sufficient warm up. The colder the environment, the longer and the more important the progressive warm up needs to be. An injured athlete is good to no one, and sustaining a muscular or tendon tear because of insufficient time and thought to complete an appropriate warm up is an absolutely avoidable circumstance. If approaching intense physical activity or competition in the next 30 to 60 minutes, faster and more intense short-burst efforts are recommended in the prescribed warm-up to present a "memory" of speed and power for the neuromusculature. To allow sufficient time for the body to recover from this increased movement, an absolute minimum of 20 minutes must be factored into the protocol. If less time is allotted, the body cannot recover sufficiently to have it pristine and ready to go. We see a buildup of a muscular acidic (lactic) environment and a depletion of *glucose* and ATP which presents as a concomitant diminished immediately-available energy reserve... all athletic hazards.

This building into speed is important for another reason. There is a small, but growing segment of the athletic world, especially swimmers, who would benefit greatly from a certain type of warm-up: the exercise-induced asthmatic who needs to lessen certain irritating chemicals released into the bronchiole tree upon vigorous activity. We see this also in land-based asthmatic athletes exposed to cold air. Balancing short, rapid movements apropos to the specific sport with adequate rest for air-recovery allows for the secreting of these chemicals and their depletion over time. Some chest discomfort and possible coughing are typical signs of the chemicals at work but eventually the symptoms subside. This ritual, though not pleasant, could make a big difference in the ensuing athletic event if it does not negatively affect the emotions of the participant. The experienced and, or well-coached athlete can come to utilize this fleeting feeling of air challenge to his or her advantage knowing that in a few minutes the body's ability to exchange air sufficiently will be up and present. Of course, most who endure "athletic asthma" are or should already be on prescribed inhalation and oral medication. The best pharmacology and physiology dictate that the inhalation medication needs to be administered at least one hour before need. This would most often coincide with the beginning of the warm up protocol. The oral medication is usually prescribed for a single dosage every 24 hours.

Cool downs have their own importance both athletically and physiologically, which often coincide.

They can vary in intensity and duration from absolutely passive, gently active or moderately active. Passive cool downs are least efficient and effective. Just resting will eventually get your air back, but it sometimes takes extended time and won't accelerate muscular and physiologic recovery. The athlete will still be under the PROLONGED influence of the negative effects of vigorous exercise (elevated blood pressure, heart rate, and blood and muscle-fiber lactate with early soreness). Gentle recovering activity provides a bit more response to intense activity but may still not allow appropriate or desired amounts quick enough for repeated efforts. Moderate recovering activity (about 50% to 60% effort) provides the best method for bringing the body "back down to earth." The exact muscular movements must be utilized in this protocol along with other easier movement to extend the cool down procedure enough to be of benefit. Since lactic acid rarely travels more than a few cells away from the ones just used in athletic activity, they need to use the built-up acid as fuel to accelerate recovery. At the moderate percentages listed above, most of the time no more lactate will be produced but the already-in-place acid will be directed to the liver and oxidized to pyruvate for use as new fuel after the recovery. Examples of this type of cool-down recovery would be: for swimmers: a straight 200 swim mixing what was just raced with freestyle. If the freestyle was raced, then only freestyle should be used at moderate pace. Then 4 x 50 yards/meters one length each of the racing stroke and freestyle and finally 8 x 25's alternating free with what was just raced... all done at MODERATE intensity so as not to create more lactate which we are trying to remove quickly. With land-based racing, it is more about time in recovery than distance. A workable time in cool down recovery mode would be between six to eight minutes. If the athlete feels he/she needs more, then, of course, more is taken until a sense of adequate *homeostasis* is retrieved.

There is also need for short bouts of recovery in between sets or with extended intervals while training. The mechanism of choice here is to bob up and down in the pool at the finish walls. INHALING while getting the HEART ABOVE THE WATER LINE (out of the water) then EXHALING while the HEART IS BELOW THE WATER LINE acts like a "poor man's" CPR... the body responds by lowering its heart rate, respiration, and blood pressure rather quickly affording the athlete a definite sense of quick recovery. Some of my swimmers would not be able to satisfactorily complete certain demanding intervals without this mini-cool down protocol.

Moderately-active recovery is the most complete and allows for the best return to base-line. Allowing an easy few laps after the bobbing-up-and-down ritual affords even more complete recovery for even more demanding upcoming sets. This is emphasized over and over to my athletes to reinforce the importance and absolute need for a proper cool-down. I also recommend that if the athlete is to include stretching in his training and competing regimens, it produces even more benefit AFTER the exercise bout than before.

Every one of my training sessions concludes with at least a 200 yards/meters cool-down at moderate intensity. As we age this protocol has another serious physiologic benefit. In swimmers and runners and cyclists, blood tends to pool in the legs which can create a blood volume deficit or slight vacuum through the heart. Cardiac irregularities with *syncope* (fainting) have been seen because of this. Moving muscle for several minutes will push pooled blood from the lower extremities back to the heart to obviate this potential for serious cardiac involvement.

CHAPTER 8

ANOTHER LOOK AT: TO SUFFER PAIN... "EVEN MY EYEBROWS HURT"...

Just about everyone who strives to be the best they can develops sore muscles at some time, so it is amazing that this condition is still mostly a mystery. Consider this: we don't really understand the main source of pain, we don't understand why it takes so long to show up, most of the treatments suggested don't work consistently, and there is no absolutely reliable way to prevent the problem except taking it easy.

If we overdo any kind of physical effort... working out longer than usual or harder than usual... about 12 to 48 hours later we stand a good chance of developing very stiff, sore muscles. In the medical field everything needs a name and category; in the sports medicine community, then, this is called **D**elayed **O**nset **O**f **M**uscle **S**oreness, or **DOMS** for short. Those of us who taper for the big meets, swimming or running faster than usual, can attest to the fact that everything hurts...even the eyebrows! This can bring on disconcerting feelings of "I'm in trouble; I don't feel good even in the taper. How can I ever do well at the meet?!" Fortunately for most athletes most times, if they hit their taper appropriately, this discomforting feeling morphs into a solid perception of strength and power by the time they have to present their best. But not always... this sensation of DOMS seems to be the price we pay for having our muscles help us move quickly and forcefully. Keep in mind that pain is still a signal that something is wrong, so let's see what we can do to minimize the problem.

MUSCLE DAMAGE

Hard exercise causes muscle damage; that is nature's way. In fact, this is the principle we have to follow to increase muscle size, strength, and power. "Muscle damage must precede size increases. The repair process leads to increased muscle size," says William Evans, PhD, at Penn State University. If we looked under a microscope at our sore muscles after a hard or fast workout, we would see ruptured individual muscle cells and breakdown of the membranes between them. There are some components of cells that are too large to escape from normal intact cells; but when the cells are "beaten up" and have broken membranes, the large molecules escape into the bloodstream. This brings about a useful physiologic tool for researchers with which to analyze muscle damage. Blood samples are much easier to perform than muscle biopsies and much less painful for the recipient of the

224

procedure. An enzyme called **C**reatinine **K**inase **(CK)** is an example which is often used as an index of muscle damage. Another enzyme called **L**actate **D**ehydrogenase **(LD)** is a prime example of a molecule that comes from the breakdown of the lipid cell membranes around muscle cells themselves, and it also leaves its "footprints" in the blood.

Muscle cell damage not only leaves us stiff and sore, we also lose some muscle strength; we usually are not able to move as well as normal, and we may even have swelling in the musculature due to broken blood vessels leaking fluid into the surrounding area. Another factor to consider is the kind of exercise we perform affects how we feel. Sometimes our muscles elongate and return to their original size; this is called ECCENTRIC movement. Other times the muscles contract and return to their original size; this is called CONCENTRIC movement. Since muscle fiber tissue is made to contract to produce force, this last type of movement is natural and is not as likely to produce tissue damage and pain as the elongation after the contraction. Though elongation is necessary to bring the contracted muscle back to neutral or normal position, if it is forced into this position repeatedly, that is what usually brings about the discomfort; the eccentric movement is much more the cause of DOMS. When we curl our upper arms, for example, to contract the biceps muscle, that is concentric movement; when we relax and let the arm straighten out, that is eccentric movement.

High-intensity speed workouts can also affect how we feel. Muscles become sore after faster movement, even if the force and work levels were higher at slower speeds according to studies from East Carolina University and the University of Wyoming. It has been stated that protein loss is a factor in sore muscles, but this is really not the case. It is true that exercise increases protein turnover because some is broken down and then replaced during repair… a natural process. But the amount is much less than most would believe.

Most Americans get around 15% of their total calories from protein which, for the average non-athlete, is more than they need for muscle repair. Athletes or people who enjoy a vigorous lifestyle, on the other hand, need that daily 15% caloric intake from a good protein source. In fact quality, muscle-friendly protein (whey, casein, and soy) is the smart choice for those who rely on their musculature to be nourished and repaired to carry them through intense prolonged training and, or competition.

PREVENTING DOMS IS TOUGH

Researchers have diligently tried to prevent muscle soreness, but their ideas usually haven't worked. For example, when we push a workout, our bodies respond naturally by breathing faster and more deeply because more oxygen is needed to help burn muscle fuel faster and to blow off (rid the body of) the concomitant buildup of (CO_2). Some of the extra oxygen causes an increase in the number of reactions that produce free radicals which can damage cells and genetic material. Several studies have shown that we can reduce this kind of damage with antioxidant vitamins and minerals, yet they don't reduce muscle soreness. Vitamins C and E and beta-carotene made no difference to the aftereffects of intense training of rowers at the University of California, Berkeley. They suffered the same amount of DOMS whether they took the antioxidants or not.

Physiologic studies have shown a similarity between sore muscles and inflammation which causes its own characteristic cascade of events to occur: pain, redness, heat, stiffness, and swelling. It would be a logical extension of thought to use anti-inflammatory medication in this situation to prevent or at least lessen muscle damage. The results have been inconsistent. Sometimes they seem to help, but often they do not. Topical products that contain counter-irritants, such as menthol, seem to stimulate blood flow which can present as soothing. Other topicals contain anti-inflammatories such as *trolamine salicylate*, a relative of aspirin. Both kinds of products may help a little by making you temporarily "feel" better, but there is no hard physiologic evidence that they promote muscle healing. Cold applications also provide no healing though they do have a place with immediate trauma by delaying swelling and slowing the attendant damaging cascade of events that usually follows moderate to severe injury. Also, cold can bring about muscle spasm and contraction which is counterproductive for recovery.

On the other hand, adding warmth such as with a heating pad (moist heat being better than dry heat due to better tissue penetration) does provide for muscle-relaxation and increased blood flow, allowing for accelerated muscle repair in many instances.

MINIMIZING DOMS

Good training habits help. First, start with a slow warm-up. Cold muscles suddenly put to work are more likely to become damaged than warmed-up muscles. In addition, the fast-twitch fibers (what I call the "Hustle Muscle") are more easily pulled (torn) than the slow-twitch fibers. Warm-ups help us to relax and put us in the right frame of mind to tackle a challenging workout or competition.

Warm-ups gradually increase our heart and breathing rates and increase the flow of oxygen and nutrients to our muscles before we begin to work them hard. They also allow for a gradual increase in the speed and strength of muscle contractions and a decrease in joint stiffness. At least 15 minutes should be allotted to each workout session for this most important of "rituals." But keep in mind that on some days more time may be needed to loosen up the body. Taking the time to prepare for intense muscular contraction is extremely important especially as the athlete gets older and develops more muscle. Short change this part of the exercise bout, and the athlete will usually pay the price later on with discomfort he or she didn't bargain for.

Wise athletes also take the time to cool down after workouts or races. Though absolutely not recommended for sound training principles, suddenly stopping from intense activity does allow the body to slow down the heart rate and breathing but the muscles will still retain by-products of strong physical activity such as lactate (which is the salt of dissociated lactic acid that is produced when not enough oxygen is available to keep up with muscle contraction over time). If not properly warmed down, the muscles will most likely begin to feel tight and lose some **R**ange **O**f **M**otion **(ROM)** within a few hours. For the older, or masters, athlete, this is just asking for physiologic trouble since blood pressure and cardiac stress need to be lessened in a logically-decreasing amount. Any athlete of any age not warming down is a mistake because the muscles need bathing by the blood to draw away the resultants of intense muscular contraction. Exercising at low intensity does two things: (1) it keeps the heart pumping at slightly higher than resting levels which keeps the supply of nutrients coming to help clean out the muscles, and (2) it causes the muscles to contract moderately to help squeeze out the by-products of intense contraction.

Since the main causes of DOMS are sudden increases in intensity or duration of muscular work, building a good training program dictates that any increase in the above parameters are kept to no more than 10% each week. It is also highly recommended to NOT increase both intensity and duration during the same week. These guidelines will allow the body to recover properly and adapt slowly to improved performance levels. I cannot over-emphasize the importance of adequate recovery from one workout to the next. Following hard workouts with easier ones is one way in implement this. Hydrating adequately and eating a moderately high complex carbohydrate low fat diet so the muscles will have enough fluid to bathe the fibers and lessen the attendant friction between them and have plenty of quality fuel to burn is the correct way to eat to compete. In fact, there are now products that are specifically designed to help in this reparative process; they have a 4:1 ratio of quality carbohydrate to muscle-friendly protein which not only fuels the muscles but lessens their damage.

HANDLING SORE MUSCLES

If you follow the ground rules but end up sore anyway, what then? Conventional injury treatments don't seem to work well for DOMS, and there is now some evidence that, though the anti-inflammatories (*Motrin, Advil, Aleve*, etc.) do keep inflammation under control and often act in consort to help the body deal with injury, they may actually retard healing due to their *prostaglandin* inhibition (*prostaglandins* allow the body to trigger natural responses to infection and injury). Relief provided by these medicines seems to come mainly from their analgesic (pain-relieving) properties.

Active sports massage has become an important accepted protocol for helping intense athletes recover between workouts or races. Whether it is the soothing psychological benefit of "hands-on" sore tissue or the potential of actual reparative processes, massage in the hands of qualified practitioners seems to provide at least perceived moderate benefit.

Even though massage hasn't proven to be absolutely cause-and-effect for the healing process or the lessening of DOMS, a series of tests have shown that when athletes worked out hard and followed up two hours later with 30 minutes of massage, their blood CK levels were lower (less damaged cell membranes); also, a type of white blood cell called a neutrophil, which helps fight inflammation, increased in number, and the athletes reported lower levels of perceived DOMS compared to a placebo treatment with "medication." Best results are usually seen in the hands of certified massage therapists, but self-massage and the use of hand-held massagers provide some benefit.

Small amounts of moderate exercise (active recovery) are much better than inactivity (passive recovery). The idea is to give the body a prod to stimulate natural healing processes, but not enough to cause more damage. Usually, one recovers in a few days from intense activity and is the better for it. Hard races need more caution, but in a multi-day championship, recovery must be timed to allow for repeat competitions. A prescribed warm-down after each intense effort would be the first procedure of benefit, followed by massage at the end of the day's events.

Ask anyone who has weathered the multi-event battles at a national competition… they are usually so beat-up at the end that EVEN THEIR EYEBROWS HURT!

PAIN AS A BARRIER TO EXERCISE FOR SUCCESSFUL AGING

It is practically a given that regular exercise, increasing from mild to moderate to vigorous, has proven absolutely beneficial in so many ways. From emotional to cognitive to physical for almost everyone partaking, that to abstain is courting eventual disastrous health. The body is an amazing adaptive machine that craves dedicated movement with enhanced air-exchange. Since our ancestors progressed to walk upright, human physiology has been geared to adapt to, and properly function with, recurrent motion, much of it vigorous. Those who choose the way of activity choose the way to better withstand most of life's challenges. Where the brain gives feedback such that it perceives: "I feel okay… I don't feel okay… I think I am going to die," this conditions the mind to permit the body to expand its ability to adapt to higher and higher levels of condition and the ability to move at ease even as we age.

Years of physical training and physiological assessment with various ages, abilities, and motivations have shown repeatedly that the mind almost always "caves" before the body. Nature provides for our relative safety by doing this. Evolution has developed a particular segment of the brain, the **amygdala,** which is sensitive to the build-up of carbon dioxide in the blood from activity. When $CO2$ reaches an increase to vascular threshold concentrations, very strong impulses are directed right to this cranial segment which can then quickly and dramatically send out its own impulses, building the sensation of air-starvation. This perception of increasing air-deprivation overwhelms everything else, almost always dictating the immediate cessation of vigorous activity in the uninitiated or untrained. Since humans are born land-based inhabitants where becoming accustomed to heavy breathing while standing or sitting after vigorous exercise is commonplace, having this sensation arise in water can easily be perceived to be much more daunting where the intense feeling of imminent drowning can overwhelm anyone.

In recent months, there has been a dramatic increase in focus and study on dealing with pain. Pain has always been with man but it appears to be growing in sufferers. The reputable Institute of Medicine has decided the numbers demand action. Government, schools of medicine, and various physician specialty groups have been requested to plan out a workable strategy to treat and manage the various causes-and-effects of pain. Almost one third of the US population, 100 million sufferers, have to deal with pain every day in various degrees at a staggering cost of $635 billion annually.

Attending physicians more and more feel that the body suffering chronic pain has been forced to deal with a medical entity separate and different from the original cause. Enduring chronic exposure to pain, nerves can become "hard-wired" to create a neurological memory. When the primary cause of the pain is gone in this situation, the pain remains. Several pain clinics have now taken the combination of ingredients approach, adding various physical activities and procedures to the administration of analgesics, not the least of which is working with the mind. Medical hypnosis and even just focusing on feeling better has proven to lessen pain and to enhance the perception of being in control of one's well-being.

Of course, everything here is relative. What might be truly challenging to the long-time unconditioned with multiple medical problems (e.g. simply getting out of bed and walking across the room), very mild exercise will not even register on the body's activity Richter scale in one who fits vigorous extended movement into a daily routine. There is also the mind-set of dealing with discomfort into pain whether from the physicality of chronic debilitating conditions like osteoarthritis or the mentality of repeatedly pushing seriously through the comfort zone. With an appropriate approach and plenty of adequate guidance, every person can improve his physical tolerance to movement which most often leads to a higher quality of life.

EXERCISE FOR PAIN MANAGEMENT

For those not restricted to a no-movement protocol but willing and able to partake of a progressive regimen, exercise is currently a major component of most pain management programs, either alone or in tandem with pharmacologic (analgesics, anti-inflammatories, etc.) and non-pharmacologic interventions (stretching, relaxation techniques {yoga}, acupuncture, massage, etc.). With physiologic adaptation to appropriate exercise, the body builds adequate supporting structures (muscle, tendons, ligaments) for movement and functionality. Having a totally stronger body enables movement and other functions of life to become accessible and available at will. Increasing strength from progressive resistance with weights has repeatedly proven quite effective in the elderly by adding safety to their daily activities. The increased ability of supporting muscles and concomitant connective tissue lessens instability and the potential for falls. Elevation of mood from endorphin release is often an appreciated tag-along with dedicated exercise along with the positive feeling of freedom to move about and complete daily tasks more easily. A building sense of confidence to handle what living demands usually has a very strong effect on lessening the negative effect of pain.

But with self-managed pain tolerance, especially as the patient ages, barriers to exercise, mostly emotional, can often derail all good intentions. Several studies have shown that when pain management is repeatedly perceived as ineffectual due to lack of emotional fortitude or support from either a coach, care-giver, or others partaking, an increasing anticipation of discomfort with movement will produce avoidance of exercise. The mind caving in before allowing the rest of the physical body to deal with the challenges of exercise is most often what limits success in this area.

EXERCISE: A SELF-MANAGEMENT STRATEGY

As we age, exercise must be classified a self-management strategy for many chronic conditions that can arise over time. If the individual is truly fortunate enough to have been spared the effects from a poor lifestyle, mounting unabated emotional or physical stress, accidental or athletic trauma, or a poor genetic inheritance, then enjoying relatively "good health" is still not the end-all to high quality longevity. The body craves movement. Just ask anyone who has had to endure being bound up to support or immobilize a damaged body part for even just a few hours to days. The muscles become so tight as to cause the sufferer to strongly seek some type of stretching or movement around the damaged area.

Our bodies are designed for movement. Unfortunately, many of us, as we age, choose not to do that. It is perceived to be less important and more of a burden, both physical and mental, and of less and less enjoyment. As time progresses, and the longer one is immersed in this mind-set, the harder it is to change.

Extra poundage, selecting reduced movement throughout the day, and the desire just to "settle in" on the favorite chair, couch, or lounge inevitably add up to reduced activity of any sort. The stresses of life can easily overwhelm us if we let them and cause depressive and, or anxious moments to take over more and more of our waking hours. These emotional "adulterants" have the ability to often cause excessive consumption of "feel-good foods" that would cause us to consume needless calories. There is a commercial for a well-known analgesic/anti-inflammatory that I like very much: **"there is a physical law: a body that remains at rest will stay at rest while a body that is able to move will stay in motion"** reinforces my point. Though it is touting a prescription medication that can present with serious side effects, the points of dedicated movement and the appreciation for an active life are well taken.

EXERCISES APPROPRIATE FOR THE AGING POPULATION

The first rule in medicine rings absolutely true for the aging athlete: *DO NO HARM!* Recommended activities should present a varied approach to increased physical fitness at any age, most certainly to those advancing in years. There have been many well documented studies and meta-analyses of several studies comparing the physiology of aging in athletes and non-athletes in various decades of their lives. Overall, the studies prove that the body can adapt and increase its physicality no matter what the age. Speed, strength, and endurance of movement are all benefited by dedicated sessions of activity. The organs of import (heart, lungs, musculature, joints, connective tissue, mind) brought into play for vigorous exercise, can and do adapt to increasing demands as long as an appropriate approach is applied over time.

The mix of training sessions that work best include water-based, machine-based, and land-based activities lasting from one to two hours or more, three to four times per week. Building from two to three sessions per week produce increases in strength, endurance, and power but after several weeks, a plateau is reached. Adding the fourth weekly session allows for continued improvement over several months. And with intelligence, training up to six days per week can produce even higher levels of condition. The key here is to NOT totally deplete energy reserves. Youth seems to provide its own "magic elixirs" for energy to live. But as we age, a more intelligent doling out of what energies we have stored in our bodies is the smartest path to follow. Energy expenditure coupled with rest and recovery allows for protracted participation in vigorous activity. It is advised that the interpretation of "vigorous activity" be participant-dependent.

The main organ of concern, and obviously the one key to immediate survival is the heart. It has definite energy reserves; deplete them, and the myocardium (heart muscle) can go into failure, either electrically, or muscularly. In fact, this is what some medical historians think happened to the first (and historically most famous) marathon runner. Phydippedes, a professional long-distance runner who acted as a courier, still in his 30's, was chosen because of his physical prowess to carry messages. He was commissioned to run to Athens to relate that the Greeks defeated the Persians on the invasion beach at Marathon. Marathon was about 26 miles away. But Phydippedes was asked to run and get help from the Spartans the two days before this invasion, covering about 150 miles. He obviously had no real time to recover. He was given water and some provisions and told to live off the land but he was to absolutely strive to deliver the message. History tells us that he did arrive, gave the good news of victory, but then collapsed and died right after. What happened? He didn't have the sophisticated nourishment we know of today to allow his heart to work so hard so long. He most probably fell due to his heart muscle being depleted of ATP and then go into failure. The heart simply ran out of energy to function adequately even in a young vigorous man. As we age, the lesson of Phydippedes is a very important one indeed. Total energy-depletion can prove very dangerous, and it can certainly inhibit recovery.

Another must-protect region of the body usually bears the brunt of gravity during vigorous physicality: the articular joints. Allowing us to change direction and force at will, these segments are often put under intense pressure with serious movement such that the laws of momentum can wreak havoc on the aging (or even young) body. Knees, hips, ankles, shoulders, elbows... if it bends or rotates or twists, it is at risk of dislocation, tearing, or sizable inflammation, any and all of which interferes with appropriate movement.

A. Water-based Exercises:

Since being submerged in water up to various levels of the body brings with it the physical property of being relatively weightless, it presents an almost ideal medium in which to train and spare the joints. With a strong positive feeling of being "one with the water" much energy (mental and physical) can be directed toward improving the ability to move. Often, constant, nagging pain seems to dissipate and "float" away from the body as an active water session progresses. The better the body adapts to increasing movement, the more this positive outcome directs the whole body to keep on trying. This cycle of positivity can build if allowed, to become an established way of life, day-to-day. Pain gets pushed into the back burners of the mind and no longer dominates thinking.

One doesn't have to be a champion swimmer to make water work. But it should be known that water presents as 1,000 times more dense than air, and it has a physical property of increasing its resistance to movement the faster or more intense one moves through it. Any increase in turbulence causes a multiple increase in resistance. Fatigue and breathlessness can set in quickly and dramatically, so if trepidation comes with movement through a liquid environment, realize that the benefits of a water workout listed above can be obtained by the simple act of moving through it in any way. If touching the bottom of the pool in the shallow end provides adequate emotional fortitude to partake, then that is where the workout should take place. Water-walking has its absolute benefits, and there are many variables that can be tried to keep the challenge fresh and stimulating. Floatation jackets, basic swim lessons, and even just a simple infusion of courage by a training partner or coach can all play a role in making time spent in water the goal to a better quality of life.

Water up to the waist allows for about 50% of total body weight to be supported.

Water up to the nipples reduces body weight by 75%.

Water up to the jaw-line supports 90% of original body weight.

Lying horizontal, floating, or actually swimming (as long as the bottom of the pool is not supporting you) provides for total body weight displacement. Whatever the person weighs, that amount of water is displaced. The swimmer doing this no longer weighs anything... gravity-free.

Osteoarthritis is the most prevalent remnant of years of physical incidence to the body. Whether from past participation in contact sports, gymnastics, accidental trauma, or physical over-indulgence in almost anything vigorous, the medical rule that "the body never forgets" seems to almost always take hold. Inflammation followed by calcium deposition and adhesions produce the condition called osteoarthritis. It is the body's ready response to the above especially if it is either acute or prolonged, forming at the injured or supportive areas. Whereas movement within a joint should be smooth and slick and not noticeably compromised, in damaged condition it becomes rough, interrupted and painful as inflammation's artifact (calcium) builds over the years. Unless one has been fortunate to lead a charmed life avoiding the slings and arrows of being physical, somewhere, somehow, sometime, pain with effort becomes de rigueur. And, unless highly motivated and appreciative of its benefits, any concerted movement against gravity magnifies pain and will most often drive away participation in physical activity.

B. Machine-based Exercises:

Land-based movement forces the body to withstand gravity and pounding against hard surfaces where as much as five times total body weight with vigorous running over hills and rough terrain is thrust upon joints of support (knees, ankles, hips), any damaged tissue comprising and supporting said joints lose their ability to permit smooth pain-free movement. For all intents and purposes the human body is a machine... our own "personal machine." And utilizing progressive resistance machines in the weight room to guide and support our "personal machines" through prescribed guided movement while allowing for gains in strength and power causes the body to work against gravity to build muscle and strengthen connective tissue. Working against gravity is not to be avoided totally. It just needs to be instituted wisely. The body evolved having to deal with gravity almost every moment. And with proper instruction in the weight room as to form and technique, desired increases in total body "functional strength" can arise outside of the water. This is good cross-training, and the body needs several approaches to gaining strength to sort of keep it 'guessing" as to what next must it withstand. Gravity also provides the necessary constant resistance that builds strong bones... makes them thicker with more calcium deposited. This, of course, prevents or at least delays the onset of *osteoporosis*.

The "machine" I most often use and recommend is the bicycle. The pounding against pavement is taken up by the rubber tires. The actual cycling activity, with the rider properly fitted to the bike, provides for smooth, rapidly-continuous movements around the knee, hip, and ankle joints. Various speeds and level of ground provide diversified stress challenges that bring in the heart, lungs, and vascular circulation to handle the demands of vigorous movement. Varying the speed and intensity of a bike session allows all the benefits sought but spares the body's supporting structures from overuse and the cumulative "hits" against the unforgiving ground that gravity brings. Swim training the legs in water has a 4:1 benefit ratio of effect and challenge over a bicycle. Anything done in the water is at least four times more challenging than on land and expands out even more as distances increase.

C. Land-based Exercises:

As stated previously, we are all born land-based inhabitants. Our anatomy and physiology have developed and are centered around the constant influence of gravity. But as we age and deal with the day-to-day and cumulative contact incidents that cross our paths, our ability to withstand all that gravity puts before us diminishes. Except for relatively rare unforeseen acute trauma or the result of suffering serious inflammatory or wasting diseases, it seems the young rarely have aches and pain of consequence or at least none that linger. Their energies and exuberance for life seem to put most minor to moderate medical conditions on the back burner. The back burner, that is, to maybe rear their ugly heads several decades down the road. For those who come to suffer the pains and pangs of life as they accumulate years almost always have to now deal with movement restrictions that never came to mind nor to the fore of daily living when in early life. For those who have a history of strong dedicated physicality and, or those who want to partake of the adventure of vigorous movement again in their advancing years there most likely is the constant reminder of the squeaky wheel needing the oil. Considering all this, the wise person wanting to experience activity needs to make wise choices on how and when to do this.

There are lots of choices on land to move in varying intensities, distances & duration, and elevation. The water provides limited variability through which the swimmer must navigate where swimming in a pool is mostly in a horizontal motion with surface tension often seen as the main drag force for constant resistance in a pool. If open water is the venue for training then waves, currents, lack of guide lines and water clarity come into play to magnify the challenge. But with land-based exercises, you have very hard ground (concrete, macadam), moderately hard ground (grass, dirt), and soft ground (sand and special composition tracks at schools). Pushing off ground provides for a much better consistent bounce-and-jounce effect than trying to grab a moveable resistance like water.

If a beach is nearby or making time and effort to get to one a desirable possibility, sand is best. Variable consistencies provide variable resistances. Soft sand is more "giving" upon push-off and causes the leg muscles and feet to work much harder over time. But it also provides a very body-friendly medium on which to move in that it gives enough each time to lessen the "hits" the body's articular system must take with each step. Walking on harder sand near the water's edge provides an easier track on which to move but is still body-friendly. Safe, effective, productive, stimulating... everything you could want in a bi-pedal activity to strengthen mind, body, and spirit, and lessen the thoughts and perceptions of pain.

CHAPTER 9

MORE METHODS FOR DEALING WITH PAIN

My take on life. "Pain... if you have it, you must still be alive." Maybe a bit Spartan, but one that has some veracity. Obviously the transmission of a painful stimulus and its perception prove that nerves and receptors and the brain's ability to decipher are intact. But when it becomes so pronounced and relentless that everything else is inhibited or diminished, or when it simply does not go away even at moderate levels to constantly remind the victim that something is medically and, or physically wrong, pain can morph into the realm of the psychological which can present its own deleterious interjection.

There is acute, chronic, and intermittent pain, each of which has its own characteristics causing the body to react in various, sometimes characteristic, ways. You name the body part or organ system; it can cause us to suffer pain.

DESCRIPTION AND MECHANISM OF PAIN

Pain can be divided into three major categories: type *(a) nociceptive,* type (b) *neuropathic,* and type (c) *intermittent.* The first is more commonly known to describe **acute pain** and the second **chronic pain.** The third classification brings in the elements of threshold, latency, individual awareness and distraction throughout the day. Type *(a) nociceptive* pain is further categorized as *somatic* and *visceral. Somatic* pain usually arises from muscle or tissue injury most probably from an *exogenous* (outside the body) source. It is usually well localized and is often described as presenting as aching, throbbing, or shooting sensations. Dental pain would fall into this category. Visceral pain is often referred from deep inside the body *(endogenous)* as from an internal organ (e.g. appendicitis, usually smooth muscle spasms as with kidney or gall stone attacks). This type of intense pain usually present as diffuse, deep, achy, and colicky and is difficult to localize. It may be sensed as a feeling of pressure but can also be sharp. It is usually treated heroically with traditional pain medications such as natural opioids, semi-, and completely-synthetic opioid-class analgesics and NSAIDS.

Neuropathic (type b), or **chronic pain,** has a more complex mechanism and is not as well understood as that for acute pain. It is theorized that this type of pain occurs as a result of a dysfunction in or damage to both the central and peripheral nervous systems. New research has shown that inflammation can actually be carried along an afferent sensing nerve root to the spinal column quite a distance from the affected body part. Once at the spinal column, the inflammation can set up house and cause continuous pain medication to travel up the spinal column to the brain and even back to the offending area allowing for constant pain sensation. The many descriptive interpretations of chronic pain present as burning, shooting, tingling, numbness, and even itching. There is one main characteristic with this type of pain: there is always something going on to inform the sufferer that all is not right. Inflammation, infection, scar tissue (*adhesions*), or re-injury or re-infection can all play into manifesting this type of pain causation. If the threshold of pain from noxious stimulation is crossed for whatever reason, and the neural components sense this, pain will be sensed even after it has been caused to subside. Re-treatment of a problem is often more difficult to resolve than originally. And if the patient is unfortunate enough to sustain residual long-term damage, then EXPECTATION of pain can even lead to negative psychological manifestations which sometimes progress to addiction behavior. [*Addiction* is the psychological component where the sufferer plans ahead to try and obtund the pain before it is actually sensed. This behavior differs from *physical dependence* which is a predictable pharmacologic effect that is manifested by the development of a withdrawal syndrome after abrupt discontinuation of therapy.]

MECHANISM OF PAIN

Acute pain is mechanistically different from **chronic** or **intermittent pain** warranting different pharmacologic agents and procedures for treatment. The process of pain transmission involves several neural pathways and neurotransmitters within the peripheral and central nervous systems. **Acute pain,** as mentioned above whether from an exogenous or endogenous causation, activates the *nociceptive* pain receptors known as *nociceptors* to produce an electrical action potential which is transmitted to the spinal cord along *afferent* (toward the spinal column and brain) nerve fibers. Different types of fibers transmit different types of pain. Sharp, well-localized pain is transmitted along "A" fibers, whereas dull, aching, poorly-localized or deciphered pain travels along "C" neural fibers. {An example of where one becomes the other occurs when a very young person touches something very hot. If it is the first time, there usually is a "delay" in pain transmission all the way to the brain (along "C" fibers) with a relatively slow draw-back of the body part from the heat source. But once this uncomfortable sensation is "recorded" into the central nervous system "memory banks," and a repeat performance with excessive heat occurs, a very rapid withdrawal is elicited each and every succeeding time in a normally-functioning person (along the "A" fibers).} The action potential then travels to the dorsal horn of the spinal cord where pain neurotransmitters, such as *glutamate* and *substance P,* are released. This transmission then continues up the spinal cord via **ascending pathways** to higher areas of the brain where pain is perceived and deciphered.

With **chronic and intermittent pain** the malfunction in the **C**entral **N**ervous **S**ystem **(CNS)** can be the result of inflammation actually traveling to the spinal column as mentioned above and, or several different processes: increased CNS cell firing, decreased inhibition of neuronal activity, and inappropriate sensitization. *Neuropathic* pain is often described as burning, shooting, tingling, and possibly accompanied by numbness. Two

236

types of conditions often occur where *neuropathic* pain is manifest: *hyperalgesia, (the exaggerated response to normally noxious stimuli,* and *allodynia, the painful response to a normally non-painful stimulus.* Chronic pain can also present as a manifestation of both *nociceptive* and *neuropathic* pain, suggesting the need for a combined pharmacological approach for optimal treatment.

Once the brain senses the painful stimulus regardless of source and cause, it releases inhibitory stimuli through the *descending* pathways *(efferent)* back to the spinal cord to inhibit the sensation of pain. The modulation of pain *endogenously* is achieved through a variety of neurotransmitters, including endogenous opioids, *serotonin* (5-HT), **N**or-**E**pinephrine (NE), and **G**ama-**A**mino**B**utyric **A**cid (GABA). The role of these inhibitory neurotransmitters has led to the rationale of using anti-depressants and anti-convulsants to treat chronic pain, but that is not within the scope of this presentation.

TREATMENT OF PAIN

Does pain serve any good purpose? Is it a cause for great concern? What if there is no frank pain with probable pathology; is there then less reason for worry? Pain is usually the first sign the body affords us that something is not right. If severe enough, pain is a prime cause for visiting the family physician or the ER, and it certainly can disrupt much-needed sleep when most of the day's distractions have subsided.

ACUTE PAIN

This is usually a matter of degree and duration. It is where and when the body means business. If the pain in intense enough and the sufferer not accustomed to same, he may also experience *sympathetic nervous system* signs such as tachycardia (rapid heartbeat), hypertension, sweating, or *mydriasis* (wide open pupils). Some patients, whether from intense physical or psychological training or severe challenges to same, will perceive various degrees of discomfort before they admit to acute pain when asked to quantify. As the intensity rises the brain finally signals enough troublesome sensation is occurring to bring the issue to the fore. There becomes no doubt about it; the victim's ability to continue functioning as before is greatly reduced or eliminated. All thoughts and most functions center around locating the area of the body involved and the possible causes. And absolutely obtaining relief ASAP becomes the driving force of action.

When dealing with the skeletal musculature which has sustained an athletic injury either directly to it or to surrounding supportive tissue, for example, a cyclic cause-and-effect produces muscle spasms which can induce intense pain which can produce more spasms, which, in turn, can keep generating pain. In this circumstance, we need to break the cycle to get on the road to pain reduction and then elimination.

Of course, we could bring out the big guns and administer strong opioids to act centrally to quickly deaden the sensation of pain or try some ancillary pharmacologic (e.g. skeletal muscle relaxant) to obtain the same end result. Most times this "combination of ingredients" will produce more profound relief more quickly. But since prescription medications are outside the scope of this chapter, my approach to pain relief will entail medications and procedures available without a physician's supervision.

CHAPTER 10

THE AUTHOR'S TRAUMATIC SHOULDER INJURY

Most traumatic injuries come unexpected and always unwanted. What the victim must do is have the injury analyzed as quickly and thoroughly as possible by the appropriate medical specialist. Once evaluated and choices laid out for the procedural repair, rehabilitation, and the road back to functionality, it is left to the one sustaining the injury to devote the time, the physical effort, and the emotional energies to complete the picture back to health and physical ability. This chapter is centered around the author's totally unexpected encounter with a very large, very heavy advertising sign that was thrown against him by way of a strong-wind, quick-approaching storm. It is presented in the first person narrative as best as the victim's memory recalls.

I was on an errand to purchase several items from my local home improvement store. They always had a large untethered sign on wheels by the front entrance that advertised the day's specials. I would glance at the sign with every entrance into the store to see if a match with what I needed were listed as a daily special. As I saw severe dark clouds forming behind the store with very strong gusts picking up all around me, I pointed my face towards the ground as most instinctively would and hustled my gait towards the front door to get out of the weather, but to my shock and great misfortune, about 15 feet from the entrance I had the frightening sensation of being lifted off the ground, carried in the air several yards and then smashed to the ground. I remember thinking I must have just been hit from behind by a truck, and I am about to die. When I hit the ground, I heard my right shoulder crack, smacked my lower jaw to the ground and was too stunned to move.

Several people came over to see if I was in need of help. I could not answer their question if I were okay. I could not move on my own. Help from the store was sought, and several more men came out to move me. This lead to the first major mistake made. They did not evaluate my condition. They did nothing to protect me in my supine state and were only motivated to get me up off the ground. Since I was too stunned to talk, they simply picked me up by both shoulders that proved later to further damage internal tissue. I remember a deep feeling of warmth in my shoulder (blood spilling into my shoulder girdle from the trauma) when they stood me up but I had no ability to move it on my own. No pain, and absolutely limp. Now my wits were returning, and I quickly realized I had sustained a serious injury. Instead of questioning me if I could move on my own or did I feel anything to be damaged, I was lifted off the ground and quickly walked to the front door out of potential parking lot traffic and the imminent weather.

Unbelievably, the store manager did not think to call 911 for medical help. All he was concerned with was me filling out an accident report. I could not even talk because when my face slammed the ground, my jaw was badly bruised and started to swell; a few back teeth were cracked from the hit, and my right knee was badly bruised and began to hurt like hell. After about 20 minutes I realized there was no ambulance. I remember asking when will the EMT people be here. As I stated, the manager had never called for medical help. He did so only on my insistence that immediately put me in a combative mood as to his either abject stupidity or total ignorance in handling this kind of emergency. Either he was totally without sense or certainly poorly trained by his company for this type of situation. If the latter, then another major mistake. Key business personnel, dealing with the public, should have at least a basic sense of the immediate when faced with medical emergencies.

During the 15 minute siren-and-light show to the hospital ER, pain started to envelop me. I mentioned what I had endured, and the EMT personnel all shook their heads in disbelief. Once in the ER, there was another 20 minute wait to be attended. The pain was rising now; I was getting very uncomfortable and started to speak in loud irritated tones as to when I would be evaluated and treated. They long ago took my medical insurance information, contact information, and accident information. Though I tried to stay in command of my situation and was thankful that I was still alive, I had to really work my emotions to control panic that was beginning to envelop me lying helpless on the gurney.

After about an hour, I was able to call a family member to come get me at the hospital. Meanwhile, I was given a shot of morphine, written a few prescriptions for expected muscle pain and spasms and something to help me sleep. X-rays showed no broken bones but could not tell the damage inside the shoulder girdle. Then I was fitted for several braces and slings and finally bandaged around my face. I looked like the poster boy suffering through combat for either the Revolutionary or Civil Wars. If it were not so serious, it looked almost comical in a Halloween-costume sort of way how they dressed me with the medical supports and bandages and pointed me to the exit.

After two days at home to get on top of the situation, I checked around for the best orthopedic surgeon in the area. When I called his office, the receptionist asked several questions, one of which was my age. I knew the reason for this because, in trauma situations like mine, surgical repair needed to be done quickly, namely in one week or less. If any torn ligaments, tendons, and muscles were not elongated and stretched back to original dimensions within that amount of time in someone my age (64 years old) they could not be brought back to original condition. I most likely would forever have to endure a functionally-damaged right shoulder which would have ended my swim training and competition at the high level I had worked so long and hard to achieve. I dared not dwell on that much negativity which would have sent me into a hell-dive of despair.

Six days later getting me to the surgical center was my daughter's job. Her early-morning drop-off, and wish for good luck were the prelude to recovery as she drove out of the surgical center's parking lot to work. My wife, who was always at my side for comfort and strength, was in the terminal stages of her battle with Multiple System Atrophy, a variant of Lou Gehrig's Disease. All she could do was hope for my best and suffer in sympathy and silence at home (she could no longer speak) with what I next had to endure. In the grand scheme of things, nothing I had waiting for me compared to her 10 year losing battle with one of the most terrible afflictions one could contract.

Well, my 24 minutes in a supposedly-open type of MRI near-coffin examination tube three days earlier proved no more beneficial than if I were spared the whole claustrophobic process in that mind-clawing torture chamber. And to top it off, the technician stated that I moved just as the last minute was approaching. In a state of building emotional frailty, I had to endure under a not-so-nice verbal protest another several minutes. You'd have thought I had to do the 200 breaststroke all underwater, I felt so engulfed in my immediate surroundings.

Being prepared in the "ready room" (as I likened it to the small room swimmers are placed before they are called out to compete in the next immediate race) there were five of us undergoing various orthopedic procedures by our respective surgeons. We were on gurneys lined up in a row; I was number four out of five. The anesthesiologist came in to offer up his services as if at a bazaar or auction. He had this "Star-Wars" weapon with three large syringes mounted vertically, each filled with a different anesthetic. He tried his spiel on all five of us stating that we would face prolonged intense pain when the general anesthetic wore off and that the next several hours would be extremely uncomfortable. What made me uncomfortable was his almost insistence we partake of his triple hand-gun of pain relief or we will be sorry. He was obligated by law to add, which he did parenthetically, that, of course, with these very potent pain killers, there was the chance we would stop breathing during the operation and would have to treated heroically to prevent asphyxia. And that these monstrous syringes with needles that looked long enough to penetrate an elephant's hide would be injected into our necks with concomitant pain. The first three patients bought into the "no-pain-after-surgery" claim and said okay. Naturally, they were not injected so the rest of us could watch; the sight of this assault-and-battery would have been very difficult to bear causing maybe more than one of us to need cardiac care more than orthopedic. Once they left the "ready room" and were set in the OR Dr. Pain Killer would ply his trade. When he came to me, I told the anesthesiologist I would pass. The last guy who was to my left must have felt my emotional vibes and also declined. I was not panicky about the surgery at this point; I just wanted it done and be on the north side of the healing grid. Get it done, and start getting better as soon as possible. That was the overriding thought as I was carried into the OR I threw out a few humorous remarks which I am want to do when I am nervous; everyone chuckled which made me feel at least I hoped they would be rooting for me to have things go well.

The surgeon's upfront prognosis was that since I chose the intelligent thing to do by having the surgery within a week of the trauma, and for what he could read in the MRI: about 45 minutes under the knife with excellent results. There may be an outside chance of a few permanent staples left in place to anchor tendons to muscle, but only if the trauma warranted it. Once I felt the pinch of the needle only three seconds counting backwards is all I can remember.

Well, my family must have thought I died on the table because after inquiring many times, they were told I was finally out of surgery and in recovery four and half hours after being wheeled in. I was feeling nauseous from the general anesthetic with a dry mouth and soreness at the back of my throat... probably from the intubation to protect me from swallowing my tongue and to keep an open airway. When I broke out of the grasp of the anesthetic, I was immediately reminded of another major surgery I had undergone many years ago for kidney stones. There was an absolute loss of time; no dreaming I could remember, just dead to the world. Was this like real death? No ability to do anything; no mental awareness, and yet time kept moving forward but not to my realization. When this thought dissipated, and I became more aware of my immediate surroundings, all I could think of was "thank God, it's over. I am alive to start my recovery." Boy was I in for a long, difficult road back.

There wasn't just one small incision for the doctor to enter the shoulder. There were two. The smaller was about an inch and a half. A little more than an inch above this must have been the main entrance into the theater. This baby was over four inches long with the look of bad intentions. I told the doctor I swim, cross-train, and do weights almost every day with serious intent. The repair must be able to withstand this type of day-to-day for as long as I am able. He obviously understood.

"Normal" physical therapy for a shoulder trauma like mine: twice weekly for eight to 12 weeks; me: three times weekly for the first six weeks, then twice weekly to a total of 18 weeks, and I needed every bit of it! Remnants of the surgery: most of the connective tissue found in my entire inner space of the right shoulder girdle had to be repaired. The labrum (cartilage that fills in the ball-and-socket joint and helps support its movement) was totally destroyed and had to be rebuilt. Seventeen nylon staples were left in place for my remaining time on earth.

I was out of the water for two weeks until the two surgical scars healed enough to prevent infection. I needed my chlorine "fix" and the comfort of warm, inviting water surrounding me. Once able to get wet again I did as much as I could with one good arm, two good legs, and the rest of my intact anatomy having to work to get me on the road back to "swim shape." Once released from therapy and after a few more follow up visits with the surgeon, I began to push in the water, rode my bike with an altered body position to lessen stress on the shoulder, and enveloped myself in a modified weight program that removed much of my overhand stressful exercises against heavy resistance.

What I have learned from all this:

- I was not the coach barking out instructions and taking charge at first, I was the patient. Then I worked to became my own coach. I developed a deeper understanding of what processes through which the body has to go, and how we can steer the mind to help handle it.

- I am somewhat damaged goods, this occurring in my mid-sixties and all, and fully understand the medical statement that when it comes to trauma, at least, "The Body Never Forgets!"

- I gave special attention to breaking up the adhesions that occurred with the serious trauma by stretching regularly, gradually increasing my range of motion in what I did to train and intelligently increasing weight resistance in the weight room, and my intensity in the pool.

- I cannot swim butterfly as well as I used to; in fact, if I try too much, the shoulder puts out warning signals to stop. When I delve too deep into my training regimen, the right shoulder "beeps" a warning to back off, so I listen or suffer the consequences of increasing pain and weakness. I can feel the staples pulling and ardently remember the surgeon telling me with a serious face that if I re-damage this shoulder, he could not fix it to my liking.

- I have been well, and I have been sick... I like well better. I have learned that everything is a matter of attitude. If you think you can, or you think you cannot... you are right. The four magic words have often come into play during my rehab and continues to this day: I CAN DO THIS!!

THE DILEMMA

To laugh is to risk appearing a fool.
To expose feelings is to risk rejection.
To weep is to risk appearing to sentimental.
To reach out for another is to risk involvement.
To place your dreams before the crowd is to risk ridicule.
To go forward in the face of overwhelming odds is to risk failure.

But risks must be taken because the greatest hazard in life is to risk nothing.

He may avoid suffering and sorrow, but he cannot learn, feel, change, grow, or love.

He has forfeited his freedom.

Chained by his certitudes, he is a slave
Only a person who takes risks if free.

CHAPTER 11

DEALING WITH THE MOST INTENSE IMMEDIATE CIRCUMSTANCE OF LIFE AND DEATH: THE NEED AND USE OF AN AUTOMATIC EXTERNAL DEFIBRILLATOR (AED)

As a coach, masters swimming competitor, and general participant in vigorous exercise, I have eye-witnessed or was in close proximity, over a 30-year period, to several sudden deaths upon those partaking in competition, vigorous training, or informal intense athletic involvement. In all the cases but the last, there was no or very little warning something devastating was about to happen. This is a dark topic and one not comforting about which to write, but it needs to be brought forth and expounded upon so all who either partake in vigorous physical endeavors, administer same, or simply view them first hand will no longer be ignorant of the most important available life-saving procedures. We call these **"the chain of survival."** This refers to a series of critical interventions that can reduce the absolute mortality from sudden cardiac arrest. But if one of these actions is neglected or poorly executed, it is unlikely the victim will survive. Saving a life is as responsible and serious an act as one can perform. Most hope never to be put in such a traumatic situation, but we also never know what life has in store and places directly before us. Being prepared to correct sudden cardiac arrest is the greatest service one can provide our fellow man when circumstance presents.

What takes down a person almost immediately in these cases is **Sudden Cardiac Arrest (SCA).** Most occur when the electrical impulses in the dysfunctional heart become rapid (*tachycardia*) or chaotic (*fibrillation*) through the more muscular segments (*ventricles*) assigned the task of blood circulation throughout the body. This irregular heart beat *(arrhythmia)* may cause the heart to suddenly stop beating, producing a precipitous drop to critically-low levels in arterial blood pressure. Death, if left to the natural cascade of events, usually ensues within 10 minutes due to the lack of oxygen supply to several vital organs. Less than five minutes of deprived oxygen at normal room temperature usually brings about some form of lingering brain damage.

Sudden cardiac arrest is a major health problem worldwide and is the leading cause of death in many developed countries. In the United States alone, there have been as many as a quarter million cardiac deaths in a single year; most arise from the high-risk segment of the population exhibiting several strong contributory factors of imprudent lifestyle which produce obesity, high blood pressure, coronary inflammation, excessive circulating fats in the blood, non-defusing of unremitting stress, and cardiac vessel constriction from smoking. And there are the very unfortunate who have inherited the dangerous genes which can produce cardiac anomalies that can crossover into pediatrics and the athletic world.

Cardio-Pulmonary Resuscitation (CPR) was developed around 1960 with closed-chest cardiac massage the key element. The "chain of survival" was fully described and delineated in the 1992 guideline for CPR and emergency cardiac care by the American Heart Association (AHA). Over the years, the actual hands-on procedures have modulated into what is taught today where it is deemed more important to keep compressing the chest rather than interrupt this to give "rescue breaths."

In fact, new research from the department of cardiology at the University of Arizona School of Medicine has shown that the procedure of just vigorous chest compressions at the rate of 100 per second will allow for perfusion of blood to the heart and brain. But, unlike the traditional procedure for compressions where the hands were always in contact with the chest, the Arizona researchers found that in this new protocol the hands should rise slightly above the chest NOT having continuous contact with the body. On the up movement, the hands come off the chest to augment the body's ability to create a vacuum in the lungs, allowing them to more easily fill with ambient air... thus, no need for rescue breathing.

The "chain of survival" has four interdependent links: (1) early access, (2) early basic CPR; (3) early defibrillation, and (4) early advanced cardiac life support (ACLS). Notice the one common word in each link: EARLY. The guidelines were again revised in 2005 to create a single international version of evidence-based, scientific resuscitation guidelines. There must be an unbroken continuation in the rescue process to ensure the greatest possibility of survival. But the obvious most critical point is the immediate recognition of the emergency and initiation of the "chain" by those surrounding the victim. If no one recognizes the signs of an emergency, and no action is taken quickly, the possibility of survival plummets to zero.

Early Access: This refers to the actions taken from the time the victim collapses until Emergency Medical Service (EMS) personnel arrive. When someone suffers sudden cardiac arrest, the most important actions a bystander can take are to recognize the critical nature of the situation, have an emergency service number called, and to start procedures on the victim for resuscitation. Recognition of early warning signs, such as chest pain, shortness of breath, and patient activation of the emergency response system can significantly increase the rate of survival. This is the compelling reason the American Heart Association stresses education concerning the importance of recognizing the signs and symptoms of cardiac arrest, acute myocardial infarction and stroke, and initiating the action plan for survival.

Early CPR: Statistics and logic confirm that the survival rate is much higher in victims who receive early CPR than in those who get delayed attention. The physical procedures involved in CPR (chest compressions pushing blood circulation through to the vital organs) help preserve cerebral and myocardial viability, but it cannot stand alone as the sole important link to increased survival mainly because of the complexity of administration and the variability of the competence of the administrator. The main cause of failure to adequately resuscitate in this chain of survival is the delay in initiating defibrillation when needed.

Early Defibrillation: The survival rate from sudden cardiac arrest, according to many studies, is poor if the victim does not receive electric-shock therapy within a few minutes to restore normal electrical cardiac activity. Studies have shown that the most critical factor for survival from ventricular fibrillation is the time difference between onset of fibrillation and administration of defibrillation. By the numbers, **the probability of survival is reduced by about 50% for each three-minute delay in administration of defibrillation.** Further, **survival rates for sudden cardiac arrest can rise to as high as 90% when immediate electrical cardiac shock is administered.** Because of this fact, **the immediate correction of *fibrillatory* cardiac beating is recognized as the most critical component in the chain of survival.** But, as stated previously, early defibrillation is not the only important aspect of treatment; all the factors in the chain of survival must be interconnected, attended to, and applied.

Early **A**dvanced **C**ardiac **L**ife **S**upport **(ACLS):** Defibrillation works best when CPR is provided right up until the electrical shock is applied, followed by rapid advanced care to prevent fallback to the previous dangerous cardiac conditions. ACLS is enhancement of **B**asic **L**ife **S**upport **(BLS)** and is provided by professional EMS personnel. It includes airway and breathing management, medications, and, in some cases, inducing dropping the body's temperature (hypothermia) to reduce onset of oxidative inflammation and destruction in cardiac and cerebral tissues. But since EMT personnel are almost never the first responders, it has been discussed with some persuasion that if the victim does not receive immediate adequately-provided CPR and fruitful defibrillation with an **A**utomated **E**xternal **D**efibrillator **(AED)**, advanced life support will prove to be disappointing and of limited or no value.

AUTOMATED EXTERNAL DEFIBRILLATOR (AED)

A defibrillator (first developed in the early 1900's) is a device that applies a therapeutic electric shock to the dysfunctional heart in order to restore normal beat rhythm. It can be utilized before the heart actually comes to sudden arrest while suffering the deadly chaotic beating of fibrillation. These devices can be external, *transvenous*, or implanted. One type of external unit, developed in 1979, is known as an **(AED)** and is capable of accurately analyzing cardiac rhythms and advising about, and delivering, therapeutic electric shocks when appropriate.

These AEDs use internal computer algorithms to analyze cardiac beating and detect for ventricular fibrillation. The modern units deliver effective low-energy waveform shocks in strengths of 120 to 200 joules. The AEDs, themselves, are safe, effective, lightweight, easy to use and maintain, and relatively inexpensive (about $1,500). **They require only four simple steps: 1) turning on the device, 2) attaching two electrodes, 3) pressing a button for rhythm analysis, and 4) pressing another button to administer the shocks.** If further shocks are required, the AED will instruct accordingly. However, the operator must carefully follow all instructions.

Many studies show positive outcomes with early defibrillation in public places, as it saves precious minutes and improves survival rates for cardiac arrest victims. This positivity relies critically on the fact of having many trained lay rescuers with readily-available AEDs in public places that attract large crowds such as public transportation, shopping malls, hotels, venues that host sports competitions, high-rise buildings, and manufacturing plants. Of course, having a private-home unit is also a wise decision especially if there are cardiac patients residing. Such a unit exits by the name of **Philips HeartStart Home Defibrillator.** It comes with a training video that can be used to familiarize the viewer with the device.

As part of the **Public Access Defibrillation (PAD)** program, a federal law was enacted in 2002 to provide AEDs to states and localities at places where circumstance might provide a need. Funds from this law also provide training for those wanting to learn to recognize symptoms of severe cardiac distress and the subsequent use, if need be, of AED's. The primary goal of a program of this type is simply to sustain the patient's previous quality of life by preserving normal neurologic functioning. The program seeks to enable rescuers to deliver early defibrillation to victims within three to five minutes of collapse, the first critical moments after sudden cardiac arrest. However, this program should not replace the care provided by EMS personnel, but rather provide a lifesaving bridge in the chain of survival during the several critical minutes it takes for advanced life support to arrive.

CHAPTER 12

THE BENEFITS OF DRINKING COFFEE

OVERVIEW

The smell of brewed coffee, no matter what time of day, is one of the most pleasurable "hits" to our senses. Studies have shown that the two most comforting aromas during stress of cold weather is the smell of chocolate baking (e.g. brownies) and the brewing of coffee. Every morning many sip their coffee with no real thought given to what the beans bring to the brew. These little bundles of taste are extraordinarily complex, containing over 1,000 compounds, only a handful of which have ever been individually investigated by scientists. Not only is coffee packed with a beneficial group of compounds called *polyphenolic antioxidants* and the familiar **caffeine** (unless processed out), but it is the single greatest source of antioxidant in the American diet.

The average American coffee drinker consumes about 3.1 cups per day, but extensive research has found that higher volumes (as much as four to 12 cups daily) can help prevent or lessen the effects of many major killer diseases: cardiovascular, cancer, diabetes, liver, and Alzheimer's. As examples, in case-controlled studies, compared to non-coffee drinkers, those women who drank the most coffee cut their risks of breast cancer by up to 57% and type-2 diabetes up to 67%. But the potential downside is that many who have consumed several cups of coffee daily whether due to habit, need, or desire have experienced various unpleasant effects: coronary palpitations, psychic hyperactivity with shaking from excess caffeine, on-and-off gastrointestinal difficulties with either caffeinated or decaf brew or sleep disturbances from a caffeinated selection.

Researchers have long wanted to test for coffee's positivity and to lessen all or most of the manifested untoward side effects. Lab tests show that not all coffee products provide the same powerful protection against chronic disease. The important polyphenol antioxidant content varies with how long the beans are roasted and the roasting method itself. Unfortunately, all roasting acts to destroy some amount of the polyphenols, the most important of which is *chlorogenic acid.* But since roasting is the necessary process to prepare the beans for brewing, tinkering with the "order of events" in the process can provide what we want and need. But for those unable to tolerate any coffee or simply don't enjoy it, pure chlorogenic acid and **"green coffee beans"** are now being standardized and are becoming increasingly popular as consumers learn of their existence and benefits.

In a new patented roasting process, the coffee beans are first soaked in water and then drained prior to being heat-roasted. Once roasted, the beans are deposited back into the same water in which they were originally pre-soaked, and are thus able to absorb back much of the previously extracted polyphenols. This process simply by-passes the direct exposure of polyphenols to the destruction of roasting.

A comparison of **Chlorogenic Acid (CA)** content with the new and old roasting methods shows what makes it to the brew. Since more chlorogenic acid is presented in the newer brewing process, less cups of potential distress need be consumed:

- Conventional coffee roasting: 92 mg CA/cup
- Polyphenol-retaining process   172 mg CA/cup-186% more chlorogenic acid
- Conventional decaffeinated coffee: 52 mg CA/cup
- Polyphenol-retaining decaf coffee: 132 mg/CA/cup-254% more chlorogenic acid

HOW THE INGREDIENTS IN COFFEE AFFECT THE BODY'S PHYSIOLOGY

Despite coffee's powerful antioxidant punch, the mechanism for coffee's protection against a host of diseases involved a lot more than a fierce battle between antioxidants and free radicals. Scientists are revealing the facts of coffee's **phytochemistry** and how this exerts direct biological action on the body which may underpin a web of indirect, protective effects against many diseases that attack the human condition.

It was early studies that suggested the **polyphenols** in both coffees (caffeinated and decaf) could modify key enzymes that would improve intracellular signaling by which vital cells could be "instructed" to enhance tissue repair, immunity, and preserve the healthy status quo (*homeostasis*). Then specific lab study in 2008 and 2009 began to show poor cell signaling as looking more and more like THE troublemaker that brings about dangerous physiologic changes that cause the most devastating diseases: plate aggregation and clots, cancer, diabetes, neurodegenerative diseases and overall aging. This in depth analysis brought about new revelations which showed that by modulating specific cell-signaling pathways, known as ERK1/2 and JNK, the various polyphenols in coffee, especially chlorogenic acid, help prevent the degeneration of specific human cells rich in lipids: mainly brain tissue. This provides for only a short leap to the conclusion that explains coffee's neuroprotective effects against cognitive decline and many neurodegenerative diseases such as Parkinson's, Lou Gehrig's (ALS), Multiple System Atrophy, and a whole host of related devastating central nervous system maladies.

An important recent study in 2011 suggests that polyphenols from coffee can affect cellular responses and sensitivity by interacting with *nuclear receptors*. These internal cellular segments pick up intracellular signals which determine whether a cell gets the right "instructions" to divide, die, or release molecules that can regulate various body functions to fight disease.

Coffee compounds also act to raise levels of *detoxifying enzymes* that act to protect against DNA damage. One advantage to this is the likelihood of reducing the susceptibility of *lymphocytes* (**W**hite **B**lood **C**ells{WBC}involved in the immune response) to damage from **R**eactive **O**xygen **S**pecies (ROS). This provides a major activity whereby coffee is able to protect DNA from oxidative damage and consequently reduce the potential for disease.

Looking into other mechanisms of helpful activity, a 2009 study discovered that just three cups of coffee daily for only three weeks increased the number and metabolic activity of beneficial *gastrointestinal bifidobacteria.* These can act in a host of good ways to boost immunity, lower blood pressure, and increase mineral absorption. Coffee's phenolic compounds have also shown (with consumption of four to eight cups daily) that they possess a direct action on **dampening inflammatory activity throughout the body**. This is key to reducing chronic low-level inflammation and its causation to aging and the breakdown of vital physiologic pathways leading to several debilitating diseases.

Involving another avenue of physiology, we see that consumption of either caffeinated or decaf coffee shows specific improvements in the function of the liver and of *adipocytes* (fat-storing cells), both of which are essential to a healthy metabolism all around, and especially important in controlling the tendency to diabetes.

And, of course, with caffeine, itself, a 2011 study confirmed that this famous ingredient in coffee is a potent scavenger of oxygenated free radicals and can work synergistically with other coffee antioxidants to function in a manner unrelated to its antioxidant action. It seems caffeine protects the integrity of the *blood-brain-barrier (BBB)* which suggests that it may reduce the risk of some diseases by limiting the transport of blood-borne pathogens, drugs, cells, and other substances into the brain chamber where they can adversely affect the functioning of brain *synapses.* The study also showed that caffeine defends against the specific blood-brain-barrier dysfunction linked to Alzheimer's and Parkinson's diseases.

COFFEE CONSUMPTION ASSOCIATED WITH THE REDUCTION IN DEATH FROM ALL CAUSES

Researchers at the National Institutes of Health in association with the **A**merican **A**ssociation of **R**etired **P**eople (AARP) explored coffee drinking and its impact on "all-cause mortality"... Dying for any reason at all. Allowances and exclusion were made for those entering the study already suffering from serious illnesses and deleterious habits like excess alcohol consumption and smoking. Hundreds of thousands of men and women were studied for 13 years to give a sample of over five-million person-years with very strong statistical significance. What was established after accounting for the above negative situations, was that there was a remarkably strong association between coffee consumption and survival. The more coffee the subjects drank, the less likely they were to die. Further analytical breakdown of the study showed that to a greater extent, specific maladies were prevented from emerging with coffee drinking: heart and lung disease, stroke, type-2 diabetes, and various infections. It even had influence in lowering the risk of dying from injuries and accidents. And this protective effect was evident whether subjects drank caffeinated or decaffeinated brews that begged the question as to what else from the coffee bean presented life-saving effects.

A Statistical Analysis from a Study in the New England Journal of Medicine:

<u>Cups of Coffee/Day</u>	<u>% Lower Risk of Dying (Women)</u>	<u>% Lower Risk of Dying (Men)</u>
Less than 1	No Reduction	No Reduction
1	5%	6%
2 or 3	13%	10%
4 or 5	16%	12%
6 or More	15%	10%

The last listing above shows reduced benefit where the max threshold of positive result was exceeded.

In addition to caffeine, as mentioned above, natural coffee beans contain more than 1,000 different compounds that could affect health and the risk of dying. Of all the compounds present, the **polyphenols** are the best candidates for several reasons. As a group, they are powerful antioxidants with all the health benefits that implies. But they also manifest other activities that include the surprising ability to modulate gene expression that translates into how much and how often a particular gene is "switched on." This allows the gene to directly influence many of a particular cell's most basic processes, including signals that control when a cell dies, when it replicates, when it can release or respond to other chemical signals and stimulation. The net effect of this impact on basic cellular function was mentioned above and includes all the physiologic activities at the cellular level which keep us going strong. When we suffer impaired cellular signaling for any reason, functionality with bad intentions usually arises with a dangerous prognosis in the offing.

The alpha chemical, both in presence and activity, of the polyphenols is chlorogenic acid. Coffee beans are the major source of this amazing compound in the American diet. Along with other polyphenols, chlorogenic acid provides its overall benefits by driving down the chronic inflammation that is the hallmark of many diseases of aging including type-2 diabetes and atherosclerosis. The acid acts preferably within cells with high fat content as such that make up the brain, helping to explain observations that coffee sustains cognition with aging. Also specifically positively affected/protected are the fat cells of the liver and the overall impact of obesity. Protecting DNA from all sorts of potential damage is the likely mechanism by which coffee consumption may lower the risk for many cancers.

DIABETES MANAGEMENT

Worldwide, it has been ascertained by scientists and confirmed by the *International Diabetes Federation* that diabetes has exploded in numbers to over 366 million. Regular coffee, with its most active and beneficial ingredient, chlorogenic acid, lowers the risk of developing type-2 diabetes by up to 67%. The acid's activity seems to stem from its ability to reduce levels of blood *glucose* formation by directly interfering with its synthesis and release in the body. The pathway of this inhibition is by blocking the activity of the major ubiquitous *glucose*-regulating enzyme, *glucose-6-phosphatase,* which results in a pronounced reduction of sugar levels traveling around in the blood. One large lab study showed that imbibing one cup of coffee per day protects against developing type-2 by 13%; consuming four cups per day protects by up to 47%, and if the consumer can handle the gastrointestinal potential for distress and the likelihood of excess neurological stimulation, drinking 12 cups daily affords protection against type-2 diabetes by up to 67%. Another large study of over half a million people showed that each additional cup of coffee added protection against type-2 by another 7%.

Chlorogenic acid also lessens the **hyperglycemic peak** (blood sugar elevation) associated with carbohydrate ingestion that results in a downturn in insulin activity and a reduced accumulation of *adipose* (fat-storing) tissue. Lessening the after-meal *glucose* surge and aiding its return to a normal level is very important in protecting against potential negative cardiovascular risks in diabetics and other with heart disease. Various compounds in coffee as well as caffeine, itself, are now being tested to see if they boost the diabetic-preventative effect of chlorogenic acid. Early lab results are showing that these chemicals are able to lower carbohydrate storage by as much as 35% while improving insulin's activity.

Dedicated coffee consumption has shown to inhibit iron absorption and storage, and in 2004, scientists found a direct link between reduced iron storage in the body and a lower risk of type-2 diabetes independent of other risk factors.

THE CONSUMPTION OF COFFEE TO PROTECT AGAINST CARDIOVASCULAR DISEASE

As the leading cause of death in our country, cardiovascular disease kills over one third more Americans than cancer, so anything that can lower this somber statistic warrants intense scientific scrutiny. Though a strong dose of coffee can briefly raise blood pressure right after consumption, its compounds have a longer-term benefit: **daily consumption actually decreases blood pressure readings after just a few weeks** due mainly to chlorogenic acid. A long-term (15 years) study of over 41,000 women (and confirmed by other studies on men and women) found that the risk of death from cardiovascular disease was 24% lower among those consuming one to three cups of coffee daily.

At the cellular level, the tendency to cardiovascular disease can be lessened by consuming just one cup of coffee due to its ability to **inhibit platelet aggregation within one hour regardless of its caffeine content.**

For year's coffee was thought to increase the risks for high blood pressure and cardiovascular disease, mainly due to effects of caffeine. But like everything else related to coffee consumption, these misconceptions have change dramatically in recent years due to intense investigative studies. The stigma of coffee drinking has also included the association of consuming enough coffee to try and overcome the toxic effects of too much alcohol, the one-two-punch of coffee and cigarettes, or the attempt at overcoming sleep deprivation with continuous caffeine ingestion. Some religions have even applied the guilt of association of coffee with alcohol and tobacco and certain food with evil-doing.

But the main "secret ingredient" of a positive nature, once, again, is the chemical now showing remarkable positive activity in the body: *chlorogenic acid.* This compound, which can be enhanced in concentration with new brewing protocols, acts to lessen the potential for endothelial (the inner lining of arteries) inflammation, keeping it smooth and with less chance for circulating fats in the blood to adhere. It is dose-dependent but comes with a threshold, above which increases in consumption provide less of a helpful consequence. It also increases the availability of artery-expanding *nitric oxide* which reduces any potential increase in blood pressure from caffeine. And more studies have found that regular coffee consumption improves the formation of (HDL)... the "good" cholesterol... which draws out the (LDL) from artery walls and decreases coronary artery calcification... all to lessen the potential for heart attacks and strokes.

A large 2011 study has shown that there is no correlation between long-term coffee consumption and increased blood pressure or cardiovascular disease. The beneficial effects of chlorogenic acid (and other coffee components) are evident from several recent large studies. Deaths from cardiovascular disease overall, and in particular from coronary heart disease and stroke are all significantly reduced by coffee consumption.

Cardiovascular Risk-Reduction From Coffee Consumption In Diabetic Adults at Increased Risk for all Causes of Death

Cups of Coffee/Day	Total	Cardiovascular	Coronary Heart Disease	Stroke
0-2	no reduction	no reduction	no reduction	no reduction
3-4	23%	21%	22%	23%
5-6	32%	30%	30%	36%
7+	30%	29%	37%	10%

COFFEE CONSUMPTION'S BENEFICIAL EFFECTS ON BRAIN FUNCTION

Coffee consumption has been documented as providing impressive benefits regarding cognitive function during the aging process. In several studies, the greatest benefit (least cognitive decline) showed with an average of three cups of coffee consumed per day that provided an astounding 4.3 times smaller level of decline in cognitive function compared with non-consumers of coffee. Enriching coffee with polyphenols, especially chlorogenic acid, produces still greater benefits, even more so than green (not yet roasted) coffee beans as proven by a study that provided an increased brain cell survival rate by an impressive 78% in the face of severe oxidant stress. But with enriched roasted coffee from enhanced beans, brain cell survival increased by an amazing 203%. Even decaffeinated coffee from enhanced chlorogenic acid beans enhanced mood and improved attention to a greater extent than with regularly-processed decaf. Of course, greater enhancement was seen with caffeinated brews. These benefits are likely to be of special importance in the face of the growing epidemic of Alzheimer's disease and other neurodegenerative conditions. Though it has been recently estimated that more than 40% of people over 84 will be stricken by Alzheimer's, moderate consumption of coffee (three to five cups per day) has been tied to reduced cognitive difficulty of all kinds in the aged.

Special animal studies with mice have recently shown, first, that caffeinated coffee consumption (the equivalent of five + cups per day in a human) not only protects the brain's primary neuronal cells against damage of Alzheimer's, but can even reverse some of that damage in as little as five weeks. Just dealing with caffeine, itself, it has been shown reproducibly in lab work that it can reduce the levels of the protein enzymes *beta-* and *gamma-secretase*, substances used to build the main damaging protein, **amyloid-beta (A-beta)**, in Alzheimer's. The proteins that go into the manufacture of **A-beta** are reduced to such low levels in the blood and brain itself as to afford definite protection and even begin to reverse some of the disease's damage. Further research is showing that there is a synergistic beneficial effect from as yet unknown chemicals in coffee that augment caffeine's ability to increase blood levels of a factor known as **Granulocyte Colony-Stimulating Factor (GCSF)** which further acts to improve cognitive function in Alzheimer's.

There are also several well-established lab-tested relationships between elevated coffee intake and protection from Parkinson's disease, the second most common neurodegenerative disorder after Alzheimer's. What has been revealed is that consumption of one to four cups of coffee per day can lower the Parkinson's risk by 47% over non-coffee drinkers, and for those who consume greater than five cups per day, risk-reduction is lowered by an impressive 60%. Increasing the concentration of GCSF by ingesting potent drugs like *Neupogen* has demonstrated efficacy in animal models of established Parkinson's treatment much as has been seen with simple coffee ingestion. More and more studies are piling on the exciting results showing the sought-after inverse dose-dependent relationship where the greater the number of daily cups of caffeinated coffee, the lower the risk of Parkinson's disease.

CANCER RISK-REDUCTION WITH COFFEE CONSUMPTION

Coffee brews with their attendant chlorogenic acid can protect the DNA of cells against damage from many sources. This can go a long way to ward off the various debilitating effects of aging and the development of many types of cancer. This was specifically and dramatically proved by a meta-analysis of thousands of women and their susceptibility to developing endometrial cancer. Those who drank the most coffee had shown a tendency of up to 30% less in developing this very dangerous cancer with an even greater protective effect among obese women.

DNA damage is characterized as a physical abnormality within the genetic makeup of a cell such as a break in a DNA strand. It usually occurs to a greater extent within cells that frequently divide. And we know for sure that DNA damage, if not quickly repaired, can lead to genetic mutations that cause diseases such as cancer. When DNA damage occurs within cells that divide less frequently, the results can promote premature aging. DNA injury can be sustained from many causes. The most common of which at the cellular level are the oxidizing agents produced by normal metabolic processes. Also, DNA defects can be triggered by numerous external agents such as ultraviolet light, ionizing radiation, chemotherapy, many industrial chemicals and their pollution into the ambient air by way of **polycyclic hydrocarbons** found in emitted smoke. But the simple consumption of a few cups of coffee can negate the DNA damage from all causes and provide up to an 18% decreased risk from a long list of cancers: of the prostate, breast, *colorectum, pharyngeal, esophageal, hepatocellular, pancreatic, bladder*, and *endometrial*.

The reduction in incidence of breast cancer, the second leading cause of cancer death in American women, appears to show a cause-and-effect response to coffee consumption. A 57% reduction to the risk of contracting **E**stroge**n**-**R**eceptor **N**egative (ER-negative, high risk) breast cancers was shown among women who drank five or more cups of coffee daily. The oft-mentioned polyphenols, especially chlorogenic acid, according to several lab studies, are the likely beneficial agents in these instances.

Men also receive important cancer protection from coffee. With prostate cancer as the second leading cause of cancer death in men, consumption of more than six cups of coffee per day is associated with an 18% reduction in risk for the disease, and a 60% reduction in risk of other aggressive or fatal cancers. Those who drank more than six cups of coffee per day have experienced as much as a 57% reduction in colon cancer incidences. The chemicals in coffee seem to target specific cancer-cell signaling systems to suppress colon cancer formation and metastasis. And cancers elsewhere in the digestive system are reduced by coffee consumption. A mere one cup daily was associated with at least a 42% reduction in risk of developing liver cancer even for those with confounding risk factors such as hepatitis-C infection. For those with no liver ailments, a single cup of coffee reduced the risk of death due to liver cancer by an astounding 50% compared to nondrinkers. And consuming more than three cups daily produced a 40% reduction in the risk of cancers of the mouth, throat, and esophagus.

COFFEE'S EFFECT IN PROTECTING AGAINST NON-CANCEROUS LIVER DISEASE

Chronic liver disease and cirrhosis cause 35,000 deaths per year in the United States making it the ninth leading cause of death in America. However, scientists have found that the risk of liver cirrhosis, and the dying from it can be greatly reduced by coffee consumption. Those drinking up to four cups daily exhibited a full 84% lower risk of cirrhosis according to a study in the *Annals of Epidemiology*. This is consistent with an earlier eight-year study of over 120,000 people that found that EACH CUP of coffee daily lowered the risk of death from cirrhosis by 23%. Also, patients with hepatitis-B or C have been shown to be less likely to develop nonalcoholic cirrhosis if they are also coffee drinkers.

SUMMARY OF BENEFITS

After years of suspecting coffee of having negative impacts on health, scientists have now concluded that it has rather remarkable health benefits. Most strikingly, a major study has revealed dramatic reductions in the risks of dying from any cause in direct proportion to the amount of coffee consumed. This comes on the heels of numerous other studies that demonstrate reduced risk of dying from specific ailments such as heart disease, stroke, cancer, diabetes, and the growing list of neurodegenerative disorders as well as controlling obesity to some extent.

Detailed analyses of coffee's many components reveal that polyphenols, especially chlorogenic acid, are the main contributors to the various brews' beneficial effects. These chemicals influence key enzymes in a positive way such that improved intracellular signaling prevents potential physiologic disaster which could lead to the major deadly diseases.

While traditional medicine fights a near-impossible battle against a tidal wave of devastating maladies that include diabetes, cancer, Alzheimer's, and other age-related diseases, extensive research now suggests that coffee, far from being a guilty pleasure to avoid, is actually **an all-natural** and inexpensive elixir of health.

Since conventional roasting processes readily diminish these compounds, it is good to know, and wise to seek out, coffees that retain the maximum amount of polyphenol content, allowing for enhanced health benefits without over-consumption and enduring the downside of potential untoward effects. There are now available supplements of concentrated chlorogenic acid and "green beans" for just such reasons.

CHAPTER 13

GASTRO-ESOPHAGEAL REFLUX DISEASE (GERD)... FEELING THE BURN

Have you ever felt the discomfort of heartburn, indigestion, or acid reflux on a recurring basis and realized something's not right? Although many Masters swimmers have experienced "feeling the burn," many do not know about the possible harmful effects of **G**astro**E**sophageal **R**eflux **D**isease (GERD), and how to deal with this situation as a swimmer.

HOW IS GASTROESOPHAGEAL REFLUX DISEASE (GERD) RELATED TO MASTERS SWIMMING?

A majority of the **U**nited **S**tates **M**asters **S**wimming (USMS) membership is represented by a determined, yet ever-aging group of people seeking the path to a healthy lifestyle. Not only does GERD increase in frequency with age, but swimming forces us into a prone position, which places pressure on the gastrointestinal tract, and allows an easier path for stomach acid to go back up the esophagus.

WHO SUFFERS FROM GERD?

Up to 15 million Americans experience heartburn and other discomforting symptoms daily. Studies have reported that across the general population 36% to 44% of adults experience heartburn at least once a month, and 67% of those over 65 have symptoms of GERD (though not necessarily heartburn) at least monthly. Just two years ago, the largest selling prescription drug of the year was Prilosec, an acid inhibitor.

WHAT ARE THE SYMPTOMS OF GERD?

The most common symptoms are heartburn (a burning sensation radiating from the stomach to the chest and throat) and regurgitation. Up to half of GERD sufferers experience dyspepsia, seen as heartburn, fullness in the stomach, and nausea after eating. The symptoms are aggravated by bending over, lifting a heavy weight, or lying down (particularly on the back), which may result in nausea and vomiting.

Chest pain can be a common symptom of GERD, and is sometimes difficult to differentiate from angina or an impending heart attack. Since both GERD and angina affect the same populations, you should see your physician if you experience chest pain.

Other symptoms of GERD include:

- Difficulty swallowing or choking
- The feeling of a lump of food trapped behind the sternum, which could be an esophageal spasm or a tumor
- Chronic sore throat
- Hiccoughs
- Asthma

Diagnosis by an experienced physician should prevent complications from long-term untreated GERD. If symptoms are relieved with a one week trial of any of the stomach acid-inhibitors (*Prilosec, Nexium, Protonix, Prevacid*), it is probable that the patient is suffering from GERD. However, caution must be used, because underlying cellular changes may have occurred already.

The state-of-the-art method for determining the condition of the patient's esophagus is to perform an upper endoscopy. Biopsies are taken either from the esophagus and, or the stomach to rule out dangerous cellular changes and look for possible infecting organisms. Another diagnostic test examines the acid contents by using a probe called a pH monitor, which is inserted into the esophagus for 24 hours. This test can be especially useful when looking for a cause of nighttime asthmatic symptoms (such as wheezing, coughing, burning throat), while suffering from GERD.

WHAT CAUSES GERD?

Mild, temporary heartburn can happen to anyone. However, persistent *gastroesophageal* reflux may be due to abnormal factors. The most common scenario involves the band of smooth muscle tissue at the base of the esophagus, the **L**ower **E**sophageal **S**phincter **(LES)**, which is responsible for closing and opening the lower end of the esophagus. The LES is essential for maintaining a pressure barrier against contents from the stomach. If it loses tone, it cannot close up completely after food empties into the stomach, thereby allowing digestive enzymes and acid to travel back into the esophagus. This situation causes the irritation found in GERD. With aging, the esophageal lining can become less sensitive to this irritation, and may sustain moderate to severe damage. If the esophagus becomes intensely inflamed, it can then lead to strictures, ulcers, and even cancer.

Other physiological factors leading to GERD include defects or injuries in the lining of the esophagus, poor motility of the stomach and duodenum, over-acidic stomach contents, and sensitivity to the other elements of digestion (enzymes, etc.).

Various substances can affect the LES, causing it to lose its tone. Examples include:

- Foods such as spearmint, peppermint, onions, garlic, chocolate, acidic citrus and tomato products
- Coffee produces a double whammy. Certain aromatic oils in coffee (whether caffeinated or not) increase stomach acidity, and the caffeine acts to relax the LES
- Alcohol relaxes the LES muscles and can also irritate the mucous membrane of the esophagus
- Smoking relaxes LES muscle function, increases acid secretion, reduces the intestinal-lining's protective substances such as *prostaglandins* and bicarbonate, and decreases mucosa] blood flow
- Medications, such as asthma inhalers, sedatives, common pain relievers, some blood pressure medications, and certain heart medications such as calcium channel blockers, can increase the symptoms of GERD. *Adrenaline*, or medications that stimulate *adrenaline* release, such as pseudoephedrine, can also increase the symptoms
- If used frequently, non-steroidal anti-inflammatories (NSAIDS) can inhibit the protective *prostaglandins* and produce ulcerations in mucous membranes lining the stomach and the esophagus

About half of asthmatic patients also have GERD, although it is not clear why. For most athletes, exercise-induced asthma does not appear to be related to GERD. However, many Masters swimmers do suffer from exercise induced asthma and GERD.

HOW CAN ONE TREAT GERD AND LESSEN ITS OCCURRENCE?

The treatment for GERD includes lifestyle changes and medication. Lifestyle and dietary changes alone can lessen the effects of GERD.

- Avoid food that relaxes the LES: caffeinated foods, chocolate, mint-flavored foods, carbonated drinks, and most spices, condiments and flavorings
- No alcohol or smoking
- Chew gum after eating, or when you sense reflux may be about to begin. This action produces more saliva, a known acid-neutralizer and protector of the esophageal lining
- Avoiding tight-fitting clothing around the waist
- If recommended by your health care practitioner, lose weight. A large belly puts undue pressure on the stomach

- Avoid full bending at the waist, especially while lifting or moving heavy weights
- Avoid ingesting a large amount of food before physical activity, such as swimming

- Never go to bed right after ingesting large amounts of food and, or drink. The rule of thumb is that three hours must pass between food ingestion and bedtime.
- Elevate the head of the bed at least six inches utilizing a wedge-shaped block. Do not make the mistake of just adding a few pillows to the head, as this can actually worsen the situation.
- Sleep on your *left* side. This positions the opening of the esophagus into the stomach higher than the bulk of the food contents.
-

THERE ARE TWO MAIN TYPES OF MEDICATIONS:

- **112-blockers** interfere with the receptor sites of *histamine* in the gut tissue), which indirectly reduces acid production. There are four I12-blockers marketed in the U.S. for over-the-counter purchase: *famotidine (Pepcid AC)*, *cimetidine (Tagamet)*, *ranitidine (Zantac)*, and *nizatidine (AXID)*. These medications do not need to be taken with food, and are appropriate to take for night-time protection against GERD. The acid-suppressing activity lasts from six to 24 hours (Pepcid is the strongest acting), and is very useful for people who need persistent acid suppression. These medications may also prevent heartburn in people who are able to predict its occurrence. With mild symptoms, this class of drugs works in about 70% of patients. With moderate symptoms, the efficacy declines to 50%.
- **Proton-pump** or **acid-pump inhibitors** directly reduce acid by shutting down the enzymatic activation of the acid-forming cells in the lining of the stomach. These medications are stronger than the 1-12-blockers, and are the major league players that keep GERD manageable. They work best when there is food in the stomach. Studies have shown that at least 93% of GERD patients are benefited by this class of drugs. The products available are *omeprazole (Prilosec)*, *lansoprazole (Prevacid)*, *pantropazole (Protonix)*, *rabeprazole (Aciphex)*, and *esomeprazole (Nexium)*. These medications require a prescription from your physician, and several similar new products are presently becoming available. Although these drugs can virtually eliminate many of the distressing symptoms of GERD, they cannot fully control regurgitation; that has to be controlled by lifestyle modifications.

Antacids are also very important, because they help lessen the effects of excess acid in the GI tract. Readily available, inexpensive, and mostly without negative side effects, antacids, can be utilized to coat the esophagus and stomach a few times per day, and specifically, when trouble may be anticipated. *Gaviscon* is a drug that can provide a unique beneficial function. This tablet foaming agent must be chewed and taken with water to put a protective barrier between the stomach and the esophagus; it works quite well to temporarily keep the acid in its place.

So, if you're 'feeling the burn' in a bad way, you may wish to make some of the recommended lifestyle changes outlined above. If the symptoms of GERD persist, you may wish to ask your physician about it. Resolving reflux and heartburn symptoms will not only allow you to focus on "feeling the burn" in your muscles, but it will make your swimming experience much more productive and enjoyable.

CHAPTER 14

THE MOST IMPORTANT CARBOHYDRATE YOU CAN CONSUME

OVERVIEW

Although it is a rather simple molecule, and most have never even heard of it, **D-RIBOSE** could quite possibly be the single most important supplement consumed by anyone partaking in vigorous exercise on a regular basis. The more it was studied, the greater the remarkable scope of benefit *d-ribose* was shown to have... to the point of assuring that vital body processes won't be starved of essential energy molecules even into aging (1,2). New discoveries about *d-ribose* make it one of today's hottest topics in the context of how we understand the relationship of energy management and chronic illness.

There is nothing extraordinary about its physical appearance... water-soluble, fine white crystalline powder, a bit sweeter than table sugar, and only a five-carbon backbone *(pentose)* instead of the usual six carbons found in the basic sugars *(mono-saccharides,* e.g. *glucose)* usually derived from the diet. The "D" moniker is used to signify a *dextro* (right-sided) *spacial* formation of the molecular structure which possesses the stronger biochemical and physiologic activity. But its biochemistry and subsequent physiology fuel interactions that power the very essence of life. And the more of it placed *in situ* (in the actual site of use) the more we are able to do, the better we are able to recover, and the stronger we are able to withstand. (3,4,5) This brings in the concept of **cellular energy management** that has been increasing the interest of late of cellular biologists and physicians caring for patients with progressive cardiovascular disease and many other age-related deteriorations. Reductions in cellular ability to utilize available energy sources or decreased ability to utilize deep-seated available energy stores already in place exposes tissues to increased risk of damage by oxidants and inflammatory reactions; this reduces efficiency of most organ activity. And since *d-ribose* is chemically central to cellular energy metabolism by forming the main-frame of what actually feeds the cells: ATP, any lessening of its concentrations can allow for cellular damage and disease by a host of causes. Planned, deliberate supplementation with *d-ribose* is showing remarkable protective and restorative activity at the cellular level to such a point that beneficial effects have been elicited following heart attacks, heart failure, strokes, and other organ dysfunctions.

On balance, we must also be aware and understand that in the natural order of living things, as the aging process manifests, the human body becomes more easily fatigued with continuous effort, the major organs do not perform up to youthful ability, and the all-too-familiar signs of aging become prominent, which all translate simply into affording less than optimal functioning all around. But the consumption of d-ribose can allow for a dramatic modification in this cascade of physiologic deterioration, in one case, being strung together in long chains to form **RiboNucleic Acid (RNA)**, the DNA-like structures essential to copying our genes and translating them into highly-functioning proteins (6) for enhanced **antioxidant** protection (7) and increased **immune** activity (8).

CARDIOVASCULAR INVOLVEMENT

Heart disease usually has multiple and inter-related causes (9). This is probably why, for the most part, no single medication or therapy usually works optimally to either prevent or repair cardiovascular damage, and the reason most heart patients undergo the "poly-pharmacy" (multiple medication protocol) syndrome to treat the complexity of the problem.

D-ribose, taken as a supplement, is an excellent cardio protective because it serves to aid multiple tissue targets as it provides defense against heart disease along the entire continuum of events that can lead to cardiac catastrophe. In regards to the heart muscle proper, *d*-ribose has a powerful protective effect against the dangerous sequence of events that allow for **ischemia-reperfusion injury.** This serious condition arises in the minutes to hours following a heart attack or stroke when *ischemic* (oxygen-starved) tissue is suddenly flooded with oxygen-rich blood as circulation is restored (reperfusion) (9). The sudden and intense availability of oxygen to previously oxygen-deprived and already-damaged tissue, though something that the main treatment strives for, sets off a deadly chain of events that culminate in release of free oxygen radicals and harmful inflammatory responses. But if high levels of ribose are made available before and immediately after the reperfusion occurs, most of those dangerous changes can be prevented or at least lessened to a great degree through ribose's activity on **inflammatory blood cells.** (10) This procedure is so potent and effective that many innovative anesthesiologists and surgeons have suggested and implemented using IV infusions of ribose during surgical procedures in which ischemia-reperfusion injury is a likely *sequela.* (11)

Ischemia, however, is not always an acute event with immediate consequences. More often in medical disturbances, low-level ischemia occurs on a continuing basis in people with advancing artery disease to various organs. With specific advancing Coronary **Artery Disease (CAD)** symptoms such as *angina* (chest pain) with exertion can build to an almost every day occurrence and to the point of causing pain even at rest. Each episode of chest pain represents steady depletion of cellular energy levels with less and less ability to support work due to frank depletion of the main energy molecule **ATP (adenosine triphosphate)** from coronary muscle cells (12, 13). These events consume the heart's normally-available supply of <u>d-ribose</u> which forces it to become a *conditionally-essential nutrient.*(14)

If allowed to continue unabated, this cellular energy starvation becomes a major contributor to **Congestive Heart Failure (CHF)** where the heart muscle simply can't "squeeze" strong enough to move blood efficiently and according to immediate demands and needs (15). *Sequalae* include fluid retention in tissues throughout the body from what is called "backward cardiac failure" where the heart loses its ability to keep circulation at optimum and move blood forward. We see the development of swollen ankles, bloating *(ascites)* in the abdominal cavity, fluid buildup in the lungs *(pulmonary edema)*, etc., all due to this poor cardiac contractility. This leads inevitably to progressive exercise intolerance and labored breathing even with simple body positioning that permits fluid gathering. It is the pulmonary edema that many times proves the deadly end result of (CHF)... the victim, in essence, "drowns" in his own fluids.

Many people with congestive heart failure find themselves on multiple medications aimed at reducing fluid accumulation or chemically increasing the heart's ability to move blood forward. While these drugs can provide a modicum of success, none are curative, and most have substantial side effects that limit their utility. Fortunately, congestive heart failure can be partially *reversed,* especially if it is diagnosed and properly treated early.

POTENT CARDIOPROTECTANT

Increasingly, scientists are "connecting the dots" with several in depth investigations linking the *ischemia-energy-content in situ relationship* to the severity of heart muscle damage where the actual supply of energy-mediating nutrients can modify the extent and duration of cardiac disability. And *d-ribose* is the leading substance being studied. (16-17)

A leading cardiologist and researcher, Stephen T. Sinatra, MD, has written extensively on the cardiac benefits of *d-ribose*. His comment that "many physicians are not trained to look at heart disease in terms of cellular biochemistry"(18) has added to the searching for viable mechanisms where safer and more effective therapy with cardiac energy preparations have arisen, utilizing *d-ribose* as metabolic support for ailing cardiac muscle right at the tissue level. (12)

The benefits of *d-ribose* began to interest researchers in earnest in the early 1990s. Those early studies were mainly focused on *d-ribose* as an aid in radiology techniques such as thallium scanning, which indicate areas of insufficient blood supply (ischemia) in the heart. Those running the tests found that infusing *d-ribose* intravenously during the scan increased the "visualization" of the heart tissue because **much more blood was permeating the tissue of the heart.** (6,19) Both the cellular biochemistry and physiology proved that cardiac muscle obviously preferred the most energy-laden molecule, Adenosine Tri-Phosphate **(ATP).** It can still function somewhat adequately for moderate duration and activity utilizing the single-phosphate depleted energy molecule, Adenosine Di-Phosphate **(ADP).** But we see trouble form and cardiac insufficiency develop when the heart's deep energy reserves become depleted over time while the immediate demand for physicality is still elevated. Heart muscle can NOT function appropriately relying on the most energy-depleted single-phosphate molecule, Adenosine Mono-Phosphate **(AMP).** We start to see the developing dysfunction of **cardiac-insufficiency** with all the attendant sequelae if the energy reserves and attendant concentrations of **ATP** and **ADP** are not quickly replenished.

The biochemistry plays out quite simply: the limiting section (moiety) of the ATP molecule is *d-ribose.* (See molecular formula below). Adenine is easily harvested from an adequate protein-rich diet, and phosphates are ubiquitous throughout what we eat. But *d-ribose* has to be biochemically manufactured by splitting off a carbon atom from *glucose* or fructose which had to be further metabolically produced from more complex carbohydrates consumed. When energy is needed NOW, the delay in producing sufficient *d-ribose* can definitely cause sputtering at high levels of demand. But if supplemental *d-ribose* is consumed, there is the biochemical and physiological advantage of immediate presence of ATP for immediate muscle-powering energy.

Too often, individuals with coronary disease also have such limited mobility that they are unable to engage even in simple exercise due to a pronounced limitation of available energy. In the late 1990s, Italian researchers found that they could use *d-ribose* **to increase exercise tolerance** in patients with severe coronary artery disease and chronic ischemia. They gave these patients an oral dose of **60 grams daily** in four divided doses for just three days to achieve gains in endurance. (9) More recently, a German group showed that *d-ribose* could **improve heart function** (as seen on echocardiograms) while also improving quality of life in patients with congestive heart failure. (20)

Through the regeneration of ATP energy molecules and an increase in the heart muscle's total energy level, *d-ribose* has shown to improve heart muscle contractility... the "squeeze" needed to pump blood efficiently to the lungs and the body in general. (21,22) When *d-ribose* was given intravenously to patients who have suffered one or more heart attacks, scientists found that the pentose increased the number of heart segments with good contractility, a visible marker of improved function. (23)

D-ribose's replenishment of heart muscle energy levels has additional benefits, as was shown in a recent study of patients with advanced congestive heart failure and extreme exercise intolerance. (24) These people were given *d-ribose* at **15 grams daily** in three divided doses. They all had impressive improvements in their abilities to breathe more deeply to ventilate their lungs along with a 44% improvement in their heart failure classification. This proved clinically significant since these severely-impaired patients could now move about more freely and with increased comfort.

[History tells us of the first recorded marathoner: Phydippedes. He was in his early 30's and considered a "professional courier." He was trained and lived his professional life as a deliverer of messages over long distances. It so happens that when the Persians were coming to invade Greece, Phydippedes was sent to fetch the aid of the battle-tested Spartans a few days before the anticipated historic clash. He had to travel about 75 miles each way to obtain this help that no doubt depleted his energy stores. He completed this task but was then required to inform the powers-that-be that the Greeks defeated the invaders. Historians provide conflicting stats on this effort. Did the courier actually run 42 miles in two days or the now-accepted 26-mile distance in one day? No matter which, Phydippedes had to be severely energy-depleted (truly d-ribose depleted) from both long distance assignments. It is reported that he expired almost immediately after delivering the good news of victory. This may be medical conjecture on my part, but I feel he succumbed most likely to heart failure. His heart was most probably depleted of ATP and ADP, and as stated above, if all that remained to power the cardiac musculature was AMP, he was done in by severe cardiac insufficiency.]

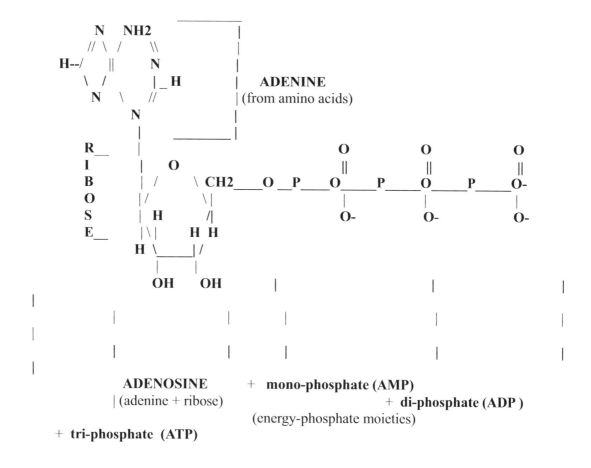

ADENOSINE + **mono-phosphate (AMP)**
| (adenine + ribose) + **di-phosphate (ADP)**
(energy-phosphate moieties)
+ **tri-phosphate (ATP)**

PROTECTING THE CENTRAL NERVOUS SYSTEM

The central nervous system can also derive extensive benefits from *d-ribose*. Several cardiologists revealed that they found, as a tremendously-positive secondary effect when given to heart attack victims, that not only did *d-ribose* improve heart functionality and blood flow, it also had a profound impact on *brain tissue* during the period of low blood pressure that can follow a coronary attack. The **pentose** reduced the presence of a protein that triggers cell death in brain tissue deprived of blood flow; mechanism obviously can also act as a life-saving defense mechanism in the case of a stroke. (22)

This *d-ribose* neuro-protective effect has major implications because heart attacks and strokes contribute enormously to the age-related cognitive decline so prevalent today in seniors. This brain-tissue protection from *d-ribose* is generating mounting enthusiasm in neurological-research scientists and is partly due to the generalized **antioxidant effects** it provides throughout the body (7,24) and partly the result from *d-ribose's* remarkable ability to **restore energy-depleted tissues** back to near normal.

Supplementation with *d-ribose* has shown to increase the available amounts of ATP in brain tissue, just as it does in heart muscle. (26) The importance of this ancillary effect cannot be over-stated since the brain consumes an enormous proportion of our daily total energy resources.

OTHER TISSUES AND ORGANS ADVERSELY AFFECTED BY DEFECTIVE PRODUCTION OF ATP

There are two conditions that often occur together with similar underlying causation. **F**ibro**M**yalgia (FM) and **C**hronic **F**atigue **S**yndrome (CFS) are now believed to become manifest due to a **defective production of ATP.** (27,28,29) This, of course, leads to the direct use of *d-ribose* as a prime candidate for therapy. Due to the **energy-enhancing capabilities of d-ribose** and since it is usually the limiting factor in the production of ATP, tests and specific studies have shown that moderate dosages of the pentose have proved beneficial in most instances of trial where other traditional medications failed. (27) The administration of **5 grams/3 times daily** over a period of three weeks produced significant improvements in all the categories of the syndromes (energy, sleep, mental clarity, pain intensity, and well-being) for all the subjects.(27) On average, patients reported a **45% increase in energy levels.** Though fibromyalgia and CFS remain complicated and often perplexing to researchers, the positive results with *d-ribose* offer real hope for a definite solution.

Restless Leg Syndrome (RLS) is a relatively common disorder that affects up to 15% of the US population, and it becomes severe enough in more than one-third of these cases to warrant medical treatment. (30,31) The condition involves an uncontrollable urge to move the legs, accompanied by uncomfortable sensations in the lower-extremities, usually felt to be worse at night. (31) Only a few medications offer even partial relief of RLS, and many make the condition worse, not giving much recourse to the sufferers.(30,31) Since **disordered energy metabolism** has been suggested as one possible cause of RLS, **low levels of *adenosine (see formula), the d-ribose-containing central molecule in ATP, has been a hallmark of this ailment.*** (32) Based on this observation, a demonstrative study has been carried out in which daytime symptoms were eliminated, and nighttime symptoms significantly reduced on **daily doses of 15 grams** *d-ribose* split as **5 grams at breakfast, lunch,** and **dinner.** (25). It is too early to claim complete cure of RLS with *d-ribose* but these encouraging findings, coupled with complete absence of untoward effects, warrant further investigation.

PROTECTING KIDNEY FUNCTION

As with the heart and brain, the human kidney receives a high proportion of the body's total blood flow which makes it virtually equal in vulnerability to damage by ischemia-reperfusion mechanisms (the loss and restoration of blood supply). This interference with renal blood supply can occur as the result of trauma or during any major surgery; it can be sometimes worsened by chronic conditions such as cardiovascular disease and diabetes. (33-36)

Several studies suggest that an **immune activation** and **inflammatory response** following this kind of kidney injury creates the bulk of the damage, especially in those with diabetes.(11,36) **Adenosine**, which is partly made from *d-ribose,* is an important regulator of kidney function, and is especially vital during times of injury (37) These observations, coupled with what we already know about *d-ribose* as an antioxidant and anti-inflammatory, have peaked considerable interest among kidney researchers.

Japanese scientists have led the way in investigating *d-ribose* as a kidney protector. They have found that, in rats subjected to renal ischemia-reperfusion, as can happen in major surgery in the human, *d-ribose* significantly reduced the release of *inflammatory cytokines.* (11) Both the function and appearance of the kidneys following injury were improved substantially. They also brought out that *d-ribose* reduced activation of *neutrophils,* the ubiquitous **W**hite **B**lood **C**ells (WBC) that are the first to arrive at the scene of an injury but that also release toxic chemicals and oxygen radicals that can cause additional harm.(10) Clearly, researchers are only beginning to realize the substantial potential of *d-ribose* for protecting and restoring kidney health.

RIBOSE AS THE "RACE CARB"

Short-duration, high-intensity muscle contractions that are involved in power movements (heavy-weight lifting, sprinting, leaping, and movement involving intense proprioception... controlling the body's movements through its immediate environment) all demand the immediate availability of only one type of carbohydrate to produce sufficient concentrations of appropriate fuel (ATP): *d-ribose.*(7)

The body manufactures its needed ATP from food, but this takes time through various biochemical pathways. Not much total ATP is normally stored in the musculature, only about **85 grams** in total, which can power the body for only about 10-15 seconds at maximum push. As intense activity progresses stored, ATP in muscle tissue is depleted steadily and readily. In most athletes on standard diets, ATP normally stays markedly depressed at least one day (24 hours) after intense exercise, and may take as long as 96 hours to fully bounce back to capacity after prolonged or multiple training bouts in those not re-fueling to optimum. With a regular training-day schedule, supplemental administration of *d-ribose* should to be taken continuously to optimally remake and refill ATP stores to training needs.

D-ribose also acts to facilitate the "salvage pathway" where breakdown products from all energy metabolism, rather than become scattered throughout in a non-beneficial way, are gathered for recycling and re-combining to expedite the replenishing of ATP concentrations in the needed muscles and organs. Physiologic evaluations show that re-creation of ATP is enhanced with regular *d-ribose* consumption and that **fast-twitch muscle fibers** (explosive force) are positively affected more than slow-twitch fibers. Many challenging physiological tests have demonstrated that those athletes supplementing with *d-ribose* develop more power and endurance than those on placebo dosing. And those subjects with cardiac conditions lasted, on average, 24% longer on treadmills before redeveloping myocardial ischemia, all demonstrating *d-ribose's* ability to enhance exercise tolerance to fatigue. (9,13)

ARE THERE ANY UNTOWARD EFFECTS OF RIBOSE

We know the good *d-ribose* can do, but several recent publications have raised the question of whether it, because of its simple carbohydrate structure, could possibly contribute to the development of harmful **advanced glycation end products.** (38-41) **Glycation** is the denaturing of protein by chemical combination (cross-linkages) with sugar molecules. This combined protein/sugar formulation cannot function properly and can, thus, cause an interfering with organ function and vital chemical processes.

Like any sugar, *d-ribose* can indeed produce protein glycation, with resulting damage to tissues. (40) And when *d-ribose* is administered experimentally at the same high challenging doses as with *glucose*, it quickly causes the protein-denaturing cross-linking that is the outcome of glycation. (38) But all the challenging studies have utilized extreme concentrations of *d-ribose;* levels never found in humans, even with high-dose supplementation. As an example with this high dosing in humans, at amounts of 20 grams and 53 grams over a 4-hour period, peak serum *d-ribose* levels rose to only 4.8mg/dl and 81.7 mg/dl respectively. (42) While challenging doses in glycation experiments were significantly higher, up to **30 times higher** than achievable in human blood. (40, 41) Other studies tried to bring about definite glycation but could only do so with massive doses of *d-ribose* that would never happen in functional life occurrences. Even direct injection of *d-ribose* into joints could not produce enough glycation to damage cartilage at the site. (43,44) To further prevent the remote possibility of *d-ribose*-induced glycation, it is recommended that daily dosages be split up to keep concentrations way below possible trouble.

SUMMARY OF TAKE-HOME POINTS

D-ribose is an essential component in our bodies' **cellular energy management** systems. Additionally, it provides antioxidant, anti-inflammatory, and gene regulatory capabilities. Together, these characteristics make it of compelling interest to forward-thinking clinicians, patients, and serious athletes.

Supplemental *d-ribose* demonstrates cardio-protection, even late in the disease process when heart attacks have already occurred, and when heart failure is developing. *D-ribose* helps ailing heart muscle maximize its effort, and allows for improved blood flow to oxygen-starved cardiac tissue.

D-ribose supplements are only just being explored for similar benefits in brain and kidney tissues, but recent studies offer great hope in these areas. Even perplexing conditions

270

such as fibromyalgia and restless leg syndrome seem to be yielding to the energy-related benefits of *d-ribose.*

Evidence garnered from several sources indicate that supplementing with *d-ribose* in split doses throughout the day will enhance physical capacity throughout the body. The more the body is pushed to train, the more *d-ribose* it needs to consume within reasonable dosing.

As long as moderation in dosing is followed, there have been no untoward side effects within any of the challenging experiments or with any of the real-world usage in strenuous exercise.

[History tells us of the first recorded marathoner: Phydippedes. He was in his early 30's and considered a "professional courier." He was trained and lived his professional life as a deliverer of messages over long distances. It so happens that when the Persians were coming to invade Greece, Phydippedes was sent to fetch the aid of the battle-tested Spartans a few days before the anticipated historic clash. He had to travel about 75 miles each way to obtain this help that no doubt depleted his energy stores. He completed this task but was then required to inform the powers-that-be that the Greeks defeated the invaders. Historians provide conflicting stats on this effort. Did the courier actually run 42 miles in two days or the now-accepted 26-mile distance in one day? No matter which, Phydippedes had to be severely energy-depleted (truly d-ribose depleted) from both long distance assignments. It is reported that he expired almost immediately after delivering the good news of victory. This may be medical conjecture on my part, but I feel he succumbed most likely to heart failure. His heart was most probably depleted of ATP and ADP, and as stated above, if all that remained to power the cardiac musculature was AMP, he was done in by severe cardiac insufficiency.]

PROTECTING THE CENTRAL NERVOUS SYSTEM

The central nervous system can also derive extensive benefits from *d-ribose.* Several cardiologists revealed that they found, as a tremendously-positive secondary effect when given to heart attack victims, that not only did *d-ribose* improve heart functionality and blood flow, it also had a profound impact on **brain tissue** during the period of low blood pressure that can follow a coronary attack. The **pentose** reduced the presence of a protein that triggers cell death in brain tissue deprived of blood flow; mechanism obviously can also act as a life-saving defense mechanism in the case of a stroke. (22)

REFERENCES:

1. Available at http://naturalmedicinejournal.net/pdf/NMJ_FEB10_NP. Accessed July 23, 2012.

2. Kohlhass M, Maack C. Interplay of defective excitation-contractions coupling, energy starvation, and oxidative stress in heart failure. *Trends Cardiovasc Med.* 2011, Apr; 21 (3); pp. 69-73.

3. Available at http://naturalmedicinejournal.net/pdf/NMJ_FEB10_NP. Accessed July 23, 2012.

4. Barsotti C, Ipata PL. Pathways for alpha-D-Ribose utilization for nucleobase salvage and 5-fluorouracil activation in rat brain. *Biochem Pharmacol.* 2002 Jan 15; 63 (2); pp. 117-122.

5. Omran H, McCarter D, St Cyr J, Luderitz B. D-Ribose aids congestive heart failure patients. *Exp Clin Cardiol.* 2004 Summer; 9(2); pp. 117-118.

6. Perlmutter NS, Wilson RA, Angello DA, Palac RT, Lin J, Brown BG. Ribose facilitates thallium-201 redistribution in patients with coronary artery disease. *J Nucl Med.* 1991 Feb; 32 (2); pp. 193-200.7.

7. Seifert JG, Subudhi AW, Fu MX, et al. The role of ribose on oxidative stress during hypoxic exercise: a pilot study. *J Med Food.* 2009 Jun; 12(3); pp.690-693.

8. Freeman ML, Mertens-Talcott SU, St Cyr J Percival SS. Ribose enhances retinoic acid-induced differentiation of HL-60 cells. *Nutr Res.* 2008 Nov;28 (11); pp.775-782.

9. Ferrari R, Pepi P, Ferrari F, Nesta F, Benigno M, Visioli O. Metabolic derangement in ischemic heart disease and its therapeutic control. *Am J Cardiol.* 1198 Sep 3;82 (5A); pp.2K-13K.

10. Sato H, Ueki M, Asago T, Chujo K, Maekawa N. D-ribose attenuates ischemia/reperfusion-induced renal injury by reducing neurtrophil activation in rats. *Tohoku J Exp Med.* 2009 May;218 (1); pp.35-40.11.

11. Nishiyama J, Ueki M, Asaga T, Chujo K, Maekawa N. Protective action of D-ribose against renal injury caused by ischemia and reperfusion in rats with transient hyperglycemia. *Tohoku J. Exp Med.* 2009 Nov;219 (3); pp.215-222.

12. Pauly DF, Pepine CJ. D-Ribose as a supplement for cardiac energy metabolism. *J Cardiovasc Pharmacol Ther.* 2000 Oct;5(4); pp249-258.

13. Pliml W, von Arnim T, Stablein A, Hofmann H, Zimmer HG, Erdmann E. Effects of ribose on exercise-induced ischaemia in stable coronary artery disease. *Lancet.* 1992 Aug 29;340(8818); pp. 507-510.

14. Kendler BS. Supplemental conditionally essential nutrients in cardiovascular disease therapy. *J Cardiovasc Nurs.* 2006 Jan-Feb;21 (1); pp. 9-16.

15. Sinatra ST. Metabolic cardiology: an integrative strategy in the treatment of congestive heart failure. *Altern Ther Health Med.* 2009 May-June;15(3); pp. 44-52.

16. Lopaschuk GD. Treating ischemic heart disease by pharmacologically improving cardiac energy metabolism. *Presse Med.* 1998 Dec 12;27(39); pp.2100-2104.

17. Pauly DF, Johnson C, St Cyr JA. The benefits of ribose in cardiovascular disease. *Med Hypotheses.* 2003 Feb;60(2); pp.149-151.

18. Sinatra ST. Metabolic cardiology: the missing link in cardiovascular disease. *Altern Ther Health Med.* 2009Mar-Apr,15(2); pp.48-50.

19. Hegewald MG, Palac RT, Agnello DA, Perlmutter NS, Wilson RA. Ribose infusion accelerates thallium redistribution with early imaging compared with late 24-hour imaging without ribose. *J Am Coll Cardiol.* 1991 Dec:18(7); pp.1671-1681.

20. Omran H, Illien S, MacCarter D, St Cyr J, Luderitz B. D-Ribose improves diastolic function and quality of life in congestive heart failure patients: a prospective feasibility study. *Eur J Heart Fail.* 2003 Oct;5(5); pp. 615-619.

21. Omran H, McCarter D, St Cyr J, Luderitz B. D-Ribose aids congestive heart failure patients. *Exp Clin Cardiol.* 2004 Summer;9(2); pp. 117-118.

22. Schneider HJ, Rossner S, Pfeiffer D, Hagandorff A. D-ribose improves cardiac contractility and hemodynamics, and reduces expression of c-fos in the hippocampus during sustained slow ventricular tachycardia in rats. *Int J Cardiol.* 2008 Mar 28;125(1); pp. 49-56.

23. Sawada SG, Lewis S, Kovacs R, et al. Evaluation of the anti-ischemic effects of D-ribose during dobutamine stress echocardiography: a pilot study. *Cardiovasc Ultrasound.* 2009;7:5

24. MacCarter D, Vijay N, Washam M, Shecterle L, Sierminski H, St Cyr JA. D-ribose aids advanced ischemic heart failure patients. *Int J Cardiol.* 2009 Sep 11;137 (1)' pp.79-80.

25. Chigrinskiy EA, Conway VD. Protective effect of D-ribose against inhibition of rats testes function at excessive exercise. *J of Stress Physiolog and Biochem.* 2011;7(3); pp.242-249.

26. Barsotti C Ipata Pl. Pathways for alpha-D-ribose utilization for nucleobase salvage and 5-fluorouracil activation in rat brain. *Biochem Pharmacol.* 2002 Jan 15;6(2)' pp. 117-122.

27. Teitelbaum JE, Johnson C. St Cyr J. The use of D-ribose in chronic fatigue syndrome and fibromyalgia: a pilot study. *J Altern Complement Med.* 2006 Nov;12(9); pp. 857-862.

28. Eisinger J, Plantamura A, Ayavou T. Glycolysis abnormalities in fibromyalgia. *J Am Coll Nutr.*
1994 Apr;13(2); pp. 144-148.

29. LeGoff P. Is fibromyalgia a muscle disorder? *Joint Bone Spine.* 2006 May;73(3); pp. 239-242.

30. Martin CM. The mysteries of restless legs syndrome. *Consult Pharm.* 2007 Nov;22(11); pp. 907-924.

31. Bayard M, Avonda T, Wadzinski J. Restless legs syndrome. *Am Fam Physician.* 20008 July 15;78(2); pp.235-240.

32. Guieu R, Sampieri F, Pouget J, Guy B, Rochat H. Adenosine in painful legs and moving toes syndrome. *Clin Neuropharmacol.* 1994 Oct;17(5); pp. 460-469.

33. Laisalmi-Kokki M, Pesonen E, Kokki H. Potentially detrimental effects of N-acetylcycstein on renal function in knee arthroplasy. *Free Radic Res.*2009 Jul;43(7); pp. 691-696.

34. Siems W, Quast S, Carluccio F, et al. Oxidative stress in chronic renal failure as a cardiovascular risk factor. *Clin Nephrol.* 2002 Jul;58 Suppl 1;S12-S19.

35. Yan SF, Ramasamy R, Schmidt AM. The receptor for advanced glycation endoproducts (RAGE) and cardiovascular disease. *Expert Rev Mol Med.* 2009;11:e9.

36. Jang HR, Ko GJ, Wasowska BA, Rabb H. The interaction between ischemia-reperfusion and immune responses in the kidney. *J. Mol Med. 2009* Sep;87(9); pp. 859-864.

37. Vallon V, Osswald H. Adenosine receptors and the kidney. *Handb Exp Pharmacol.* 2009 (193): pp. 443-470.

38. Mentink CJ, Hendriks M, Levels AA, Wolffenbuttel BH. Glucose-mediated cross-linking of collagen in rat tendon and skin. *Clin Chim Acta.* 2002 Jul;321(1-2); pp. 69-76.

39. Kuo TY, Huang CL, Yang JM. The role of ribosylated-BSA in regulating PC12 cell viability. *Cell Biol Toxicol.* 2012 Aug;28(4); pp.255-267.

40. Wei Y, Han CS, Zhou J, Liu Y, Chen L, He RQ. D-ribose in glycation and protein aggregation. *Biochem Biophys Acta.* 2012 Apr;1820(4); pp.488-494.

41. Han C, Lu Y, Wei Y, Liu Y, HeR. D-Ribose induces cellular protein glycation and impairs mouse spatial cognition. *Plos One.* 2011;6(9); pp. E24623.

42. Gross M, Zollner N. Serum levels of glucose, insulin, and C-peptide during long-term D-ribose administration in man. *Klin Wochenschr.* 1991 Jan 4;69(1); pp.31-36.

43. Vos PA, Degroot J, Barten-van rijbroek AD. Elevation of cartilage AGEs does not accelerate initiation of canine experimental osteoarthritis upon mild surgical damage. *J Orthop Res.* 2012 Mar 2.

44. Willett TL, Kandel R, DeCroos JN, Avery NC, Grynpas MD. Enhanced levels of non-enzymatic glycation and pentosidine crosslinking in spontaneous osteoarthritis progression. *Osteoarthritis Cartilage.* 2012 Jul;20(7); pp 736-744.

CHAPTER 15

DEALING WITH INFECTIOUS DISEASES

In addition to the mental and physical effects of overreaching and overtraining, vigorous training also involves the risk of immunologic breakdown, which leaves the athlete open to infectious diseases. When the swimmer is exhausted from training hard and working in close physical proximity to the rest of the team, it is easy to become sick and to suffer from it.

There is a 3-foot rule in public health: if you can separate yourself from someone who is sick with a cold or other **Upper Respiratory Infection (URI)** by at least 3 feet for the short time that you may share proximity, your chances of coming down with the infection are reduced. I want to emphasize the fact that a short time of exposure means just a few minutes at best. Double the distance, and you cut the risk to at least a quarter. If you are walking behind someone who is sneezing or coughing during cold season, take a detour off to the side so as not to breathe in his trailing effluence, spreading germs. If forced to share space with someone exhibiting symptoms of a cold or URI for longer than an hour, try to get as far away as practical and have as many people fill in the space between you two, and, if at all possible, open the windows to circulate fresh air. Spraying a Lysol-type product through the air in a contaminated space will help to reduce virus and bacteria load. The air ducts and accompanying filters in the home and car should be sprayed at least once a week. Years ago it was discovered that the infecting bacteria for Legionnaires' disease in hospitals found a "home" in the hot water pipes and air ducts heating the rooms. A cough or sneeze in a car can cause several thousand infecting organisms to linger for days in the A/C ducts, a major cause for relapse or reinfection.

At the pool, we can take a logical approach to prevention. Even though swimmers are surrounded by water, they, too, can sweat. In fact, most swimmers, if they do not replenish liquid during practice, will lose up to 2 pounds of weight. This is water weight equivalent to about two pints (32 oz.) of fluid. Replacing this is not only important for more efficient muscle contraction during practice but also vital for overall well-being. Logically, and with good public health in mind, if there are any swimmers exhibiting URI symptoms, they should not be at practice, infecting the rest of the team. To help control infectious spread, swimmers should not all be bunched up in the same tight area after each set; they should be spread out a bit and breathing in different directions. Remember, even a 3-foot separation can make a big difference.

In terms of the viruses and bacteria that cause the vast majority of URIs, there are three main components to consequential infection: (1) the infecting load or total amount of initial exposure; (2) the length of time exposed, and (3) the condition of the body and its immune system at the time of exposure. The absolute simplest yet most important procedure to keep the spread of infection down is to prevent potentially contaminated hands from coming in contact with mucous membranes (eyes, nose, and mouth). Carrying gel-type disinfectants to use on the hands before eating out (if no access to a rest room), for example, is a smart move.

Another simple but very important procedure is to blow the nose after exposure to airborne germs, or better yet, at the end of every day, to help eliminate many of the infecting organisms caught in the nasal passages and in the upper respiratory tract before they can "dig in," since it takes up to several hours for most infecting organisms to penetrate the mucous linings of the body. The body's coating of mucus, which it produces to lay down a protective layer over all the linings opening to the environment, gets thicker as it dries out, so I recommend blowing the nose while taking a hot shower, as the moisture from the hot water works to hydrate and loosen. You should also keep hydrating the body with fluid intake throughout the day, you should never wait to get thirsty to drink. It is extremely important to keep up hydration when the seasons change from the humid summer to the cooler, drier fall and winter months. Regular intake of sufficient liquid is especially important in extreme climates—both hot and cold—since they can each dry out the body's portholes to its surroundings. If the relative humidity in your home is less than 50% during the dry, cold winter months, then the air is too dry.

Chlorinated water is very drying and irritating to all mucous membranes, but it is not just the chlorine. It is more what chlorine has combined with— body fluids interact with free chlorine to produce *hypochlorites*. This is what we smell at pools and what burns our eyes and makes us cough. Symptoms include sensitivity to the smell of chlorine, burning eyes, and coughing with exertion at some pools. Along with lack of rest and overtraining, reactions to chlorine can put the swimmer in a run-down, less protective condition. The thick mucus that is caused by a negative reaction to chlorine is not helpful at all to the body and hinders its ability to breathe, especially under duress. To help correct this and some of the other negative effects on the respiratory tract, I highly recommend using a hot steam vaporizer in the bedroom each night. The benefit comes from a sterile, soothing, warm mist that helps heal an irritated respiratory tract and ward off infection. In addition, each morning, the room should be aired out and sprayed down with a product like Lysol to prevent mold growth on rugs, drapes, blankets, and blinds. It is worth all this extra work to prevent illness that could prove detrimental to a swimmer who needs to train hard and breathe unimpaired.

CHAPTER 16

THE DAMAGE-REPAIR CYCLE: MUSCLES FAIR BETTER THAN TENDONS

When you exercise, bodily movement vigorous enough to produce muscle soreness is causing structural damage to the contracting muscle fibers and their surrounding membranes. This allows for increases in muscle enzyme leakage into the blood, which act as easy markers for detecting tissue damage directly related to trauma. Inflammation usually follows quickly and surrounds the traumatized area as the body tries to protect the injury from becoming more intense by making movement painful and difficult. It helps to know just what is occurring when you damage muscle versus *tendinous* tissue, in order to understand that the recovery process should never be short-changed, in particular when tendons are involved.

WHAT EXERCISE DOES TO DAMAGE MUSCLE

Some exercises and movements are more damaging to intact muscle tissue than others. Activities that cause a forceful lengthening of the fibers (eccentric movement) will usually produce more concerted damage than those only requiring contraction since that is what muscle tissue was fabricated to do: contract forcefully.

Another way of looking at this is: Abnormally lengthened fiber undergoes increased tension because the elongated fiber must endure an increased load-to-fiber ratio; that is, there is not enough tissue acting against a resistance. Conversely, a contracted muscle has an increased fiber-to-load ratio and can more easily handle the load because much more tissue is available to move a resistance.

A popular activity utilizing mostly concentric movement is cycling. Compare this type of movement to activities that produce extraordinary lengthening of muscle tissue—running or hiking downhill, descending stairs, lowering weights back to a starting position—and it's easy to see why in eccentric movement micro- Increased swelling produces increased pressure against nerves in the immediate area, signaling discomfort, pain, weakness, and reduced range of motion. tears occur. This then begins a cascade of events starting with bleeding at the site. Bleeding adds leaked fluid volume to the already crowded area of swelled fiber tissue. An injured muscle also fatigues more readily than an intact, fully-functioning muscle.

WHAT EXERCISE DOES TO DAMAGE TENDONOUS TISSUE

Tendons can become irritated and inflamed, leading to fraying of the fibrous material if they are caused to rub against hardened surfaces in a crowded joint capsule, for example, in the shoulder of a swimmer or baseball pitcher. An inflamed tendon then swells, taking up more room than nature intended in areas not designed to accommodate lots of tissue. Tendons, all of which attach muscle to bone, can also become overly-stressed and even torn from insertion into the muscle if too great a resistive load is placed on the muscle fibers. And finally, tendons can be damaged simply by applying repeated pressure against them, as with someone constantly leaning on their knees, causing the main connective tissue running over the kneecap, the patellar tendon, to become inflamed.

This condition, from the constant pressure of excessive force against the knees, can develop in high jumpers, participants in basketball and volleyball, weightlifters who excessively and incorrectly stress their knees with deep knee bends and leg lifts at the wrong angle of attack, and anyone else having to endure the force of body weight transmitted through the knees against gravity and immoveable ground.

Tendonous tears, as with muscle tears, come in various degrees of severity. It is usually an easier road to healing if a muscle sustains a minor to moderate tear than a tendon.

Muscle has more tissue to help it sustain a resistive load. Appropriate rest and physical rehabilitation can help the damaged tissue rejoin together, though scar tissue and calcium deposits can ensue. However, a tear in a stringy tendon, even one somewhat enhanced due to the adaptive processes in training, could much more easily produce a complete or near-complete separation requiring surgical repair.

SECTION IV:

RISING ABOVE... A MAN'S GOT TO KNOW HIS LIMITS... OR DOES HE?!

The psychology of competition is much more important than many would allow. Thousands of hours of focused and intense participation through prescribed and demanding movements to direct correct neuro-muscular adaptations; hundreds of hours in the weight room to become as powerful as possible; serious nutrition becoming a full-time necessity... even bordering on the exotic, all take a secondary position as the athlete approaches the starting point of his or her competition. The mind has to be right at the right time (The Power of the Moment, to say it in a few words) to allow for an optimum performance. Harnessing this power usually makes for successful and happy athletes.

YOU GOTTA BELIEVE!

Possibly the most important psychological factor involved in heroic athletic performance is a belief in yourself... a belief that you can achieve the most difficult objective.

Roger Bannister was the first runner to break four minutes for the mile. His 3:59.4 was "the greatest athletic performance of the century," according to sports psychologist William Morgan, EdD., at the University of Wisconsin in Madison.

Barrnister was not quite the leading runner at the time. The most consistent winner had been Gunder Haegg, but he had read that a four minute mile was not possible; it was beyond human reach. Bannister, on the other hand, believed the increasing competition between himself and Haegg would make it possible to break this barrier. And he believed that he, Bannister, was the man who could do it. He set breaking four minutes as a personal goal, trained to do it, and with his coach, Franz Stampfl, set up the race in which he would do it, on the Iffley Road track in Oxford, on May 6, 1954. A month earlier Haegg recognized Bannister's determination and wrote, "I think Bannister is the man to beat four minutes. He uses his brains as much as his legs. I've always thought the four minute mile more of a psychological problem than a test of physical endurance."

Bannister believed in himself, and he succeeded. Many have thought that Bannister's knowledge of the body and its workings (he was a medical student) gave him a scientific training advantage. Bannister knew differently. Later, he wrote, "Though physiology may indicate respiratory and cardiovascular limits to muscular effort, psychological and other factors beyond the ken of physiology set the razor's edge of defeat or victory and determine how closely the athlete approaches the absolute limits of performance."

Once the psychological barrier was down, other runners began to run under four minutes because they knew it could be done. This record has continued to fall at an average rate of more than half a second a year.

"If you think you can or you think you cannot, you are probably right," Henry Ford is supposed to have said. Bannister thought he could, and he did. Haegg thought he could not, and he didn't.

To get the most out of yourself, not just in sports, but in all your life's activities, set difficult goals that you believe you can achieve. Without that belief, all the training in the world won't work.

CHAPTER 1

EMOTIONAL BENEFITS OF EXERCISE

Up until my late 30's, life had been pretty good to us. We were a loving family blessed with an adequate income, good health, two gifted children, and the three most important words I know: PEACE OF MIND. For years I was taught to be humble, be thankful, and "don't break the bubble." I had my normal wants and disappointments and envies, but I was taught early-on never to wish harm on anyone, for it would only come back to me. I guess life does not always play fairly, for I sure got mine. One of my greatest fears as I grew older was to have a handicapped child; I whispered prayers many times to be spared such a life-long burden.

My need for exercised-induced stress release took on new and urgent meaning at 38 years of age. Our third child, Matthew, was born under severe fetal distress, complicated by inadequate medical care. From the start, we knew we were in deep trouble. I had been swimming Masters for more than two years, returning to the pool after a 20-year hiatus, and dared not stop, for I always felt a great emotional lift after each workout. I needed that lift more now than at any time in my life!

Dealing with a severely handicapped child was a 25-hour-a-day job for my wife; the kids and I had some diversion with school, work AND the pool. My daughter Lee and my son Jason were very talented age-group swimmers with national rankings. They both took Matt's condition as motivation for their own endeavors. Their important swims were dedicated to him. What kids! Eventually, my wife Eileen worked some pool time into her schedule that definitely lifted her spirits and gave some balance to her life.

As time passed, Matt was fitted with a special wheelchair, and we were able to take him just about everywhere... he was my little buddy. People used to stare, but so what; he was my son, and I loved him. At swim meets, we use to wheel him onto the decks off to the side and near the starting blocks. In time, most of the regulars got to know the Nessel's as much by Matt's presence as by Lee's and Jason's performances. This must have really psyched my kids, for they became New Jersey state champions in their respective age groups, and were even written up in Swimming World.

It is axiomatic that "FISH GOTTA SWIM." If nothing else, they are prisoners of their environment. We, on the other hand are prisoners of our minds. The body does what the mind dictates. I dare not stop swimming to keep a lid on my anxiety.

There is nothing new in the universe. What was true at society's beginning, holds for today: being anxious and fearful come free with breathing. Exercise in olden days meant escaping the man-eaters, truly "invigorating" if not adaptive. Today, exercise is just as essential, only the man-eaters are the more subtle predators of our health.

What allows for the benefits to the mind? Is it the security of a repetitive set of movements in a comfortable environment? Is it that commitment to self enhancement, knowing that something good is being accomplished physically (higher HDL's, weight control, body-toning)? Is it the totally structured involvement required to participate or maybe the intrinsic *beta-endorphins* stimulated well into each exercise bout? How about all of the above? The Nessel's know all too well the psychological bridge to good mental health that swimming provides.

That bridge crashed down on me and my family six years ago when we lost Matt. He was 7, and his cerebral palsy had made it very difficult for him to do anything including swallowing and digestion. Sometime during the early morning hours, he must have aspirated some vomitus. I remember only that I was startled awake by my wife's screams, my leaning over Matt giving him CPR and thinking "this is NOT my child in my arms, just do what you have been trained to do and he will recover." The heart started, but the cerebral damage added to his already compromised condition, was too much. We had to let him go. My greatest fear, life's greatest perversion, to see a child of mine die... came to be. Now we had to deal with this... life's final crushing blow to my little buddy. No choice here; sink or swim.

Having to endure, I "dove" into swimming with a vengeance. At first I had some trouble. When I became breathless, Matt's face would come before me, and I would panic and stop dead in the water. My team knew I was suffering and offered sympathy and concern. But it was up to me to deal with this. I was determined to beat this. To break these panic attacks, I would rush to the locker room and stare at myself in the mirror and would talk to the "guy" in there; eventually I would calm down and return to the pool. The attacks came less frequently in the water, but my torment in the wee hours of the morning was not eased. Recurring nightmares of that terrible morning mercilessly tortured my wife and me.

Fortunately, summer was upon us, and we were able to rise early for the 6AM Masters workout at the near-by county long-course pool. These proved to be the most enjoyable and beneficial. Obvious contributors were warm, bright days, clean air, the 50-meter pool itself with the sun coming over the trees lining the deck, garnished with our shared team spirit. The dawn of a new day allowing for another chance at doing ourselves some good. They say time heals; I do not know about that. I would rather say it mitigates; makes less painful, allowing one to go about the new day-to-day...

My daughter Lee has gone on to become a High School All-America and the Captain of the University of Miami Swim Team. My son Jason gave up swimming after Matt's death; I guess the demands of the sport on someone with his talent were more than his personality would allow. But he is still active in sport, playing on his high school's baseball and football teams. My wife and I are devoted Masters swimmers. So much so, that I gave up practicing

Pharmacy and became a full-time swim coach, running an age-group, senior, and master's program nearby. My involvement with the youngsters stems from the fact that I want to give them a chance to reach their potential... something Matt never had. My involvement with the Masters should be obvious: it was there when I needed it, and pay-back is oh! so sweet!

CHAPTER 2

THE PSYCHOLOGY OF COMPETITION; IF YOU THINK YOU CAN OR YOU THINK YOU CAN'T... YOU ARE RIGHT. THE FOUR MOST IMPORTANT WORDS YOU CAN MUTTER: "I CAN DO THIS."

It is well established and universally accepted that "the body follows the head." Whether it be physically, emotionally, or mentally, what comprises about 10 percent of our mass absolutely controls the other 90. Integration and correlation of body functions are so complex that there need be various segments of the contents of our skulls... a division of labor if you will. This "specialization" was developed and has been honed since we first arose as a species. Specific functional activity is all geared to allow us to understand and learn and then remember what is constantly happening around us. No matter what the energy requirement or physical demand, if bodily movement is sought, it is initiated by signals from the brain.

No matter what the chosen effort, correct movement demands proper head positioning appropriate for each sport. This is the physical aspect mentioned above but not the focus of this chapter. The message here is to elucidate the centers of the brain intimately involved in learning, storing, analyzing, and interpreting what messages are sent north through the body which nobody sees, and what resultant messages are sent south to move the body that everyone sees. But there is more, much more, to learning how to harness the power of the mind to bring all systems to "go" when physical demands present themselves. I've spent years studying deeper into the functions of the body when it is placed under vigorous physical and emotional stress. We know that stress damages, even kills, especially unrelenting stress. And we know that when placed in situations we cannot completely control; it is usually our minds that are impacted first and foremost and which signal distress and "yell" for help.

The day-to-day training for any sport physically conditions the body and causes it to adapt to greater and greater demands that are required for success. But it is also during this time that the mind and all its vital segments need conditioning. I proved this several years ago with a simple but emphatic test when I brought land-based athletes (varsity college football players) into water too deep for them to secure footing.

These land-based "lab rats" were asked to move across the pool (75 feet) in any fashion they could. As fatigue and breathlessness set in, almost to a man, they began to panic and fight the water. The more they fought, the more the water "fought" back, magnifying their fatigue and sense of air-deficit. Most could not make it across and had to either grab for the lane guides or the side of the pool or, even more dramatic, jump on the backs of their teammates. When they finally did struggle their way to the perceived security of the far wall, almost immediately they began to relax and gain some measure of control over panic. What they could do all day long on land where they were used to vigorous activity, they could only do for a few seconds in a medium foreign to them. Their perceptions changed quickly from "I'm okay" to "I am NOT okay," ending with "I THINK I AM GOING TO DIE!" Being varsity scholarship athletes meant nothing during this perception of impending doom.

The statement: "What we perceive is what we believe" comes alive due to a specific part of the brain called the *amygdala*. Nature provides this almond-shaped segment of the inner brain to protect us from dangerous situations that could do us in. It registers intense experiences both good and bad and stores them for immediate retrieval when we place ourselves in corresponding situations.

If training is to be thorough and productive, conditioning, the mind is absolutely as important as working the body. I am talking here about the physical segments of the brain that play the major roll in trying to keep us in a stabilized state. Quality movement through any vigorous exercise unequivocally demands specific training to produce "mental toughness" or "mental conditioning." This brings in the segment called the *amygdala* almost constantly. Appropriately-designed training sets (where air-exchange is challenged while holding technique) cause the build-up of both *carbon dioxide (CO2)* and the *hydrogen ion* (H+) of acid. It is mainly carbon dioxide which activates special receptors in the circulatory system that, in turn, send strong signals to the *respiratory centers* (controlling inhale and exhale) located in the *brain stem.* These centers dictate how fast, how deep, how thorough our respiration becomes to help us recover from vigorous exercise. The body is always playing catch-up with air and exercise. The *amygdala* also is bombarded with these signals of physiologic distress and further influences our intense desire to breathe along with bringing out the emotion of fear. The secret here is not trying to inhale excessively, though that is the overriding thought for the uninitiated. Rather, extra mentality and the benefit of proper physiologic coaching are called for to work the focus on only one thought: EXHALE. Blow out as much CO2 as possible. This produces two conditions that are beneficial: removal of CO2 and the lessening of the H+ concentration in the blood. It is an interesting physiologic occurrence that pharmacological testing of the efficacy of anti-anxiety, anti-panic medications encompasses the injection of pure lactic acid in varying concentrations.

There is a prime law in physics that states that "two things cannot occupy the same space at the same time." The goal of getting oxygen-laden air into the lungs (which function by having the lungs' air sacks fill by negative vacuum) can only come about by first ridding (exhaling) them of "stale" air laden with carbon dioxide. The take home point here is to **concentrate on the exhale rather than the inhale.** You want to keep forcefully blowing out as the perception of becoming air-challenged increases. This all seems crazy to those not trained to handle it: being asked to keep the body moving fast, yet to concentrate on exhaling rather than inhaling. To train against this fearsome sequence, as a swim coach, I have instituted Navy SEAL challenges to my athletes with underwater streamlines motivated by crisp snappy submerged kicking across the pool, intentionally allowing CO2 to build up; I then ask for strong swims, strong kicks, or both with racing finishes. As a group, my triathletes are weaker in the water than on the bike or the run and have found these challenges more daunting than my swimmers, but once they adapt to this type of training, all three segments of their event seem noticeably easier.

The *amygdala* and the *respiratory centers* are constantly bombarded with impulses signaling distress. Eventually, with the proper mind-set (four "magic" words come into play here: "I CAN DO THIS!"), the distressing signals become more easily handled by the mind that then translates to more aggressive bodily movement. My responsibility as coach is to constantly remind my people in the water that my intention is to have them endure increasing discomfort yet have the emotional wherewithal to get their hands on the wall with bad intentions towards their competitors.

The next segment of the brain that I stimulate to our purpose is called the **R**eticular **A**ctivating **S**ystem (RAS). This group of cells is in close proximity to the *limbic system* where all these groups of tissue function to make us aware, keep us focused, and present impulses from our **perceived** surroundings that can be construed as threatening. This is the segment that gives us the negativity of jitters: pounding heartbeat, interrupted uneven respiration, "butterflies" in the stomach, the repeated flashing of negative thoughts that the task at hand cannot be completed successfully. But it can also provide just the right amount of adrenal stimulation to make us appropriately on edge so we can muster all our energies quickly. The trick here is to create the shift to just the right amount of positive stimulation without being overwhelmed by it. The great industrialist, Henry Ford, without knowing one thing about physiology or anatomy, is credited with once saying: "if you think you can, or you think you cannot... you are right." *He was* astute enough about success in life to realize the importance of winning over the parts of the brain *(RAS and the limbic system)* to have the mind positively direct the body's movements... I CAN DO THIS! Today, we can help stimulate the same area of the brain without exotic chemicals and pharmaceuticals. I called these *"benign psychic stimulants."* A flavor, a color, and the most ubiquitous ingested chemical in the world all come under this classification: mint, the color amber, and the stimulating ingredient in coffee and chocolate, caffeine.

The psychological use of aroma and taste stimulation with mint (peppermint being the most effective) has been known for several years. It has been shown to act on the *RAS* and provide for such stimulation as to definitely make a positive difference in the ability to focus on most tasks at hand. Teachers are now utilizing mint whether in gum, lozenge, or quick-dissolving strips to help their students score higher in academic achievement tests. It can certainly bring the importance of a strong start to any race into the forefront of thought and action. The same stimulant effect is elicited by having the eyes look through *bright amber color*. The visual stimulation from this particular wavelength has been proven to aid in focus and increase awareness of the immediate surroundings. I have shown that the use of both mint and amber eye-wear cause many of my swimmers to narrow their field of view and to focus on what is directly in front of them. This has helped them to enter a competition with more intensity off the start and into the race.

The last of the psychic stimulants to be discussed in this chapter is *caffeine*. This substance has diverse pharmacological and psychological properties which aid the body and mind in both quick, reflexive and prolonged movements. It can stimulate the mind to respond almost hyper-reflexively to surrounding stimulation and yet put off the use of glycogen as an energy source till the sprinting end of a race while tapping into the utilization of free fatty acids to fuel the body for endurance events. Caffeine works so well and is consumed by so many people throughout the world that international sports governing organizations have issued rules as to how much of it can be acceptably present in blood and urine.

Whenever a neuro-muscular movement is first leaned, the related impulses land in the domain of the *cerebrum*. Any stimuli that enter this highest of human brain segments must first be "digested" then analyzed and finally "understood." If it is not made to be as clear and near perfect as the desired goal at this point, the "learning" process will be adulterated. "Garbage in produces garbage out." The more complicated the movements, the more CORRECT must be the analysis. If a coach is trying to have his athletes learn a better method of movement, it is extremely important at this point in the training that extra care be taken by both the transmitter (coach) and receiver (athlete). Everything must be slowed down. All movements should be more deliberate and analyzed for correctness. As familiarity develops and facility of movement builds with repeated practice (as much as 10,000 hours to produce elite-level talent) speed is introduced. When speed and smooth, correct execution become easier to elicit with continued practice and guidance, motor impulses begin emanating from the *cerebellum,* a more rudimentary segment of the brain one step down from the *cerebrum*.

Now that we know what segments perform what functions, we need to make them earn their keep. What I call **critical thinking** is the correct way to bring training elements to the fore under the stress of competition. Just because you know that something needs to be done does not mean you will do it under stress, let alone do it correctly. And even if you know that correct things should be done and how to do them, it does not mean you will remember to do them under duress. To have **critical thinking** work, the athlete needs to be repeatedly trained such that all appropriate movement occurs in a timely fashion throughout the event. This should be orchestrated at a pace that will not totally tax the physiology. By staying relatively in the comfort zone at first and then building speed throughout the event over time, impulses TO all of the aforementioned segments of the brain can occur and be correctly analyzed while impulses FROM them can be handled appropriately through the duration of the event. Ancillary thoughts can be analyzed during training such as: "how do I feel at this point in the event" and at various points throughout. With proper analyses of how the body's physiology and mentality change during prolonged vigorous movement at faster and faster speeds, the athlete becomes better prepared to tackle the challenges of his event during competition. When he places himself deep into the scenario of his event BEFORE he actually does it, the athlete is practicing **visualization.** If executed properly (the athlete seeing himself executing everything perfectly and putting in a fine effort) this type of mental training becomes invaluable.

The final element for discussion has to do with the amount and type of input stimuli the athlete takes in from ambient surroundings. Too much extraneous input and the athlete can easily become overwhelmed and distracted from the immediate task at hand. Recent research from Stanford University has shown that too much electronic stimulation from various sources caused the participants to become "suckers for irrelevancy" as the lead author put it. Everything seemed to distract them. The researchers also found that heavy multi-taskers consistently underperformed those who preferred to complete one task at a time. Weaknesses were shown to include their inability to pay attention to detail, organize memory, and switch from one job to the next. But there is the converse to this finding.

Too little stimuli and the athlete can suffer listlessness and insufficient arousal for optimum performance. The expression for this input is called *F/1 noise.* Years ago in the 1930's and '40's, Hollywood made a certain type of movie called film noir. They were shown in black and white, were mostly well written, and usually presented a dark topic. The story line was worked out by the end of the movie with good conquering evil as the take home point. But they only had on average 230 "cuts" for the whole movie. A "cut" is what the industry calls a dramatic change in scene on the screen... something of sufficient stimulating impact that rivets the viewer; an action scene after some important dialogue along with appropriately-integrated music causes the viewer to re-focus and become submersed into the story. In today's film presentations, the average is 1400 "cuts." The story line can be weak, even poor, but the viewer is riveted to the screen with intense computer-generated images, even though he feels the film might have been frivolous. The extra cuts comprise negative *F/1 noise.* It is excessive incoming stimulation. Sometimes, as the Stanford research has shown, this is just too much to integrate properly over a set period of time as when we see people constantly working their MP3's, talking on cell phones while driving, or ear phones always worn. Excessive sensory bombardment can negatively impact critical thinking. But there is a time and place for positive F/1 noise.

To work athletes such that they have to think more during training sets is to bring in more input, more positive F/1 noise. More thinking equals more analysis; more analysis equals more conscious effort required if combination tasks are the challenge. Swimming combined with kicking and maybe another stroke with extra tight streamlines off each wall during various lengths of a prescribed distance brings in more F/1 noise than just asking people to swim a distance. Running and, or biking at varying intensities over distance with flat and hilly terrain and imagined scenarios of competition can also provide for positive F/1 noise.

The coach needs to emphasize to the athlete that all correct movement must be thought through and focused on before starting the effort and that proper execution be instituted throughout. This type of F/1 noise causes the various segments of the brain to strongly re-enforce the important elements for winning form. These types of combination sets are just complicated enough to bring in the need for extra thinking and analysis. This is the final touch for preparing athletes for quality performances. But it takes extra effort for both coach and athlete in organization, execution, and analysis. Time and energy well spent to make "I CAN DO THIS!" a reality.

CHAPTER 3

THE NEURO-BIOLOGY OF COMPETITION

The statement: "What we perceive is what we believe" comes alive due to a specific part of the brain called the *amygdala*. Nature provides two fingernail-sized almond-shaped segments of the inner brain to protect us from dangerous situations that could do us in. They register intense experiences both good and bad and store them for immediate retrieval when we place ourselves in corresponding situations.

If training is to be thorough and productive, conditioning, the mind is absolutely as important as working the body. I am talking here about the physical segments of the brain that play the major role in trying to keep us in a stabilized state. Quality movement through any vigorous exercise absolutely demands specific training to produce "mental toughness" or "mental conditioning." Since, in my opinion, there is no education and training as good as dealing with and overcoming adversity, this brings in the segment called the *amygdala* almost constantly. Appropriately-designed training sets (where air-exchange is challenged while holding technique) cause the build-up of both *carbon dioxide* (CO_2) and the *hydrogen ion* (H+) of lactic acid. It is mainly carbon dioxide which activates special receptors in the circulatory system that, in turn, send strong signals to the respiratory centers (controlling inhale and exhale) located in the brain stem. These centers dictate how fast, how deep, how thorough our respiration becomes to help us recover from vigorous exercise. The body is always playing catch-up with air and exercise. The *amygdala* is also bombarded more easily (twice as much) with these signals of physiologic distress than the highest level of our brains, the frontal lobes. These lobes that are directly causative for human physical response and intentional movement influence our intense desire to breathe along with bringing out the **emotion of fear.** They can be trained to withstand and delay panic and then to initiate the correct movements that produce desired results. The secret here is not trying to inhale excessively, though that is the overriding thought for the uninitiated. Rather, extra mentality and the benefit of proper physiologic coaching are called for to work the focus on only one thought: EXHALE. Blow out as much carbon dioxide as possible. This produces two conditions that are beneficial: removal of CO_2 and the lessening of the H+ concentration in the blood. It is an interesting physiologic occurrence that pharmaceutical companies often test the efficacy of anti-anxiety, anti-panic medications with the injection of pure lactic acid in varying concentrations.

There is a prime law in physics that states that "two things cannot occupy the same space at the same time." The goal of getting oxygen-laden air into the lungs (which function by having the lungs' air sacks fill by negative vacuum) can only come about by first ridding

290

(exhaling) them of "stale" air laden with carbon dioxide. **The take-home point here is to CONCENTRATE ON THE EXAHLE RATHER THAN THE INHALE.** You want to keep forcefully blowing out as the perception of becoming air-challenged increases. This would all seem counter-intuitive (crazy) to those not trained to handle it: being asked to keep the body moving fast, yet to concentrate on exhaling rather than inhaling. To train against this fearsome sequence, as a swim coach, I have instituted Navy SEAL challenges to my athletes with underwater streamlines propelled by crisp, snappy submerged kicking across the pool, intentionally allowing CO2 to build up; I then ask for strong swims, strong kicks, or both with racing finishes. As a group, the triathletes who train with me are weaker in the water than in their bike or run segments and have found these challenges more daunting than my swimmers, but once they adapt to this type of training, all three segments of their event seem noticeably easier.

The *amygdala,* the respiratory centers, and the frontal lobes, as mentioned above, are constantly bombarded with impulses signaling distress. What to do... how to quickly make the right choices to handle the perceived impending mounting distress. That is where the specific training of strengthening the proper mind-set come into play. The four "magic" words "I CAN DO THIS" become the overriding mantra of the moment. The distressing signals become more easily handled by the higher centers of the brain which then translates into more aggressive and appropriate bodily movement. My responsibility as coach is to constantly remind my people in the water that our goal is to have them endure increasing discomfort yet have the emotional wherewithal to push through and work to get their hands on the wall with bad intentions towards their competitors.

The next segment of the brain that I stimulate to our purpose is called the **R**eticular **A**ctivating **S**ystem **(RAS).** This group of cells is in close proximity to the *limbic system* where all these groups of tissue function to make us aware, keep us focused, and present impulses from our perceived surroundings that can be construed as threatening. This is the segment that give us the negativity of jitters: pounding heart, interrupted uneven respiration, "butterflies" in the stomach, the repeated flashing of negative thoughts that the task at hand cannot be completed successfully. But it can also provide just the right amount of adrenal stimulation to make us appropriately on edge so we can muster all our energies quickly. The trick here is to create the shift to just the right amount of positive stimulation without being overwhelmed by it. The great industrialist, Henry Ford, ignorant of physiology or anatomy, is credited with once saying: "If you think you can, or you think you cannot... you are right." He was astute enough knowing the human element to realize the importance of winning over the mind (here, the RAS and the limbic system) to have it positively direct the body's movements... I CAN DO THIS! Today, we can help stimulate the same areas of the brain without exotic chemicals and pharmaceuticals. I call these "benign psychic stimulants." A flavor, a color, and the most ubiquitous ingested substance in the world all come under this classification: **MINT**, the **COLOR AMBER**, and the stimulating ingredient in **coffee** and **chocolate...**

CAFFEINE. The psychological use of aroma and taste stimulation with mint (peppermint being the most effective) has been known for several years. It has been shown to act on the RAS and provide for such positive stimulation as to definitely make a difference in the ability to focus on most tasks at hand. If teachers are now utilizing mint whether, in gum, lozenge, or quick-dissolving strips to help their students score higher in academic achievement tests, it can certainly bring the importance of a strong start to any race into the forefront of thought and action. The same stimulant effect is elicited by having the eyes look through bright amber color. The visual stimulation from this particular wavelength has been proven to aid in focus and increase awareness of the immediate surroundings. I have shown that the use of both mint and amber eye-ware (goggles) cause many of my swimmers to narrow their field of view and to focus on what is directly in front of them. This has helped them to enter a competition with more intensity off the start and into the race.

The last of the psychic stimulants to be discussed is caffeine. This substance has diverse psychological and pharmacological properties which aid the mind and body in both quick, reflexive and prolonged movements. It can stimulate the mind to respond almost hyper-reflexively to surrounding stimulation and yet put off the use of glycogen as an energy source till the sprinting end of a race while tapping into the utilization of free fatty acids to fuel the body for endurance events. Caffeine works so well and is consumed by so many people throughout the world that international sports governing bodies have ruled as to how much of it can be acceptably present in the blood and urine.

Whenever a neuro-muscular movement is first learned, the related impulses land in the domain of the *cerebrum.* Any stimuli that enter this highest of human brain segments must first be "digested" then analyzed and finally "understood." If the stimuli are not made as clear and near perfect as the desired goal at this point, the "learning" process will be adulterated. "Garbage in = garbage out." The more complicated the movements, the more CORRECT and THOROUGH must be the analysis. If a coach is trying to have his athletes learn a better method of movement, it is extremely important at this point in the training that extra care be taken by both the transmitter (coach) and receiver (athlete). Everything must be slowed down. All movements should be more deliberate and analyzed for correctness. As familiarity develops and facility of movement builds with repeated practice (as many as 10,000 or more repetitions for good quality talent, while as much as 10,000 or more HOURS to produce elite-level talent) speed is introduced. When speed and smooth, correct execution become easier to elicit with continued practice and guidance, motor impulses begin emanating from the *cerebellum,* a more rudimentary segment of the brain one step down from, and more primitive than, the cerebrum.

Now that we know what segments perform what functions, we need to make them earn their keep. What I call critical thinking is the correct way to bring training elements to the fore under the stress of competition. Just because you know that SOMETHING needs to be done does not mean you will DO it under stress, let alone do it CORRECTLY. And even if you know that CORRECT things should be done and HOW to do them, it does not mean you will REMEMBER to do them under duress. To have critical thinking work, the athlete needs to be REPEATEDLY TRAINED such that all appropriate movement occurs in a timely fashion throughout the event. This should be orchestrated at a pace that will not totally tax the physiology. By staying relatively in the comfort zone at first and then building speed throughout the event over time, impulses TO all of the aforementioned segments of the brain can occur and be CORRECTLY ANALYZED while impulses FROM them can be handled appropriately allowing for quality movement through the duration of the event. Ancillary thoughts can be analyzed during training such as: "how do I feel at this point in the event" and at various points throughout. With proper analyses of how the body's physiology and mentality change during prolonged vigorous activity at faster and faster speeds, the athlete becomes better prepared to tackle the challenges of his event during competition. When he places himself deep into the scenario of his event BEFORE he actually does it, the athlete is practicing *visualization.* If executed properly (the athlete seeing himself EXECUTING everything PERFECTLY and putting in a FINE EFFORT) this type of mental training becomes invaluable.

The final element for discussion has to do with the amount and type of input stimuli the athlete takes in from his ambient surroundings. Too much extraneous input and the athlete can easily become overwhelmed and distracted from the immediate task at hand. Recent research from Stanford University has shown that too much electronic stimulation from various sources caused the participants to become "suckers for irrelevancy" as the lead author put it. Everything seemed to distract them. The researchers also found that heavy multi-taskers consistently underperformed those who preferred to complete one task at a time. Weaknesses were shown to include their inability to pay attention to detail, organize memory, and switch from one job to the next. But there is also the converse to this finding.

Too little stimuli and the athlete can suffer listlessness and insufficient arousal for optimal performance. The expression for this input is called *F/1 noise.* In the 1930's and '40's, Hollywood made a certain type of movie called "Film Noir"... Shown in black and white, mostly well-written, and usually presenting a dark topic. The story line was worked out by the end of the movie with good conquering evil as the take home point. But they only had on average 230 "cuts" for the whole movie. A "cut" is what the industry calls a dramatic change in scene on the screen... something of sufficient stimulating impact that rivets the viewer. An action scene after some important dialogue along with appropriately-integrated music causes the viewer to re-focus and become immersed into the story... sufficiently-appropriate input to aid focus. But in today's film presentations the average is 1400 "cuts." The story line can many times be weak, even poor, but the viewer can become riveted to the screen with intense non-stop computer-generated images. During post-show analysis he later feels the film might have been frivolous and unworthy of his time and expense.

The extra cuts comprise **negative F/1 noise**. It is **excessive incoming stimulation.** Sometimes, as the Stanford research has shown, this is just too much to integrate properly over a set period of time as when we see people constantly working their MP3's, talking on cell phones while driving, or ear phones always worn. **Excessive sensory bombardment can negatively impact critical thinking.** But there is a time and place for positive F/1 noise.

To work athletes such that they have to think more during training sets is to bring in more input, more positive F/1 noise. **More thinking equals more analysis; more analysis equals more conscious effort required** if combination tasks are the challenge. Swimming combined with kicking and maybe another stroke with extra tight streamlines off each wall during various lengths of a prescribed distance brings in more positive F/1 noise than just asking people to swim a distance. Running and, or biking at varying intensities over distance with flat and hilly terrain and imagined scenarios of competition can also provide for positive F/1 noise.

The coach needs to emphasize to the athlete that all correct movement must be thought through and focused on before starting the effort and that proper execution be instituted throughout. This type of F/1 noise causes the various segments of the brain to strongly re-enforce the important elements for winning form. This works best going from slow to easy speed to push pace to race pace. If the mechanics can be held true as the physicality increases, it means the neurology has been laid down well, going correctly from cerebrum to cerebellum. But there is a very important neurologically-related phenomenon that occurs right along with this. It has to do with how constant repetitions build skills.

What happens with repeatedly performing physical tasks is the body lays down layer upon layer of myelin (a fatty protective substance) sheathing coating along nerve fibers innervating into muscle tissue. The more the repetitions, the more the myelin sheathing. What this proves out to occur is that simply practicing a movement will only reinforce that exact movement performed. It may be anywhere from totally incorrect to absolutely perfect. This, then, brings in the learning principle that practice does NOT make perfect... it makes permanent. PERFECT PRACTICE MAKES PERFECT. The myelin sheathing needs to be laid down PERFECTLY along the neurons for elite functioning. But when an athlete seeks quality coaching to help correct imperfections in his/her movements, it is often many times much harder to achieve corrected movements than to learn them brand new with no bad habits... thanks to all the myelin sheathing laid down over several thousands of already experienced movements.

Appropriately-designed combination sets are just complicated enough to bring in the need for extra thinking (focus) and analysis. This is the final touch of finesse for preparing athletes for quality performances. But this always takes extra effort for both coach and athlete in organization, execution, and analysis, allowing for time and energy to be well spent to make "I CAN DO THIS!" a reality.

CHAPTER 4

THE PSYCHOLOGICAL NEEDS OF AN ATHLETE UNDERGOING PHYSICAL THERAPY

Those sustaining injuries severe enough to require physical rehabilitation, no matter what the sport and level of skill and competition react psychologically in different ways to what will inevitably be down time. Some can handle the setbacks logically and positively and find ways to train around them or work to strengthen other weaknesses to keep on the schedule for higher levels of physical condition while undergoing the obvious modalities for injury repair. Other athletes, just as talented and dedicated to success, often cannot muster up the mental energies or find the right attitude to go along with the planned physical rehabilitation; they cannot seem to handle the sudden, unplanned set back of a debilitating injury or illness and allow appropriate time and the medical profession to work their "magic.

In the animal world, for example, the scenario of putting down a severely leg-injured race horse has been observed by racing fans and the public at large as a matter of indigenous protocol for many years. The main reason is that the race horse's genetics and innate response to training do not allow for reason and understanding of the long-range path to rehabilitation. The animal simply can neither understand nor tolerate his/her legs needing time free from movement to heal. The two most famous instances of this happening to world class thoroughbreds were more than 30 years apart. Involved first was the filly, Ruffian, and then the colt, Barbaro. They were considered so talented and valuable that attending surgeons tried their best in both instances with extensive surgery that was successful. The problems arose after the anesthetics wore off, and a hard lesson was learned. When Ruffian's anesthetic wore off, she began to thrash about with such force as if she as if she were trying to get up and run, that all the surgery was undone, and the horse was in severe distress. The only humane resultant left was to put her down. But an important lesson had been learned. If this were tried again in the future, the horse would be place in a pool of water to keep it from thrashing about and its weight off the surgically-repaired injury. This was tried on Barbaro, and it worked. The horse was kept from incipient danger by being placed intelligently in water and appropriately sedated to prevent his innate desire to run. The surgery had time to heal, but other complications arose which eventually dictated the same fateful end as befell Ruffian.

Human athletes who react negatively to their injuries show anger, denial, depression, and self-defeating attitudes and actions. For the good of the team or themselves, these athletes must be pulled aside and explained to and reasoned with as to how this unfortunate situation can have a brighter outlook. Since everything in life is a matter of attitude, turning around negative thoughts is a very important effort to get across.

Sports injury recovery most often focuses solely on the physical rehabilitation. But to bring about the quickest and most successful therapy, the attendant staff must be ready, able, and observant enough to include sports psychology skills and techniques in the recovery program. This optimally affords the injured athlete his best chance of getting back to where he was before the set back. By making him a more confident and resilient athlete, adding psychological guidance can bolster his response to other adversity should it arise during his training or competitions. The following are some of the areas where a competent and thorough rehabilitation specialist can implement sports psychology into the comprehensive rehab program.

UNDERSTANDING THE APPROPRIATE TIME LINES FOR TOTAL REHABILITATION

The first concept an athlete needs to comprehend is the time frame involved in his/her injury rehab process. A foolish approach of trying too much too soon will likely set the stage for disaster as with the above-mention race horses. A devastating blow to the recovery process due to presumptuous inappropriate activity can sometimes permanently negate the sought-after results. The time from surgery/injury to competition needs to be broken down into easy to understand stages. For example, following an **Anterior Cruciate Ligament** (ACL) reconstruction in the knee joint, the patient needs to be told accurately how the rehab process works in four to six weeks stages:

1. weeks 1-6 allows for protection of the surgery
2. weeks 7-12 produces the regaining of full range of motion
3. weeks 13-18 afford the athlete time to regain full strength
4. weeks 19-24 presents the athlete the time to regain full functional capacities

By being made to understand the specific time line for recovery and knowing what to expect during the rehabilitation process and its stages, the athlete will feel less anxiety and develop an increase sense of control.

POSITIVE ATTITUDE/MINDSET

For an athlete to heal quickly and progress through his rehab stages, he must be committed to overcoming the injury or illness by showing up for treatments, working hard to regain appropriate movement and ROM and listening and doing what the doctor and physiotherapist recommend. They also need to monitor what the athlete is thinking and saying regarding the injury and the rehab process. Positive self-talk is a definite plus, so much so that it constantly needs to supplant any negativity that always seems able to creep into conscious thinking throughout the day. Daily benefits from prescribed rehabilitation are

296

enhanced with focus on what needs to be done to recover almost every minute during the sessions.

Physical and psychological rewards are an important and often-looked-for respite from the hard work and usually uncomfortable time spent at rehab. A sunny day at the shore, or time in a warm, soothing whirlpool or a total body massage; maybe enjoying a favorite meal and, or dessert, purchasing clothes that the athlete feels will enhance his presence: all for that feel-good sensation we deem to be so important that signals life is good in spite of the damaged state I am in.

EMOTIONAL SUPPORT STRUCTURING

A common response for the athlete after an injury is to isolate himself from teammates, coaches, and friends. Many times he feels less worthy or foolish for succumbing to the injury or illness. It is important for an athlete, as he recovers, to maintain contact with others. Concerned friends, family, teammates, and coaches, can listen when the athlete needs to vent anger, despair, frustration, and lack of focus on the prize...to enjoy good health again. Knowing day-to-day they are not alone in their recovery process becomes a sustaining bridge to successful rehabilitation. Especially important is the reliance on and the encouragement of teammates. Who better to understand the needs of the rehabbing athlete than a teammate who has suffered the same slings and arrows involved in their chosen sport?!

GOAL SETTING

This is key to long term rehab success. Each stage of recovery needs particular objective measures that the athlete is striving to achieve. These measures include joint range of motion, strength building on a weight machine, a functional field test for sport specific movement, or the overall feeling of participation in the specific sport. By striving for achievement in a rehab stage, it places the bigger overall picture into context and makes the small immediate stages to improvement more manageable.

CHAPTER 5

FISH GOTTA SWIM

To say "Fish Gotta Swim" is to say a lot. You really cannot fight Mother Nature; if you try, you will probably lose. You might find ways to enhance her, but you would be wise to realize that the natural things in life have taken millions of years to evolve and perfect. The seeker of truth, wisdom, and some modicum of perfection will work hard at finding the secret of Nature's way and how it relates to all of us.

For man to swim, for example, he must obey the rules of nature. Then, in learning to do same, along the way, he may find a certain balance and rhythm not only in moving through water, but in life itself. Although there are many good writings that cover solely the nuts and bolts of swimming, this one mainly uses swimming as metaphor to that search for meaning and beauty in life.

What we see in the rhythm of the swimmer, what we see in the dance, what we see and hear in music, is all pleasing to the senses and sensibilities and so makes all of life better: There is beauty in music with examples abounding depending on your taste... beauty in the symmetry and fine proportions of the trained athlete, beauty in the poetry-in-motion of a dancer, for example, Fred Astaire in one of his hit movies of the depression era dancing across the screen so entranced and divorced from the travails of life that he sings "I'm dancing, and I cannot be bothered now."

Imagine a world devoid of beauty, wanting in passionate music, lacking in the well-turned phrase, devoid of the fine arts, missing the symmetry and graceful movement seen in the well-proportioned body of the elite swimmer effortlessly gliding through the water, a world never to have watched Astaire dance or a Greg Luganis dive, a world that moved Shakespeare to put these words in the mouth of Lorenzo *(The Merchant of Venice)*:

> *The man that hath no music in himself,*
> *Nor is not mov'd with concord of sweet sounds,*
> *Is fit for treasons, stratagems, and spoils;*
> *The motions of his spirit are dull as night,*
> *and his affections dark as Erebus:*
> *Let no such man be trusted...*

From ancient times, the Greeks appreciated the beauty in the athlete. We can gather such from a letter by the Greek satirist, Lucian, to a skeptical friend in Scythia:

...the energy we give to athletics is not wasted. But telling you how delightful the games are will not convince you. You should sit there yourself, among the spectators, and see the fine contestants, how beautiful and how healthy their bodies are, their marvelous skill and unbeatable strength, their daring and ambition, their firm resolve and their absolute will to win. I know quite well that you could never stop praising them, clapping and cheering.

Every society in the history of man has had in common some form of music and dance. Yet as individuals, Oliver Wendell Homes once remarked that "Most of us go to our graves with our music still inside us." Still, the beauty found in the dance and music can be found in a sport that requires one to learn their essences of rhythm and smooth motion... swimming.

Indeed, all sports when performed at a high level of proficiency, is pleasing to behold. Over long periods of time, working diligently, it takes much effort to make a sport look so easy, so effortless. Yet, just what must go in to that effort so to master the secret of correct, yet seemingly smooth and facile movement? What sense of propriety must be nurtured to allow for the proper flow to come forth at will?

It is, in part, a matter of proprioception, which means knowing where your body is in relationship to its three-dimensional environment. More simply put, it is a matter of balance, that thing we look for in swimming; more importantly, the very element we seek in life itself. This attained balance that lends beauty to the action can be seen in different mediums and for varying time spans. Those athletes that have pronounced movement and balance in air, for example, high-divers and ski-jumpers, "approach" the sensation of flying, but it is short-lived and only within the action of the particular sport. Whenever the fabulous high-divers at the University of Miami perform, all who watch them leap from the 10-meter platform are spell-bound, but only for an instant or two. I am not a Winter Olympics fan, but I do enjoy watching the ski-jumpers. I am in awe of their consummate skill (and courage) which allows them to soar like eagles for hundreds of feet and set down so gracefully as if on eggshells. It makes no difference to me which country the medal winners represent; it is the beauty of their efforts that lifts my spirits.

But movement in a medium one thousand times as dense as air (water) makes for *continuous* motion in a gravity-free environment. Continuous liquid movement with rhythm and grace is possible, since you weigh nothing in water (of course you need to *have* or *develop* the aesthetic endowments of rhythm and grace to make this work). You merely displace your gravitational weight in the water. While you actually weigh nothing in it, this buoyancy effect is at once both a blessing and a scourge.

Some, having buoyancy, will produce less passive drag as they swim. What this means is that if you have the ability to float, less effort, in general, is required to move GENTLY through the water. A dense body that has a tendency to sink requires more energy to stay afloat; a buoyant body needs less energy to stay afloat. But, unfortunately, life is not that simple. TO SWIM FAST (like a fish) requires power and muscle (which is dense tissue that does not promote floatation), and a sense of "slipping through the water." Then there are forces that hinder one's movement through the water. They are collectively called active drag. A person who has high body fat may be able to float, but is usually not streamlined enough to slip through the water with grace and speed, hence a hindrance.

I have seen only a few exceptions to what an early swim coach of mine once said: "fat people do not swim fast." Not to pick on the overweight, rather this states a fact. As we double our Toward speed in water, we exponentially increase our frontal resistance to forward movement, the water "tugging" at us at ever-increasing amounts, making a more streamlined effort all the more important. We need to lessen active drag as best we can to enable a smooth, powerful—and most importantly—PROLONGED effort in the water. Most proficient and virtually all elite, swimmers have that esthetically-pleasing build: broad, powerful shoulders, well-defined arms and legs, with a tapered, yet solid torso... a truly balanced physique. in effect, the more beautiful the body, the more beautiful the swim can be, specifically if done with a sense of balance.

I think I can tell you about these things by summing up what it takes to swim fast and with corresponding aesthetic beauty. That is technique. Technique and the continual practice of that technique. Technique that simulates that which is natural. And that which is natural is usually that which transmits beauty. Think of the seemingly effortless swing of the "natural" batter, the flow of a skater or ballet dancer, the stride of the runner, the flow and rhythm of the swimmer. The swimmer in effect is mimicking the fish; the swimmer is obeying rules of nature that allow the greatest and most powerful flow of energy translating itself into seemingly effortless movement. But still, the practice of technique alone does not do it.

To take a note from music for example; Arthur Rubinstein, no slouch at technique, nevertheless with age (he played well past his 90th birthday) was wont to miss a few notes here and there. Yet he still transcended mere technique by his exquisite sense of rhythm, so that despite a few missed keys, he still would "make music." With rhythm comes that altered state of consciousness, a meditative state if you will, that intangible ingredient without which you do not make music, you do not create beauty.

To create beauty, like all great musicians, he had a teacher, and playing in a symphony he always had a conductor. So too for swimming: there has to be the coach to impart technique and rhythm and to synchronize the efforts of both the individual and the team.

A family tragedy at midlife became the final push that sent me into full time coaching (though I have coached in one capacity or other since my early 20's) and away from decades of practicing pharmacy. It has taken many years of experiencing what's important in life and in the water and how they are miscible. Swimming was there when I needed it, and I feel I owe much to the sport. So much so that at middle age I pretty much ignored pharmacy and two masters degrees to become totally immersed in coaching and competing in swimming, searching for the nuances of technique, rhythm, teaching (coaching), questing for those peak moments of beauty, those beautiful moments of clapping and cheering.

The participation in sport, even vicariously, is what I have come to believe is necessary to create that all-important balance in life. It gets the "juices" flowing; it creates interest and anticipation above and beyond the mundane or perfunctory.

Sure, making a living and dealing with family responsibilities, in our society at least, seem to occupy the lion's share of time and energy; propriety dictates such. But who can argue with the fact that, time and again, the excitement generated by a championship season, game, bout, match, or meet totally engulfs most of our lives, even for just a short while. Add the possibility of you or a family member actually participating in such a sporting event, and the emotions are treated as though they have come across a palm-lined, cool-watered oasis providing a psychic balm in the desert of our existence.

ABOUT THE AUTHOR

I am unaware of any books on the shelves that have the same approach as I am taking with KEEPING THE ATHLETE HEALTHY. Most are concerned with recover after injury or illness or the proper way to train to maximize positive adaptations, but I have not seen any works that stress appropriate public health and physiologic methods to enhance the ability to carry vigorous exercise to its logical conclusion of bringing out the best in athletes. I feel because of this; KEEPING THE ATHLETE HEALTHY would have great appeal to a vast audience.

MARKET AND READERSHIP

This book is intended to enlighten a great diversity of athletes, their coaches, their parents, and their training partners engaging in various sports and types of competition. It is be written in an engaging yet easily-understood manner, giving the reader the feeling that this is a go-to ready reference. It will be stimulating as if a coach were lecturing to his charges. Facts and figures will be presented quickly and emphatically to help enhance the impact the author is trying to make. And while the book will not be presented as entertainment, it will be loaded with enjoyable, easily-understood information the moment the reader opens its pages. My goal is for it to become a sought after addition to the personal library of anyone engaging in sports or vigorous exercise and for use by all teams and organizations.

COACH NESSEL

Coach Nessel has been involved in swimming since the age of 10 and has offered up his skills, patience, and innovative approach to coaching, teaching, and training now going on 48 years. Though a talented aquatic athlete in his own right (high school state champion, masters national and world champion, Coach Nessel's mark has been repeatedly set by his ability to bring out the best in his athletes, and he is known nationally and internationally for his attribution of importance to all details, physical and biologic. Though The Coach included segments in his first book about keeping the athlete healthy, he felt this specific topic to be of such importance as to warrant a book all its own.

The Coach has worked with six Olympians, the most recent being Cullen Jones, gold medal winner in Beijing in 2008 and a gold and double-silver medal winner in 2012 (London) and a brother and sister duo representing Puerto Rico, Kristina and Doug Lennox.

Coach Nessel has earned membership to a very select group, being chosen as one of 30 USA coaches who had the greatest influence on the 2012 Olympic Swim Team. He has also been honored as a United States Masters Swimming Coach of the Year (1998) and selected to coach at the US Olympic Training Center in Colorado Springs (2001). He is an actively contributing member of USMS coaches and sports medicine committees. He has been published in all the important swim magazines in the USA, in many medical journals, and his work has been translated to appear in periodicals throughout the world. Coach Nessel was also the USA coach at the 1997 World Maccabiah in Israel, the second largest group of world class athletes to gather at a scheduled games, and earned Coach of the Meet honors where his swimmers won 34 out of 36 possible gold medals.

His personal life has been a testament to steadfastness of purpose, his ability to rise above, and the desire to help others reach their physical potential no matter what the obstacle presented. The Coach has had to bury both his sons (who succumbed to tragic accidents) and his wife (who fought to the end over a 10-year period to battle a variant of Lou Gehrig's Disease called Multiple System Atrophy). He has a daughter, Lee, whom he coached to become a high school All-America. She later became the captain and an All-America at the University of Miami and Female Scholar/Athlete Of The Year in 1997 when she graduated. She was also Miami's representative and a finalist to the very select NCAA Woman of the Year listing.

Through all his tribulations, Ed has endured. The goal and essence of his very being: to balance the physical with the mental, the academic with the athletic, the good with the bad.

His varied academic backgrounds of chemist, pharmacist, biochemist, and physiologist have all been placed into a large "brewing pot" to stir up his consistently winning approach to life and state-of-the-art presentation of science, super-seeding traditional methods for KEEPING THE ATHLETE HEALTHY. As The Coach is fond of saying: "I've been sick, and I've been well... I like well better."

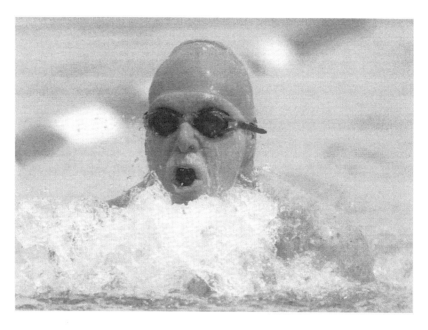

Author Ed Nessel at a Masters Swimming meet.

Edward H. Nessel, R.Ph, MS, MPH, PharmD

GLOSSARY

Academy of Dermatology (AAD)
Acetyl-Salicylic-Acid (ASA).
Adenosine Di-Phosphate (ADP)
Adenosine Mono-Phosphate (AMP)
Adenosine TriphosPhate (ATP)
Advanced Cardiac Life Support (ACLS)
Advanced Glycation End products (AGEs)
All-Out Fast Twitch Fibers (Fiib),
American Association of Retired People (AARP)
American College of Sports Medicine (ACSM)
American Heart Association (AHA)
Anterior Cruciate Ligament (ACL)
Automated External Defibrillator (AED)
Basic Life Support (BLS)
Basic Metabolic Rate (BMR)
Bemoglobin (Hb)
Bone Mineral Density (BMD).
C-Reactive Protein (CRP)
Carbon Dioxide (CO2)
Cardiac Output (CO = Heat Rate x Stroke Volume
Cardio Vascular Disease (CVD),
Carbohydrate (CHO)
Cardio-Pulmonary Resuscitation (CPR)
Central Nervous System (CNS)
Chronic Fatigue Syndrome (CFS)
Congestive Heart Failure (CHF)
Coronary Heart Disease (CHD).
Creatinine Kinase (CK)
Creatinine Phosphate (CP).
CycloOXygenase-2 (COX-2).
Delayed Onset Of Muscle Soreness (DOMS)
Electro-cardiogram (EKG)
Emergency Medical Service (EMS)
End Products (AGEs)
Estrogen-Receptor Negative (ER-negative)
Excess Post-Exercise Oxygen Consumption (EPOC).
Exercise-Induced Asthma (EIA)
Exercised-Induced Bronchospasm (EIB)
Forced Expiratory Volume (FEV)
Fast Twitch (FT)

Fast-Twitch Fibers (Fiia)
FibroMyalgia (FM)
Free Fatty Acids (FFAs)
Gamma-Amino-Butyric Acid (GABA)
GastroEsophageal Reflux Disease (GERD),
High-Density Lipoproteins (HDL's)
Hyaluronic Acid (HA)
Hypertrophic Cardiomyopathy (HCM)
Hypertrophic Cardiomyopathy (HCIVI),
Ilio-Tibial Band (ITB)
Indole-3-Carbinol (I3C)
International Center of Aquatic Research (ICAR)
Lactate DeHydrogenase (LDH)
Lean Body Mass (LBM),
Low-Density Lipoproteins (LDL)
Lower Esophageal Sphincter (LES)
Maximal Expiratory Ventilation (VE max)
Maximum Heart Rate (HR max).
Olympic Training Center (OTC)
Over-The-Counter (OTC)
Neutrophil Chemotactic Factor (NCF)…
Non-Steroidal Anti-Inflammatory Drugs (NSAIDS)
NorepinEphrine (NE)
Oxygen (O2)
Peak Expiratory Flow Rate (PEFR)
PyrroloQuiniline Quinone (PQQ)
Range Of Motion (ROM)
Reactive Oxygen Species (ROS)
Reactive Nitrogen Species (RNS)
Residual Volume (RV)…
Rest and Recovery (R&R)
Resting Metabolic Rate (RMR)
Reticular Activating System (RAS)
RICE... Rest, Ice, Compression, Elevation.
RiboNucleic Acid (RNA)
Sino-Atrial (SA)
Slow Twitch (ST)
Stroke Volume (SV max)
Sudden Cardiac Arrest (SCA)
Total Lung Capacity (TLC)
TricyClic Antidepressant (TCA)
Ultra-Violet (UV)